A NATIONAL STRATEGY FOR THE ELIMINATION OF HEPATITIS B AND C

PHASE TWO REPORT

Gillian J. Buckley and Brian L. Strom, *Editors*

Committee on a National Strategy for the Elimination of Hepatitis B and C

Board on Population Health and Public Health Practice

Health and Medicine Division

A Report of

The National Academies of
SCIENCES • ENGINEERING • MEDICINE

THE NATIONAL ACADEMIES PRESS
Washington, DC
www.nap.edu

THE NATIONAL ACADEMIES PRESS   500 Fifth Street, NW   Washington, DC 20001

This activity was supported by the American Association for the Study of Liver Diseases, the Infectious Diseases Society of America, the National Viral Hepatitis Roundtable, and the U.S. Department of Health and Human Services/Centers for Disease Control and Prevention (Contract No. 200-2011-38807, Task Order #44). Any opinions, findings, conclusions, or recommendations expressed in this publication do not necessarily reflect the views of any organization or agency that provided support for the project.

International Standard Book Number-13:   978-0-309-45729-3
International Standard Book Number-10:   0-309-45729-7
Digital Object Identifier: https://doi.org/10.17226/24731
Library of Congress Control Number: 2017942500

Additional copies of this publication are available for sale from the National Academies Press, 500 Fifth Street, NW, Keck 360, Washington, DC 20001; (800) 624-6242 or (202) 334-3313; http://www.nap.edu.

Suggested citation: National Academies of Sciences, Engineering, and Medicine. 2017. *A national strategy for the elimination of hepatitis B and C: Phase two report*. Washington, DC: The National Academies Press. doi: https://doi.org/10.17226/24731.

The National Academies of
SCIENCES · ENGINEERING · MEDICINE

The **National Academy of Sciences** was established in 1863 by an Act of Congress, signed by President Lincoln, as a private, nongovernmental institution to advise the nation on issues related to science and technology. Members are elected by their peers for outstanding contributions to research. Dr. Marcia McNutt is president.

The **National Academy of Engineering** was established in 1964 under the charter of the National Academy of Sciences to bring the practices of engineering to advising the nation. Members are elected by their peers for extraordinary contributions to engineering. Dr. C. D. Mote, Jr., is president.

The **National Academy of Medicine** (formerly the Institute of Medicine) was established in 1970 under the charter of the National Academy of Sciences to advise the nation on medical and health issues. Members are elected by their peers for distinguished contributions to medicine and health. Dr. Victor J. Dzau is president.

The three Academies work together as the **National Academies of Sciences, Engineering, and Medicine** to provide independent, objective analysis and advice to the nation and conduct other activities to solve complex problems and inform public policy decisions. The National Academies also encourage education and research, recognize outstanding contributions to knowledge, and increase public understanding in matters of science, engineering, and medicine.

Learn more about the National Academies of Sciences, Engineering, and Medicine at **www.national-academies.org**.

The National Academies of
SCIENCES · ENGINEERING · MEDICINE

Reports document the evidence-based consensus of an authoring committee of experts. Reports typically include findings, conclusions, and recommendations based on information gathered by the committee and committee deliberations. Reports are peer reviewed and are approved by the National Academies of Sciences, Engineering, and Medicine.

Proceedings chronicle the presentations and discussions at a workshop, symposium, or other convening event. The statements and opinions contained in proceedings are those of the participants and have not been endorsed by other participants, the planning committee, or the National Academies of Sciences, Engineering, and Medicine.

For information about other products and activities of the National Academies, please visit nationalacademies.org/whatwedo.

COMMITTEE ON A NATIONAL STRATEGY FOR THE ELIMINATION OF HEPATITIS B AND C

BRIAN L. STROM (*Chair*), Chancellor, Biomedical and Health Sciences, Rutgers University, The State University of New Jersey
JON KIM ANDRUS, Adjoint Professor and Senior Investigator, Division of Vaccines and Immunization, Center for Global Health, University of Colorado Denver
ANDREW ARONSOHN, Associate Professor of Medicine, University of Chicago
DANIEL CHURCH, Senior Epidemiologist, Bureau of Infectious Disease and Laboratory Sciences, Massachusetts Department of Public Health
SEYMOUR S. COHEN, American Cancer Society Research Professor, retired
ALISON EVANS, Associate Professor, Dornsife School of Public Health, Drexel University
PAUL KUEHNERT, Assistant Vice President, Program, Robert Wood Johnson Foundation
VINCENT LO RE III, Assistant Professor of Medicine (Infectious Diseases) and Epidemiology, University of Pennsylvania
KATHLEEN MAURER, Director, Health and Addiction Services, Connecticut Department of Correction
RANDALL MAYER, Chief, Bureau of HIV, STD, and Hepatitis, Division of Behavioral Health, Iowa Department of Public Health
SHRUTI MEHTA, Professor of Epidemiology, Bloomberg School of Public Health, Johns Hopkins University
STUART C. RAY, Professor of Medicine, Center for Viral Hepatitis Research, Division of Infectious Diseases, Johns Hopkins University
ARTHUR REINGOLD, Edward Penhoet Distinguished Professor of Global Health and Infectious Diseases, School of Public Health, University of California, Berkeley
SAMUEL SO, Lui Hac Minh Professor, School of Medicine, Stanford University
NEERAJ SOOD, Professor and Vice Dean for Research, Sol Price School of Public Policy and Schaeffer Center for Health Policy & Economics, University of Southern California
GRACE WANG, Family Physician, International Community Health Services
LUCY WILSON, Chief, Center for Surveillance, Infection Prevention, and Outbreak Response, Maryland Department of Health and Mental Hygiene

Reviewers

This report has been reviewed in draft form by individuals chosen for their diverse perspectives and technical expertise. The purpose of this independent review is to provide candid and critical comments that will assist the institution in making its published report as sound as possible and to ensure that the report meets institutional standards for objectivity, evidence, and responsiveness to the study charge. The review comments and draft manuscript remain confidential to protect the integrity of the deliberative process. We wish to thank the following individuals for their review of this report:

HARVEY ALTER, National Institutes of Health Clinical Center
SANJAY BASU, Stanford Prevention Research Center
JOHN BIRGE, The University of Chicago Booth School of Business
JULES DIENSTAG, Harvard Medical School
SHELLY F. GREENFIELD, McLean Hospital
RUTH KATZ, The Aspen Institute
ANNA LOK, University of Michigan Medical School
DAVID MENDEZ, University of Michigan School of Public Health
WALTER O. ORENSTEIN, Emory University School of Medicine
ROBIN POLLINI, Pacific Institute for Research
CHARLES RICE, The Rockefeller University
JOSHUA M. SHARFSTEIN, Johns Hopkins Bloomberg School of Public Health
DAVID THOMAS, John Hopkins Bloomberg School of Public Health

Although the reviewers listed above have provided many constructive comments and suggestions, they were not asked to endorse the conclusions or recommendations nor did they see the final draft of the report before its release. The review of this report was overseen by **Robert B. Wallace,** University of Iowa, and **Robert F. Sproull,** University of Massachusetts Amherst. They were responsible for making certain that an independent examination of this report was carried out in accordance with institutional procedures and that all review comments were carefully considered. Responsibility for the final content of this report rests entirely with the authoring committee and the institution.

Acknowledgments

The Committee on a National Strategy for the Elimination of Hepatitis B and C wishes to acknowledge the many people whose contributions and support made this report possible. The committee benefited from presentations made by a number of experts. The following individuals shared their research, experience, and perspectives with the committee: Jerome Adams, Sabrina Assoumou, Ryan Clary, John Coster, Ben Cowie, Jeff Duchin, Michael Fried, Nadine Gracia, Tim Gronniger, Jennifer Havens, Alicia Ifkovic-Mau, Michael Klompas, Kimberley Lenz, Steve Miller, Robin Pollini, Joshua Sharfstein, William Stauffer, Coy Stout, David Thomas, Chia Wang, John Ward, Stefan Wiktor, and Robert Zavoski.

The following individuals were important sources of information, generously giving their time and knowledge to further the committee's efforts: Anne Burns, James Kachadoorian, Dima Qato, Homie Razavi, Mitch Rothholz, Mehlika Toy, and Timothy Westmoreland.

The committee acknowledges the support of the National Academies of Sciences, Engineering, and Medicine staff, especially Daniel Bearss, Clyde Behney, Iliana Espinal, Chelsea Frakes, Greta Gorman, Hope Hare, Nicole Joy, Sarah Kelley, Ellen Kimmel, Rebecca Morgan, Tina Ritter, Doris Romero, Barbara Schlein, Lauren Shern, Elizabeth Tyson, Jennifer Walsh, Annalyn Welp, and Taryn Young. The committee and staff thank Rebekah Hutton for designing the cover art.

The committee also benefited from the work of committees of the Institute of Medicine that conducted studies relevant to this report, particularly the Committee on a National Strategy for Prevention and Control of Viral Hepatitis Infections in the United States.

Finally, funding for this project was provided by the American Association for the Study of Liver Diseases, the Centers for Disease Control and Prevention Divisions of Viral Hepatitis and Cancer Prevention and Control, the Infectious Diseases Society of America, the National Viral Hepatitis Roundtable, and the Department of Health and Human Services Office of Minority Health. The committee extends special thanks for that support.

Contents

PREFACE   xiii

ACRONYMS AND ABBREVIATIONS   xv

SUMMARY   1

1   INTRODUCTION   15
The Charge to the Committee, 17
Hepatitis and Liver Cancer, 22
References, 25

2   TARGETS FOR ELIMINATION   29
Hepatitis B Models, 32
Hepatitis C Models, 38
A Central Coordinating Office, 46
References, 49

3   PUBLIC HEALTH INFORMATION   57
Describing the Viral Hepatitis Epidemic, 59
References, 69

4   ESSENTIAL INTERVENTIONS   75
Prevention and Testing, 75
Care and Treatment, 93
References, 97

5   SERVICE DELIVERY   113
    Encouraging Compliance Among Providers, 113
    Reaching Patients, 116
    References, 134

6   FINANCING ELIMINATION   147
    An Increased Patient Burden, 147
    A Purchasing Strategy for Medicines, 151
    References, 167

7   RESEARCH   177
    Research Across the Care Continuum, 179
    References, 192

APPENDIXES
A   Population Health Impact and Cost-Effectiveness of Chronic
    Hepatitis B Diagnosis, Care, and Treatment in the United States   203
B   Modeling the Elimination of Hepatitis C in the United States   235
C   Public Meeting Agenda   267
D   Committee Biographies   271

Preface

Viral hepatitis can be a devastating disease, causing over one and a half million deaths a year. Recent developments in prevention and treatment have engendered a change in the way the world views this problem. Increasingly, we ask if there is a better, feasible alternative to the suffering and untimely mortality caused by hepatitis B and C. The National Academies of Sciences, Engineering, and Medicine's Committee on a National Strategy for the Elimination of Hepatitis B and C was charged with determining if these diseases might be eliminated in the United States and, if so, how that goal might be met. My fellow committee members and I were humbled by the philosophical and practical challenge these questions posed.

In our first report, the committee concluded that these infections could be eliminated as public health problems in the United States. (For purposes of brevity, the material in the first report is not repeated in this second one.) At the same time, the report emphasized the multiple barriers that stand in the way of this goal, all of which could be seen as consequences of another, more basic problem: viral hepatitis is simply not a sufficient priority in the United States.

The time is right for this to change. This report, which the committee hopes will be a vehicle for such change, lays out a strategy through which morbidity and mortality from viral hepatitis could be reduced by 2030 to the point that neither hepatitis B nor C commands attention as a major public health threat in the United States.

The committee's deliberations necessarily touched on other pressing topics of public health significance, such as the opioid epidemic and the problem of unaffordable medicines. Ultimately, this study deals with these topics only as they relate to viral hepatitis. I refer readers seeking a broader analysis of either question to two other committees currently convened by the National Academies: the Committee on Ensuring Patient Access to Affordable Drug Therapies and the Committee on Pain Management and Regulatory Strategies to Address Prescription Opioid Abuse.

The committee met three times to prepare this report. In closed session, the group evaluated the evidence and deliberated on the best strategy to eliminate hepatitis B and C as public health problems in the United States. Based on expert opinion and review of the evidence, the committee came to conclusions about a suitable strategy, recommending action for specific organizations to reach this goal. The committee drew on published literature and presentations from expert speakers in its deliberations. Members of the public were free to submit written testimony to the committee.

The committee is greatly appreciative of the strong and constant support provided by the study staff, who worked diligently over the many months of our deliberations and report preparation. Without their excellent and unending support we would never have been able to complete our task. We specifically wish to thank Gillian Buckley, who served as Study Director, and provided us enormous assistance and direction as the committee work proceeded, and without whom this report would not have existed. Other members of the National Academies staff who aided the study include Aimee Mead, Marjorie Pichon, Annalyn Welp, and Sophie Yang. Finally, as committee chair, I would like to thank my colleagues who served as committee members, who not only taught me an enormous amount about viral hepatitis, but served as a tremendous team, sharing expertise and (usually!) coming to an easy consensus. They also put in enormous work, providing the initial drafts of the report text.

Brian L. Strom, *Chair*
Committee on a National Strategy for the
Elimination of Hepatitis B and C

Acronyms and Abbreviations

AASLD	American Association for the Study of Liver Diseases
ACIP	Advisory Committee on Immunization Practices
ACOG	American College of Obstetricians and Gynecologists
AHN	acute hepatic necrosis
ALT	alanine transaminase
anti-HBc	antibody to hepatitis B core antigen
anti-HBe	antibody to hepatitis B e antigen
anti-HBs	antibody to hepatitis B surface antigen
CDC	Centers for Disease Control and Prevention
CHB	chronic hepatitis B
CHeCS	Chronic Hepatitis Cohort Study
CI	confidence interval
CMS	Centers for Medicaid & Medicare Services
CT	computed tomography
DAA	direct-acting antiviral
DEA	Drug Enforcement Agency
ECHO	Extension for Community Healthcare Outcomes
FDA	Food and Drug Administration
FQHC	federally qualified health center
HBeAg	hepatitis B e antigen

HBsAg	hepatitis B surface antigen
HBV	hepatitis B virus
HCC	hepatocellular carcinoma
HCV	hepatitis C virus
HEDIS	Healthcare Effectiveness Data and Information Set
HHS	Department of Health and Human Services
HRSA	Health Resources and Services Administration
ICER	incremental cost-effectiveness ratio
IDSA	Infectious Diseases Society of America
IMPACT	Improving Mood–Promoting Access to Collaborative Treatment
MRI	magnetic resonance imaging
NCQA	National Committee for Quality Assurance
NHANES	National Health and Nutrition Examination Survey
NIH	National Institutes of Health
OPTN	Organ Procurement and Transplantation Network
PWID	people who inject drugs
QALY	quality-adjusted life year
SAMHSA	Substance Abuse and Mental Health Services Administration
SEER	Surveillance, Epidemiology, and End Results
SMR	standardized mortality ratio
SVR	sustained virologic response
UI	uncertainty interval
UN	United Nations
UNAIDS	Joint United Nations Programme on HIV/AIDS
USPSTF	U.S. Preventive Services Task Force
VA	Department of Veterans Affairs
WHO	World Health Organization

Summary[1]

Every year viral hepatitis causes almost one and a half million deaths worldwide, more than HIV, tuberculosis, or malaria. Hepatitis B virus (HBV) and hepatitis C virus (HCV) account for 96 percent of these deaths, more than 20,000 a year in the United States alone. Such loss of life comes at a cost to society, both directly, through the expense of treatment, and indirectly, through the loss of adults in their prime; viral hepatitis culls most heavily from the 45 to 64 age group. It is therefore surprising how relatively little public or scientific attention viral hepatitis has garnered. In a 2016 report the World Health Organization (WHO) described it as "largely ignored as a health and development priority until recently."[2]

But because of recent advances, hepatitis C is now curable with short and easily tolerable courses of treatment; treatment can prevent most deaths from hepatitis B, and there is an effective vaccine against hepatitis B. Such developments inspired the World Health Assembly resolution in June 2016 to eliminate viral hepatitis as a major public health problem by 2030.

In the first phase of this project,[3] the sponsors[4] asked the committee to

---

[1] References are not included in the summary; please see the body of the report for references and the bulk of the discussion and justification.

[2] WHO. 2016. *Global health sector strategy on viral hepatitis, 2016-2021: Towards ending viral hepatitis.* Geneva, Switzerland: WHO.

[3] The committee's phase one report, *Eliminating the public health problem of hepatitis B and C in the United States: Phase one report*, is available for free download. Please see Chapter 1 for the full statement of task.

[4] The Centers for Disease Control and Prevention's (CDC's) Office of Viral Hepatitis and the Department of Health and Human Services' Office of Minority Health sponsored the first

consider the feasibility of such a goal in the United States. The committee's previous report concluded that hepatitis B and C could be eliminated as a public health problem, defining a public health problem as a disease that by virtue of morbidity, mortality, or transmission commands attention as a major threat to health in a community. In this report, the second of two, the committee lays out appropriate goals for disease reduction and a path to achieve these goals. The report is organized according to the WHO strategy document, which encourages countries to consider five areas (information, interventions, service delivery, financing, and research) in forming their national plans. Each report chapter deals with one of these topics; a separate chapter presents results of commissioned models informing the committee's conclusions on a suitable timeline and targets.

TARGETS FOR ELIMINATION

As a first step to identifying targets for eliminating hepatitis B and C from the United States, the committee commissioned models to estimate the effects of different interventions on disease burden. Modelers were chosen for their prior work in the field; only models that have been extensively validated and peer reviewed were considered. Given the differences in biology, epidemiology, and treatment options for hepatitis B and C, the models presented are not directly comparable, but both consider the reduction in morbidity and mortality that might be expected from different strategies for diagnosis, care, and treatment.

Hepatitis B Models

The hepatitis B model compared different levels of diagnosis, care, and treatment on the population of HBV-infected people in the United States. The modeled prevalence of chronic hepatitis B was 1.29 million cases (range: 855,000 to 2.02 million cases). It found that diagnosing two-thirds of hepatitis B cases in the United States, almost doubling the current diagnosis rate, but changing nothing else, would reduce deaths by only 4.5 percent by 2030. In order to see a meaningful reduction in deaths, simultaneous improvements would have to be made in care and treatment of chronic infection. Diagnosing 90 percent of cases, bringing 90 percent of those to care, and treating 80 percent of those for whom treatment is indicated, on the other hand, would, assuming highly motivated patients with good adherence to treatment, result in a cumulative 50 percent reduc-

---

phase of this report. They were joined in phase two by the American Association for the Study of Liver Diseases, the CDC Division of Cancer Prevention and Control, the Infectious Diseases Society of America, and the National Viral Hepatitis Roundtable.

tion in deaths by 2030 (relative to a 2015 baseline), averting over 60,000 deaths. The same level of diagnosis, care, and treatment would reduce incident cirrhosis by about 45 percent and new cases of hepatocellular carcinoma by a third.

The model has important limitations. The model cohort does not include the roughly 23,370 new cases of chronic hepatitis B that enter the United States every year from immigration (about 1 percent of the total cases) or the relatively small number of chronic infections acquired domestically.[5] When considering these cases, the prevalence of chronic hepatitis B will increase from 1.29 million in 2015 to 1.64 million in 2030. These additional cases would not, however, affect the estimated percent reduction in cumulative risk if they follow the same diagnosis, care, and treatment patterns.

The model also does not include strategies to end mother-to-child transmission of HBV or chronic hepatitis B as a result of horizontal transmission, partly because both are rare in the United States. However, work in Alaska has shown that it is possible to fully eliminate both.

Hepatitis C Models

The hepatitis C model compared four scenarios of diagnosis and treatment coverage on incidence and prevalence of hepatitis C and on liver-related deaths, liver cancer, and cirrhosis. It suggested considerable public health benefit to combining aggressive case finding with unrestricted treatment for chronic hepatitis C. In such a scenario, the total number of viremic cases would drop 85 percent and annual deaths from chronic HCV infection would drop 65 percent by 2030 (relative to 2015), averting a cumulative 28,800 deaths between 2015 and 2030. The same level of treatment and case finding would reduce incident infections by 90 percent (relative to 2015) by 2030.

The model's limitations include the assumption that only 260,000 people can be treated in a year. There is no reason why this number could not increase, especially if the capacity of primary care providers to treat hepatitis C were expanded. The model also assumes diagnosis of 110,000 new cases a year until 2020 and roughly 70,000 to 90,000 a year between 2020 and 2030. Case finding will be more challenging as time passes; the people in contact with the health system will have already been cured. Meeting the target of a two-thirds reduction in HCV-related deaths by 2030 will require special attention to testing and treatment among people who inject drugs, a population accounting for most new HCV infections in the United States, and people in prisons.

---

[5] Fewer than 2,000 a year from vertical and horizontal transmission combined.

A Central Coordinating Office

The targets presented in this report represent the committee's best effort to balance a compelling public health target against practical constraints. Meeting these targets depends on considerable improvements in testing, diagnosis, and care, as well as increased preventive measures and focused research. The actions recommended in this report all advance some part of the larger goal: eliminating the public health problem of hepatitis B and C in the United States by 2030. This program will require the cooperation of various federal and state government agencies, as well as professional societies, legislators, and private companies. With work spread among so many organizations, the opportunity for distraction is real. The leadership of a single office would help ensure efficient and harmonious work.

Recommendation 2-1: The highest level of the federal government should oversee a coordinated effort to manage viral hepatitis elimination.

Strong central leadership is a characteristic of successful disease elimination programs. The elimination strategy described in this report may have particular need for such leadership, given its emphasis on reaching people who inject drugs and novel strategies to finance medicines for Medicaid beneficiaries and prisoners.

PUBLIC HEALTH INFORMATION

Chronic hepatitis B and C are both clinically silent in most patients. Serious symptoms may not emerge for decades, and the root infection is often unrecorded on death certificates. This long latency is part of the reason why morbidity and mortality from viral hepatitis are undercounted. A better understanding of the true burden of disease will be essential when tracking progress toward elimination. Measuring disease burden is the primary responsibility of state and local health departments, but is something most health departments are not in a position to do.

Describing the Viral Hepatitis Epidemic

The Centers for Disease Control and Prevention (CDC) currently supports enhanced viral hepatitis surveillance in seven jurisdictions, and these offices are finding considerably higher disease burden than national data would suggest. Proper viral hepatitis surveillance requires tracking patients over time and processing a large amount of data for every case. The data gleaned from routine surveillance can identify spikes in new infections, give insight into patterns of access to care, help estimate disease prevalence in an area, and tailor prevention and response programs. Highly automated surveillance systems can help make this task more efficient; an investment in such systems and the human expertise to manage them would advance the goal of hepatitis elimination in the United States.

> **Recommendation 3-1: The Centers for Disease Control and Prevention (CDC), in partnership with state and local health departments, should support standard hepatitis case finding measures and the follow-up, monitoring, and linkage to care of all viral hepatitis cases reported through public health surveillance. The CDC should work with the National Cancer Institute to attach viral etiology to reports of liver cancer in its periodic national reports on cancer.**

The use of automated, electronic reporting from diagnostic laboratories holds promise to improve viral hepatitis case finding. Such systems cannot replace traditional surveillance, however. The work of managing data, tracking cases, and describing the demographics and risk factors for viral hepatitis will continue to fall on health department epidemiologists. Their work might be made easier by changes to state regulations on the reporting of HBV and HCV test results. A negative HCV RNA test result after treatment is particularly valuable as it indicates sustained virologic response or cure of hepatitis C, but such results are not reportable in many states.

Measuring mortality due to viral hepatitis could be improved by attention to cancer registries. A classification system that captures liver cancer etiology would improve understanding of the burden of HBV infection and HCV infection.

A better understanding of the incidence of viral hepatitis would come from cohort studies, especially among high-risk populations. Further, periodic cross-sectional surveys in similar populations would inform a more accurate understanding of disease prevalence and trends therein. Such studies would complement information about hepatitis coming from population-based surveys.

> **Recommendation 3-2: The Centers for Disease Control and Prevention should support cross-sectional and cohort studies to measure HBV and HCV infection incidence and prevalence in high-risk populations.**

The CDC could make use of existing contacts for sero-surveys in populations at risk for hepatitis. Serum analysis is clearly essential in any study of viral hepatitis, and researchers should be encouraged to measure a basic panel of serum biomarkers including HBsAg, total anti-HBc, and anti-HBs, HCV RNA, and HCV antibody. The new HCV immunoglobulin antibody avidity assay, which measures biomarkers that change with duration of infection, could be used with HCV RNA to identify new infections. Though validation studies are ongoing, this assay promises to improve estimates of incidence of hepatitis C, especially in high-risk groups.

ESSENTIAL INTERVENTIONS

This committee's first report reviewed the epidemiology of hepatitis B and C in the United States. With this review in mind, the committee considered specific actions with the power to interrupt transmission of HBV and HCV and prevent morbidity and mortality from chronic infection. In identifying interventions with the greatest possible effect, the committee considered a continuum of services from prevention to chronic care. As much as possible, this report separates discussion of essential interventions from strategies for improving their delivery.

Prevention and Testing

Prevention is the first step to eliminating the public health problem of hepatitis B and C.

Prevention of HBV Infection

Immunization against HBV can prevent 95 percent of infections. About 90 percent of U.S. children were fully immunized against HBV in 2013, but as of 2014, only about a quarter of adults over 19 were. Unvaccinated adults remain vulnerable to HBV infection through unprotected sex or contact with infected blood. There is not good awareness of the importance of adult vaccination however, and clinics often fail to stock the vaccine, partly because there is no funding to deliver it to uninsured and underinsured adults, and partly because they fear losing patients over the three-dose vaccine schedule.

Adult immunization does not have to be so complicated. Every year since 2009 about 40 percent of adults in the United States have received seasonal influenza vaccine. If states supported hepatitis B vaccination to the same level as seasonal influenza vaccine, great improvements could be made in hepatitis B immunization. The relative success of seasonal influenza immunization is partly a matter of making vaccination convenient, especially for hard-to-reach patients, including homeless people and substance users. Offering vaccination in pharmacies is one way to reach a wider cross-section of the population, as pharmacies have evening and weekend hours without appointment. Some states restrict the types of vaccines offered in pharmacies and the circumstances under which pharmacists may administer them, however. State laws reimbursing pharmacies for vaccines also vary widely.

Recommendation 4-1: States should expand access to adult hepatitis B vaccination, removing barriers to free immunization in pharmacies and other easily accessible settings.

Early vaccination and dosing with hepatitis B immune globulin can prevent mother-to-child transmission of HBV even among HBeAg+ women. Infants born to highly viremic women face particular risks, however. About 9 percent of infants born to women with HBV DNA greater than 20 million IU/mL contract HBV at birth despite proper prophylaxis.

Among highly viremic women, prophylactic antiviral therapy in the third trimester of pregnancy has been shown to further reduce perinatal HBV transmission. At the same time, women may experience hepatitis flare after stopping treatment, making long-term antiviral therapy necessary. The precise viral load threshold for antiviral therapy is not clear, but all HBsAg+ pregnant women should have early testing so that they and their doctors can weigh the pros and cons of antiviral prophylaxis.

Recommendation 4-2: The Centers for Disease Control and Prevention, the American Association for the Study of Liver Diseases, the Infectious Diseases Society of America, and the American College of Obstetricians and Gynecologists should recommend that all HBsAg+ pregnant women have early prenatal HBV DNA and liver enzyme tests to evaluate whether antiviral therapy is indicated for prophylaxis to eliminate mother-to-child transmission or for treatment of chronic active hepatitis.

Prevention of HBV and HCV Infections

There is no vaccine for HCV and, until there is, prevention will be mostly a matter of limiting exposure to the virus. One component of prevention is curing all chronic infections, thereby removing infected cases from the population. Stopping transmission also depends on reducing risk of HCV among people who inject drugs, a group that accounts for 75 percent of the roughly 30,500 new HCV infections every year in the United States.

Stopping HCV transmission among people who inject drugs is challenging. HCV can survive on fomites for hours, even days, and transmission by needle stick is 10 times more efficient for HCV than HIV. The best way to prevent hepatitis C in this population is to combine strategies that improve the safety of injection with those that treat the underlying addiction.

Opioid agonist therapy can relieve the symptoms of drug withdrawal and is considered part of the tertiary prevention of substance use disorder (meaning that it prevents the worst complications of the condition). However, 30 million Americans live in places where not a single provider can prescribe opioid agonists. Syringe exchange programs, similarly, do not have sufficient coverage even in cities. Rural and suburban areas, home to half of people who inject drugs, have 30 percent of the nation's syringe services and distribute only 8 percent of the total number of syringes.

Recommendation 4-3: States and federal agencies should expand access to syringe exchange and opioid agonist therapy in accessible venues.

Evidence indicates that syringe exchange programs neither encourage new users nor increase drug use among clients. Nevertheless, in some states, drug paraphernalia laws and regulations on the sale of syringes can impede the proper reach of syringe services. Expanding syringe exchange to rural and suburban areas may require modification to models developed in cities. Pharmacies may be a promising venue for syringe exchange, as they are accessible to people in most parts of the country and reasonably well equipped to provide a confidential space for counseling. Exchanges operating from a van or bus can reach more people and face less community opposition than a fixed-site exchange. They may also be more appealing to younger clients and to people concerned with maintaining anonymity.

Diagnosis of infected cases is also essential for elimination. U.S. Preventive Services Task Force guidelines recommend screening for people at high risk of HBV or HCV infection, but wider screening may be warranted. Compliance with the current recommendation that anyone born between 1945 and 1965 be screened for HCV is poor.

Emergency departments serve as safety net providers for uninsured and underinsured people, and some have explored opt-out screening for hepatitis C. As the elimination effort continues, finding cases in emergency departments and other such settings will be a key to continued progress.

Recommendation 4-4: The Centers for Disease Control and Prevention should work with states to identify settings appropriate for enhanced viral hepatitis testing based on expected prevalence.

Care and Treatment

The direct-acting antivirals that cure hepatitis C make elimination feasible in the United States. There is no comparable cure for hepatitis B, but entecavir and tenofovir are effective at viral suppression and are cost-effective. The combination of cost and demand for hepatitis C treatments has strained the budgets of many payers since these drugs came to market. Insurers responded with restrictions that create more work for providers. There is also evidence of disparities in access to treatment. A recent study found that 46.3 percent of Medicaid patients were refused treatment, compared to only 5.0 percent of Medicare patients and 10.2 percent of patients with commercial insurance.

Delaying treatment only increases a patient's risk of cirrhosis, liver cancer, and death. There are also consequences to society, as failure to treat chronic HCV infection creates a reservoir for transmission. Treating everyone with chronic hepatitis C, regardless of disease stage, would avert considerable suffering and anxiety.

Recommendation 4-5: Public and private health plans should remove restrictions that are not medically indicated and offer direct-acting antivirals to all chronic hepatitis C patients.

Without universal hepatitis C treatment, elimination of viral hepatitis will not be possible in the United States. Health plans should not stand in the way of this goal. The committee recognizes that the cost of the drugs presents an obstacle to universal treatment, but a strategy to control these costs is discussed later.

SERVICE DELIVERY

Part of the challenge of eliminating hepatitis B and C in the United States is that the people suffering from or at risk for the infections are often not engaged in care. Therefore, the elimination strategy must give as much attention to the delivery of services as to the services themselves. This piece of the strategy considers steps that could be taken to make viral hepatitis a higher priority, to support efficient care, and to reach patients who might otherwise be neglected.

Encouraging Compliance

There is often a gap between the practice of medicine as recommended by experts and what actually happens. Closing this gap is of concern to the National Committee for Quality Assurance (NCQA) which maintains the HEDIS[6] indicators, a set of measures used to monitor the performance of 90 percent of American health plans. HEDIS measures command a certain attention from providers and health plan managers. Addition of viral hepatitis indicators to HEDIS would help make these services higher priority.

---

[6] Officially, the Healthcare Effectiveness Data and Information Set.

Recommendation 5-1: The National Committee for Quality Assurance should establish measures to monitor compliance with viral hepatitis screening guidelines and hepatitis B vaccine birth dose coverage and include the new measures in the Healthcare Effectiveness Data and Information Set.

Screening and immunization measures would benefit from NCQA's attention, and they meet established criteria for inclusion in HEDIS. Increased screening could also encourage improvements to point of care assays for HBsAg and HCV core antigen.

Various measures of child and adolescent immunization are also included in HEDIS, including full immunization against HBV in the first year of life. This indicator does not take into account the relative importance of the timing of the first dose, however. Children born to HBsAg+ women or to women who have not been tested for HBV infection require vaccination within 12 hours of birth, others within 1 day of birth. Emphasis on the hepatitis B birth dose as well as the completion of the series could help direct attention to this essential intervention.

Reaching Patients

Primary care is an efficient way to provide services, and viral hepatitis services should be no exception. At the same time, treating viral hepatitis carries risks that providers in small practices may be reluctant to accept, causing a disparity where viral hepatitis care is out of reach for people in rural and underserved communities.

There is precedent for managing hepatitis C in primary care. The University of New Mexico's ECHO[7] program is one example of an ongoing training and support program between primary providers and specialists. ECHO and similar programs have transferable lessons for building capacity in primary care and could be replicated at large scale with support from professional societies.

Recommendation 5-2: The American Association for the Study of Liver Diseases and the Infectious Diseases Society of America should partner with primary care providers and their professional organizations to build capacity to treat hepatitis B and C in primary care. The program should set up referral systems for medically complex patients.

Capacity building in primary care will have to go beyond one-time training programs and include standing teleconferences to keep the lines

---

[7] Officially, Extension for Community Healthcare Outcomes.

of communication between primary care providers and specialists open. A shared patient information system accessible to all involved providers will also be important to track patients over time and facilitate shared decision making.

Eliminating viral hepatitis will also require additional work to reach patients who are not in regular contact with any primary care provider. Some of the people with the most serious need for viral hepatitis care are hard to reach: people born abroad, who are uninsured, who have substance use problems, and who are or have been imprisoned. Various federal and state agencies should give more explicit attention to bringing hepatitis services to these populations. The Ryan White Act[8] was passed in response to a similar problem with HIV. A system of the same breadth and flexibility would go far to reaching marginalized viral hepatitis patients. While building a parallel program comparable to Ryan White might not be feasible, outreach activities for viral hepatitis could be built onto existing Ryan White programs, using separate funding for HIV-negative people.

Recommendation 5-3: The Department of Health and Human Services should work with states to build a comprehensive system of care and support for special populations with hepatitis B and C on the scale of the Ryan White system.

People in jails and prisons bear a particularly high burden of viral hepatitis; CDC estimates from the early 2000s put the prevalence of hepatitis C in correctional facilities at 12 to 35 percent and chronic hepatitis B infection between 1 and 3.7 percent. Unprotected sex and needle sharing are both common among incarcerated people, making jails and prisons an amplifying reservoir for the infections. Ironically, correctional facilities are also an ideal place to test and vaccinate for HBV and to cure chronic HCV infection, as directly observed therapy is the norm and the risk of drug diversion is low.

Recommendation 5-4: The criminal justice system should screen, vaccinate, and treat hepatitis B and C in correctional facilities according to national clinical practice guidelines.

Prisons and jails have a constant rotation of inmates, sometimes living in close quarters. The mixing of people and opportunities for disease transmission make immunization important. Nevertheless, the cost of vaccines and problems with staffing make it difficult for states to vaccinate widely in jails and prisons. More attention to testing for HBV infection could help

---

[8] Officially, the Ryan White Comprehensive AIDS Resources Emergency Act of 1990.

draw attention to the related problem of immunization. If many inmates are shown to be vulnerable to HBV infection, correctional health officers might be able to make a stronger case to their state authorities for immunization support.

Screening inmates for viral hepatitis will bring many new diagnoses to light, especially cases of chronic hepatitis C. Concerns about the adequacy of treating these cases may have prevented prison health officers from screening more aggressively. The expense of testing, vaccination, and treatment is a barrier to hepatitis care in jails and prisons. Strategies to defray these expenses are discussed in the next section.

FINANCING ELIMINATION

Eliminating the public health problem of hepatitis B and C will require increasing preventive and therapeutic services. There will be an expense to this increase, but the cost of inaction is also high. By a 2009 estimate, Medicare alone stood to absorb a fivefold increase in hepatitis C expenses, and the introduction of direct-acting antivirals has only increased this estimate. U.S. payers will spend an estimated $136 billion on hepatitis C drugs between 2015 and 2020, about 45 percent of which will come from the government.

In 2016 Congress allocated over a billion dollars to treat hepatitis C in veterans. The committee commends this decision and sees complementary spending on prevention and treatment for a wider patient group as the best strategy to protect the taxpayers' investment. Congress is in the best position to marshal funds to implement the strategy outlined in this report.

A discretionary program would be one way for Congress to track the effects of their spending over time. As discussed in the previous section, it might be most efficient to use another discretionary program, the Ryan White Act, to reach viral hepatitis patients with overlapping risk factors for HIV. Any modifications to the Ryan White Act should make it clear that services for viral hepatitis patients should supplement the program's main goal of supporting treatment for poor and uninsured HIV patients. It is also important to remember that the Ryan White Act was passed out of concern for marginalized people facing a lifetime of expensive medical care. Loosening its restrictions to cover viral hepatitis treatments would be consistent with the spirit of this law and would hasten the end of a disease that poses particular risk to people with HIV.

A Purchasing Strategy for Medicines

The cost of the direct-acting antivirals that cure HCV infection is a major obstacle to elimination. These drugs have strained the budgets of public and private payers alike. Faced with the unenviable task of allocating scarce treatment, payers gave first priority to the sickest patients, those at most immediate risk of death. Many also imposed sobriety restrictions, fearing the risk of reinfection in active drug users too great to justify the expense of treatment. Such restrictions have met with criticism. Overt drug rationing offends the American public, but it is difficult to know how else to act in the face of such high prices.

Unrestricted mass treatment of hepatitis C will be necessary to eliminate the disease as a public health problem by 2030, but no direct-acting agent will come off patent before 2029. Delaying mass treatment would result in tens of thousands of needless deaths and billions of dollars in wasted medical costs. It is the government's role to avoid such suffering, while still respecting innovator drug companies' right to compensation for the risk they took to bring a valuable product to market.

> **Recommendation 6-1: The federal government, on behalf of the Department of Health and Human Services, should purchase the rights to a direct-acting antiviral for use in neglected market segments, such as Medicaid, the Indian Health Service, and prisons. This could be done through the licensing or assigning of a patent in a voluntary transaction with an innovator pharmaceutical company.**

There are times when the government must act to correct a market failure. With this in mind, the committee recommends a *voluntary* transaction between the government and the companies producing direct-acting antivirals wherein the companies compete to sell their patent rights to the federal government for use in neglected populations. The voluntary nature of this process guarantees the drug company reasonable compensation; the patent holder has the option to walk away if the price is too low. Furthermore, the government would license the patent only for use in those populations for whom the government buys *and* access is limited, such as prisoners and Medicaid beneficiaries. This limitation will also control costs; the government should not have to pay as much as if it were compromising the lucrative private market.

Calculations shown in Chapter 6 suggest that the licensing rights should cost about $2 billion, after which states would pay about $140 million to treat 700,000 Medicaid beneficiaries and prisoners. For comparison, under the status quo it would cost about $10 billion over the next 12 years to treat only 240,000 Medicaid beneficiaries and prisoners.

Critics of this strategy may maintain that it sets a dangerous precedent; they may fear the government negotiating a license for other expensive medicines. This is unlikely, as the U.S. government has never been inclined to such action. In general, the United States is extremely supportive of the pharmaceutical industry, investing heavily in the science infrastructure that supports it and paying more for medicines than other rich countries. Indeed, the government's very reluctance to interfere in the pharmaceutical market may have emboldened the industry. The Senate Finance Committee's investigation into the pricing of sofosbuvir concluded that Gilead[9] had deliberately elevated the price in an effort to raise the market floor, ensuring continued high prices for all future hepatitis C treatments. Action now might discourage other companies from pursuing this strategy in the future.

RESEARCH

The WHO identified research as one of the essential pieces of any country's viral hepatitis elimination strategy. For the United States, a comparative advantage in science and technology compels special attention to research. Yet despite being the seventh leading cause of death in the world, viral hepatitis accounts for less than 1 percent of the National Institutes of Health's research budget.

This report identified a series of key gaps in the research that would benefit from scientific attention, broadly divided into mechanistic and implementation research questions. Mechanistic research questions include the immune response and curative therapies for HBV and vaccine for HCV, as well as rapid diagnostic tests and new treatments for fibrosis, cirrhosis, and liver cancer. Implementation research questions include how to manage substance use in prisons and ways to reach key populations, as well as novel strategies for harm reduction, better understanding of networks of drug users, and prevention of injection drug use.

---

[9] The innovator pharmaceutical firm that brought the drug to market.

1

Introduction

In June 2016 the World Health Assembly set the goal of eliminating viral hepatitis as a major public health problem by 2030 (WHO, 2016a). In the first strategy document of its kind, the organization concluded, "hepatitis has been largely ignored as a health and development priority until recently," despite causing more deaths than HIV, tuberculosis, or malaria (Stanaway et al., 2016; WHO, 2016a; Wiktor and Hutin, 2016).

The world cannot afford to ignore viral hepatitis any longer. The Global Burden of Disease Study estimated 1.45 million deaths from viral hepatitis in 2013 (95 percent confidence interval [CI]: 1.38 to 1.54 million) (Stanaway et al., 2016). Together hepatitis B virus (HBV) and hepatitis C virus (HCV) account for 96 percent of these deaths (Stanaway et al., 2016), more than 21,000 of them in the United States (CDC, 2016). Such loss of life comes at a cost to society, both in the direct financial burden of treatment and indirectly through the loss of adults in their prime—most viral hepatitis deaths cull from the 45 to 64 age group (Ly et al., 2012).

There is no longer any reason to disregard these diseases. There is an effective vaccine to prevent hepatitis B, advances in treatment can prevent most deaths in those chronically infected with HBV, and hepatitis C is now curable with a short course of easily tolerated treatment (Afdhal et al., 2014; Feld et al., 2014). (Box 1-1 describes a national treatment program in Egypt.) Preventive measures against both infections abound (Thomas, 2013). Hepatitis B vaccine confers long-standing immunity in 95 percent of recipients (WHO, 2015); immunization of newborns prevents community acquisition in childhood (Mast et al., 2005). Mother-to-child transmission of HBV, once inevitable, can now be prevented in 85 to 95 percent of cases

BOX 1-1
Unrestricted Hepatitis C Treatment in Egypt

Egypt is a rare example of a country with high hepatitis C prevalence and commitment to treatment. Its hepatitis C prevalence is among the highest in the world (CDC, 2012; Gower et al., 2014; Kandeel et al., 2016). In 2015, about 10 percent of adults between 15 and 59 years old tested positive for HCV antibody and another 150,000 to 165,000 are infected every year (CDC, 2012; Kandeel et al., 2016; McNeil, 2015). In some villages of the Nile delta region, as many as half of men older than 50 test positive for HCV antibody (McNeil, 2015).

The problem is largely attributable to efforts from the 1950s through the 1980s to control schistosomiasis, a water-borne parasitic disease that causes serious organ damage (WHO, 2016b). Schistosomiasis was endemic in Egypt, about 20 million Egyptians suffered from the infection in 1980 (Abdel-Wahab, 1982; Abdel-Wahab et al., 1980; Strickland, 2006). The standard of care treatment at the time was an intravenous injection of tartar emetic, which millions of people received at community clinics and other health posts (Strickland, 2006). Syringes were frequently reused, often without adequate sterilization, spreading HCV years before it was discovered and named (McNeil, 2015; Strickland, 2006). Roughly as many people were infected with hepatitis B virus, but only about 5 percent went chronic, compared to 70 or 80 percent of those exposed to HCV (Strickland, 2006).

The Egyptian ministry of health started a hepatitis C control program in 2001; in 2007 it launched a national treatment plan, providing pegylated interferon and ribavirin treatment to about 190,000 people (CDC, 2012; Egyptian Ministry of Health and Population, 2014). The advent of direct-acting antivirals was particularly welcome in Egypt, where about 850,000 people have been cured since late 2014 (*Daily News Egypt*, 2016a; Kandeel et al., 2016).

Since 2015, Gilead has sold Sovaldi® to the Egyptian government for about $10 per pill and licensed two Egyptian manufacturers to produce generic sofosbuvir for about $4 per pill (Gilead, 2015; McNeil, 2015). The Egyptian government pays for 40 percent (about $80 million per year) of costs related to the national treatment program, with the remaining 60 percent paid by insurance companies and patients (Egyptian Ministry of Health and Population, 2014). As of July 2016, a government referendum guaranteed free HCV treatment for uninsured patients (*Daily News Egypt*, 2016b).

(Nelson et al., 2014). Direct-acting antiviral treatments with cure rates of 95 percent and higher have revolutionized hepatitis C care (Afdhal et al., 2014; Zoulim et al., 2015). Although there is no vaccine for HCV, secondary prevention measures can impede the spread of infection. In the United States, where most new HCV infections are associated with injection drug use, syringe exchange programs have particular promise to interrupt transmission (Mehta et al., 2011). Treatment of all chronic infections would do the same.

Yet this committee's previous report concluded that while elimination of hepatitis B and C in the United States may be entirely feasible, it is not likely without meaningful changes to policy and directed research (Buckley and Strom, 2016; NASEM, 2016). Like a previous Institute of Medicine committee that commented on woefully underfunded surveillance systems and inadequate public spending on viral hepatitis prevention and treatment, this committee's previous report discussed limitations with, among other things, surveillance, case detection, and access to care, as well as gaps in the current understanding of the viruses (IOM, 2010; NASEM, 2016). The report concluded that most of the barriers to preventing and treating viral hepatitis could be seen as consequences of another, more basic problem: viral hepatitis is not a public priority in the United States.

The United States is not alone in this, as the World Health Assembly resolution observed. The international movement toward eliminating hepatitis B and C as public health problems could help generate the impetus for change. A concrete action plan and clear goals could also do much to change attitudes domestically. The United States should not come late or halfheartedly to the global elimination effort. With this in mind, the Committee on a National Strategy for the Elimination of Hepatitis B and C issues this strategy document recommending actions that will hasten the end of HBV and HCV infections and deaths in the United States and advance the international goal of eliminating the public health problem of viral hepatitis by 2030.

THE CHARGE TO THE COMMITTEE

The Centers for Disease Control and Prevention (CDC) and the Department of Health and Human Services (HHS) have a commitment to fighting viral hepatitis; the CDC Division of Viral Hepatitis and the HHS Office of Minority Health sponsored the first phase of this project. In phase two, the original sponsors were joined by the American Association for the Study of Liver Diseases, the CDC Division of Cancer Prevention and Control, the Infectious Diseases Society of America, and the National Viral Hepatitis Roundtable. Box 1-2 shows the statement of task for both phase one and two of this project, though this report is limited to the phase two task.

The Phase One Report

In the first phase of this project, the sponsors asked the committee whether it is feasible to eliminate hepatitis B and C from the United States. The first publication in this series briefly reviewed the literature on the

---

BOX 1-2
Statement of Task

PHASE I

The National Academies of Sciences, Engineering, and Medicine will conduct a literature review and convene two meetings of the committee, one of which will include a two part workshop, one part focused on hepatitis B virus (HBV) and one focused on hepatitis C virus (HCV) to determine whether HBV and HCV elimination goals for the United States are feasible and to identify possible critical success factors. A brief report containing the committee's conclusion regarding the feasibility of setting elimination goals and possible critical success factors shall be prepared.

PHASE II

The committee will prepare a consensus report containing committee conclusions and recommendations, specifically identifying

1. the appropriate hepatitis reduction or elimination goal(s) and specifying a plan of action to achieve the goal(s) including, but not necessarily limited to: medical and substance abuse services, community-based services, and correctional health services;
2. barriers to achieving the goal(s) such as access to treatment and related policy issues; public health infrastructure resources for screening, education and outreach; and surveillance;
3. potential solutions to the barriers identified; and
4. specific stakeholders and their responsibilities to achieve the goal.

---

epidemiology and natural history of both infections.[1] The committee then considered the feasibility of eliminating hepatitis B and C, dividing that question into smaller questions about ending transmission and reducing morbidity and mortality from chronic infection; for hepatitis C it also weighed the feasibility of eliminating chronic infection.

Part of the challenge of this task was first clarifying exactly what level of disease control could be considered elimination. Unlike eradication, which refers to a permanent, zero-level incidence of new infections without ongoing control measures, elimination is a softer target (CDC, 1993; Dowdle, 1998). CDC definitions of disease elimination emphasize cessation of transmission, and allow for circumstances where a disease may remain,

---

[1] The committee encourages readers who are unfamiliar with the basic virology and natural history of these infections to consult the first report.

but its most devastating consequences avoided (e.g., trachoma remains, but with no further cases of blindness) (CDC, 1993). In this understanding, disease elimination can refer to a level of control where the disease is no longer considered a public health problem (CDC, 1993).

In considering the elimination of hepatitis B and C from the United States, it is important to remember that both infections are endemic abroad, making frequent importation of cases inevitable. Hepatitis C, though curable, is not vaccine-preventable. Chronic HBV infection, on the other hand, is incurable, but largely preventable with vaccination and prophylactic measures against vertical transmission. Antiviral treatment can reduce the risk of disease progression; there is no reason why people with chronic hepatitis B should not live long lives and die of unrelated causes. For these reasons, the committee concluded that, "hepatitis B and C could both be eliminated as public health problems in the United States, but that this would take considerable will and resources" (NASEM, 2016, p. 2). The report went on to define a public health problem as one that, "by virtue of transmission or morbidity or mortality commands attention as a major threat to the health of the community" (NASEM, 2016, p. 2). Tables 1-1 and 1-2 summarize the committee's assessment of these questions, as well as critical factors relating to each step, and barriers to meeting the elimination goal.

This phase of the project builds off the conclusions of the phase one report. In this document, the committee has been asked to lay out appropriate goals for hepatitis reduction over time and specific actions to achieve them, being clear about possible barriers and ways to overcome them and articulating responsibilities for key stakeholders.

The Committee's Approach to Its Charge

The committee met three times to prepare this report; see Appendix C. In closed session, the group evaluated the evidence and deliberated on the best strategy to eliminate hepatitis B and C as public health problems in the United States. Based on expert opinion and review of the evidence, the committee came to conclusions about a suitable strategy, recommending actions for specific organizations to reach this goal. The committee drew on published literature and presentations from expert speakers in its deliberations. Members of the public submitted written testimony to the committee (available from the National Academies of Sciences, Engineering, and Medicine's Public Access Records Office, PARO@nas.edu).

The World Health Organization's 2016 strategy document identified five areas in which action will be needed, referred to in the document as strategic directions. These five areas are meant to guide countries' formation of their national strategies, each area addressing a set of essential questions (see Box 1-3). This report is organized around these five strate-

TABLE 1-1 The Feasibility of Eliminating Hepatitis B as a Public Health Problem in the United States with Critical Factors for Success and Crosscutting Problems

Goal		Feasibility	Critical Factors	Crosscutting Barriers
Ending transmission	Perinatal	Highly feasible	• Identifying HBV-infected mothers • Consistent birth dosing with hepatitis B vaccine	• Surveillance is sporadic and underfunded. • Vaccine tracking across jurisdictions is poor. • Stigma keeps people from screening and care. • Foreign-born adults can be difficult to reach with screening and treatment programs. • Much of the burden for managing chronic hepatitis B falls on overworked primary care providers. • There is a need to better understand the virus and the management of chronic HBV infection.
	Children	Highly feasible	• Consistent vaccination and attention to catch-up dosing	
	Adults	Feasible	• No system for vaccinating adults • Undiagnosed, asymptomatic chronic infections a reservoir for infection	
Reducing morbidity and mortality attributable to ongoing infection	Slowing progression to cirrhosis	Feasible	• Need for physicians trained in the management of chronic HBV infection • The threat of reactivation in chronic or resolved infection	
	Reducing deaths		• No available treatment eliminates cccDNA or cures the disease	

NOTE: cccDNA = covalently closed circular DNA; HBV = hepatitis B virus.
SOURCE: NASEM, 2016.

TABLE 1-2 The Feasibility of Eliminating Hepatitis C as a Public Health Problem in the United States with Critical Factors for Success and Crosscutting Problems

Goal		Feasibility	Critical Factors	Crosscutting Barriers
Ending transmission		Feasible	• No vaccine • Reaching people who inject drugs with harm reduction programs • Comprehensive drug and alcohol programs • Treating those transmitting the virus to prevent new infection • Reducing the possibility of reinfection	• Surveillance is sporadic and underfunded. • Only about half of chronically infected people have been diagnosed. • Most new infection is associated with injection drug use, the group most affected is difficult to screen. • Poor, marginalized, and hard-to-reach populations are difficult to enroll and retain in care. • The high cost of direct-acting antiviral drugs makes universal treatment unfeasible. • Hepatitis C is not a public priority. • Stigma keeps highest risk people away from care. • The limited capacity of prison health systems to treat HCV-infected inmates.
Eliminating chronic infection		Feasible	• Increasing access to treatment • The threat of antiviral resistance • Understanding the role of treatment adherence	
Reducing morbidity and mortality attributable to ongoing infection	Slowing progression to cirrhosis	Feasible	• Problems assessing and staging fibrosis • Obesity, HIV, alcohol use can aggravate disease progression • Eradicating the virus before progression to advanced fibrosis can almost eliminate complications and risk of death • Need for reliable models of disease progression	
	Reducing deaths			

NOTE: HCV = hepatitis C virus.
SOURCE: NASEM, 2016.

BOX 1-3
WHO Strategic Directions from the Global
Health Sector Strategy on Viral Hepatitis

1. Information: *What is the situation?*
   Focus on the need to understand the viral hepatitis epidemic and response as a basis for advocacy, political commitment, national planning, resource mobilization and allocation, implementation, and program
   improvement.

2. Interventions: *What services should be delivered?*
   Describe the essential package of high-impact interventions that need to
   be delivered along the continuum of hepatitis services to reach country
   and global targets, and which should be considered for inclusion in national health benefit packages.

3. Delivering for Equity: *How can these services be delivered?*
   Identify the best methods for delivering the continuum of hepatitis services to different populations and in different locations, so as to achieve
   equity, maximize impact, and ensure quality.

4. Financing: *How can the costs of delivering the package of services be
   met?*
   Identify sustainable and innovative models for financing of hepatitis responses and approaches for reducing costs so that people can access
   the necessary services without incurring financial hardship.

---

gic directions: information, interventions, service delivery, financing, and
research. A separate chapter presents the results of commissioned models
informing the committee's goals on suitable targets, interim indicators, and
a timeline for elimination in the United States.

HEPATITIS AND LIVER CANCER

The 2016 *Annual Report to the Nation on the Status of Cancer* cel-
ebrated continued declines in cancer deaths in the United States, attribut-
ing much of this progress to public health (Ryerson et al., 2016). Tobacco
control measures have curbed the incidence of many cancers, especially lung
cancer, long the most common and fatal cancer in the country (CDC, 2011;
Henley et al., 2014; Jemal et al., 2008). Improved screening, early diagnosis, and treatment have contributed to declines in incidence and lengthened
survival time for lung, colorectal, prostate, and breast cancers (Edwards

5. Research: *How can the trajectory of the response be changed?* Identify where there are major gaps in knowledge and technologies, where innovation is required to shift the trajectory of the viral hepatitis response in order for those responses to be accelerated and for the 2020 and 2030 targets to be achieved.

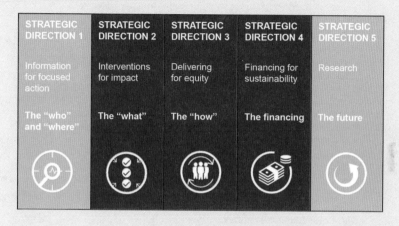

SOURCE: Adapted with permission from *Global health sector strategy on viral hepatitis, 2016-2021: Towards ending viral hepatitis. Figure 1.* http://apps.who.int/iris/bitstream/10665/246177/1/WHO-HIV-2016.06-eng.pdf (accessed July 19, 2016).

et al., 2010, 2014; Kohler et al., 2015; Ryerson et al., 2016). The recent annual report highlighted one troubling trend, however. The incidence of hepatocellular carcinoma, the most common form of primary liver cancer, increased 38 percent between 2003 and 2012, the most recent years for which data are available (Ryerson et al., 2016). Liver cancer deaths rose 56 percent in the same time, a sharper increase than that of any other cancer (Ryerson et al., 2016). Data from 2008 to 2012 indicate a disproportionate increase in racial and ethnic minorities: American Indian and Alaska Natives have the highest incidence of liver cancer (14.9 per 100,000), followed by Asian and Pacific Islanders (13.8 per 100,000) and Hispanics (12.7 per 100,000). Among non-Hispanic blacks, the age-specific rate of liver cancer has shifted over time and is now highest (around 60 per 100,000 people) at the relatively young ages of 55 to 59 (Ryerson et al., 2016). Another recent study confirmed the increase in hepatocellular carcinoma incidence,

BOX 1-4
Hepatitis Control and Elimination in Mongolia

Mongolia has the highest rate of liver cancer and liver cancer deaths in the world, mostly due to viral hepatitis. Hepatitis B virus (HBV) infection is usually acquired at birth or in early childhood, while chronic hepatitis C is more commonly due to unsafe medical injection and transfusion. In adults, HBsAg prevalence is about 10 percent, and in the general population, chronic hepatitis C prevalence is almost 7 percent. Almost every family in Mongolia is affected by hepatitis or liver cancer.

Mongolia's first national strategy on viral hepatitis covered years 2010 to 2015, and emphasized hepatitis B immunization to decrease HBsAg prevalence to less than 2 percent among children under 5. This goal was met; the most recently reported HBsAg prevalence in 4 to 6 year olds was 0.53 percent. In 2014 and 2015 experts from the World Health Organization (WHO) regional office, the Centers for Disease Control and Prevention, and the National Institutes of Health conducted a review of the viral hepatitis response in Mongolia, including clinical medicine and public health measures in the public and private sectors. Their review formed the basis for a new national strategy that will likely emphasize wider hepatitis B catch-up vaccination, increasing prevention, making better use of the private sector, and combining hepatitis and alcoholism prevention in public messaging.

With bipartisan parliamentary support, Mongolia's hepatitis elimination program has become a key government policy. In 2016 hepatitis B antivirals were added to the country's national health insurance plan, which subsidizes 80 percent of the cost of generic tenofovir. Direct-acting antivirals (four generic and one brand name) were also licensed in Mongolia in 2016, with the national health insurance plan subsidizing more than half the cost. Out-of-pocket costs after subsidies are about $1.40 a month for hepatitis B treatment and $198 for a 3-month course of hepatitis C treatment.

In the first 10 months of 2016, the WHO reported that more than 5,800 patients in Mongolia had been treated for chronic hepatitis C, with a sustained virologic response rate of 92 to 99.5 percent, depending on fibrosis stage. Costs for generic direct-acting antivirals are expected to continue to decrease, making treatment more accessible.

SOURCES: Dashdorj et al., 2014; Mongolia WHO Representative Office, 2010; WHO and Center for Disease Analysis, 2015; WHO Regional Office for the Western Pacific, 2014, 2015, n.d.

especially among subgroups such as men aged 55 to 64, and highlighted geographic variation in the trend (White et al., 2016).

Hepatitis B and C are driving this increase. Together HBV and HCV account for about 80 percent of the world's hepatocellular carcinoma (the most common form of liver cancer) (Arzumanyan et al., 2013).

Chronic hepatitis B increases odds of liver cancer 50 to 100 times, chronic hepatitis C by 15 to 20 times (El-Serag, 2012; Sherman and Llovet, 2011). Action against viral hepatitis is essential to combatting liver cancer. Box 1-4 describes Mongolia's hepatitis elimination program in response to the country's high rate of liver cancer mortality.

Much as public health measures have lessened the burden of lung, breast, colorectal, and prostate cancers over time, so can public health programs reverse troubling trends in liver cancer. This report outlines ways to reduce the burden of viral hepatitis in the United States and discusses the likely effects of such a reduction on the incidence of liver cancer and its frequent precursor, cirrhosis. The strategy of expanded screening and treatment, improved surveillance, harm reduction, adult vaccination, and ensured access to medicines would make hepatitis B and C rare diseases in the United States by 2030.

REFERENCES

Abdel-Wahab, M. 1982. *Schistosomiasis in Egypt*. Boca Raton, FL: CRC Press.

Abdel-Wahab, M. F., G. T. Strickland, A. El-Sahly, L. Ahmed, S. Zakaria, N. El Kady, and S. Mahmoud. 1980. Schistosomiasis mansoni in an Egyptian village in the Nile Delta. *American Journal of Tropical Medicine and Hygiene* 29(5):868-874.

Afdhal, N., S. Zeuzem, P. Kwo, M. Chojkier, N. Gitlin, M. Puoti, M. Romero-Gomez, J. P. Zarski, K. Agarwal, P. Buggisch, G. R. Foster, N. Bräu, M. Buti, I. M. Jacobson, G. M. Subramanian, X. Ding, H. Mo, J. C. Yang, P. S. Pang, W. T. Symonds, J. G. McHutchison, A. J. Muir, A. Mangia, and P. Marcellin. 2014. Ledipasvir and sofosbuvir for untreated HCV genotype 1 infection. *New England Journal of Medicine* 370(20):1889-1898.

Arzumanyan, A., H. M. Reis, and M. A. Feitelson. 2013. Pathogenic mechanisms in HBV- and HCV-associated hepatocellular carcinoma. *Nature Reviews Cancer* 13(2):123-135.

Buckley, G. J., and B. L. Strom. 2016. What stands in the way of making hepatitis B and C rare diseases in the United States? *Annals of Internal Medicine* 165(4):284-285.

CDC (Centers for Disease Control and Prevention). 1993. Recommendations of the International Task Force for Disease Eradication. *Morbidity and Mortality Weekly Report* 42(RR-16). https://www.cdc.gov/mmwr/PDF/rr/rr4216.pdf (accessed February 24, 2017).

CDC. 2011. State-specific trends in lung cancer incidence and smoking—United States, 1999-2008. *Morbidity and Mortality Weekly Report* 60(36):1243-1247.

CDC. 2012. Progress toward prevention and control of hepatitis C virus—Egypt, 2001-2012. *Morbidity and Mortality Weekly Report* 61(29).

CDC. 2016. *Viral hepatitis surveillance: United States, 2014*. http://www.cdc.gov/hepatitis/statistics/2014surveillance/pdfs/2014hepsurveillancerpt.pdf (accessed Setpember 22, 2016).

Daily News Egypt. 2016a. All hepatitis C patients on waiting list now treated: Ministry of Health. July 28. http://www.dailynewsegypt.com/2016/07/28/hepatitis-c-patients-waiting-list-now-treated-ministry-health (accessed September 6, 2016).

Daily News Egypt. 2016b. State council rules for free treatment of hepatitis C patients. July 18. http://www.dailynewsegypt.com/2016/07/18/state-council-rules-for-free-treatment-of-hepatitis-c-patients (accessed September 6, 2016).

Dashdorj, N., B. Dashtseren, B. Bold, and D. Yagaanbuyant. 2014. P29: Epidemiological study of prevalence and risk factors for HBV among apparently healthy Mongolians. *Journal of Viral Hepatitis* 21(Suppl S2):38.

Dowdle, W. R. 1998. The principles of disease elimination and eradication. *Bulletin of the World Health Organization* 76(Suppl 2):22-25.

Edwards, B. K., E. Ward, B. A. Kohler, C. Eheman, A. G. Zauber, R. N. Anderson, A. Jemal, M. J. Schymura, I. Lansdorp-Vogelaar, L. C. Seeff, M. van Ballegooijen, S. L. Goede, and L. A. Ries. 2010. Annual report to the nation on the status of cancer, 1975-2006, featuring colorectal cancer trends and impact of interventions (risk factors, screening, and treatment) to reduce future rates. *Cancer* 116(3):544-573.

Edwards, B. K., A. M. Noone, A. B. Mariotto, E. P. Simard, F. P. Boscoe, S. J. Henley, A. Jemal, H. Cho, R. N. Anderson, B. A. Kohler, C. R. Eheman, and E. M. Ward. 2014. Annual report to the nation on the status of cancer, 1975-2010, featuring prevalence of comorbidity and impact on survival among persons with lung, colorectal, breast, or prostate cancer. *Cancer* 120(9):1290-1314.

Egyptian Ministry of Health and Population. 2014. *Plan of action for the prevention, care & treatment of viral hepatitis, Egypt 2014-2018.*

El-Serag, H. B. 2012. Epidemiology of viral hepatitis and hepatocellular carcinoma. *Gastroenterology* 142(6):1264-1273 e1261.

Feld, J. J., K. V. Kowdley, E. Coakley, S. Sigal, D. R. Nelson, D. Crawford, O. Weiland, H. Aguilar, J. Xiong, T. Pilot-Matias, B. DaSilva-Tillmann, L. Larsen, T. Podsadecki, and B. Bernstein. 2014. Treatment of HCV with ABT-450/r–ombitasvir and dasabuvir with ribavirin. *New England Journal of Medicine* 370(17):1594-1603.

Gilead. 2015. *Chronic hepatitis C treatment expansion: Generic manufacturing for developing countries.* http://www.gilead.com/~/media/files/pdfs/other/hcv%20generic%20agreement%20 fast%20facts%2072815.pdf (accessed September 15, 2016).

Gower, E., C. Estes, S. Blach, K. Razavi-Shearer, and H. Razavi. 2014. Global epidemiology and genotype distribution of the hepatitis C virus infection. *Journal of Hepatology* 61(1 Suppl):S45-S57.

Henley, S. J., T. B. Richards, J. M. Underwood, C. R. Eheman, M. Plescia, and T. A. McAfee. 2014. Lung cancer incidence trends among men and women—United States, 2005-2009. *Morbidity and Mortality Weekly Report* 63(1):1-5.

IOM (Institute of Medicine). 2010. *Hepatitis and liver cancer: A national strategy for prevention and control of hepatitis B and C.* Washington, DC: The National Academies Press.

Jemal, A., M. J. Thun, L. A. Ries, H. L. Howe, H. K. Weir, M. M. Center, E. Ward, X. C. Wu, C. Eheman, R. Anderson, U. A. Ajani, B. Kohler, and B. K. Edwards. 2008. Annual report to the nation on the status of cancer, 1975-2005, featuring trends in lung cancer, tobacco use, and tobacco control. *Journal of the National Cancer Institute* 100(23):1672-1694.

Kandeel, A., M. Genedy, S. El-Refai, A. L. Funk, A. Fontanet, and M. Talaat. 2016. The prevalence of hepatitis C virus infection in Egypt 2015: Implications for future policy on prevention and treatment. *Liver International* 37(1):45-53.

Kohler, B. A., R. L. Sherman, N. Howlader, A. Jemal, A. B. Ryerson, K. A. Henry, F. P. Boscoe, K. A. Cronin, A. Lake, A. M. Noone, S. J. Henley, C. R. Eheman, R. N. Anderson, and L. Penberthy. 2015. Annual report to the nation on the status of cancer, 1975-2011, featuring incidence of breast cancer subtypes by race/ethnicity, poverty, and state. *Journal of the National Cancer Institute* 107(6):791-797.

Ly, K. N., J. Xing, R. M. Klevens, R. B. Jiles, J. W. Ward, and S. D. Holmberg. 2012. The increasing burden of mortality from viral hepatitis in the United States between 1999 and 2007. *Annals of Internal Medicine* 156(4):271-278.

Mast, E. E., H. S. Margolis, A. E. Fiore, E. W. Brink, S. T. Goldstein, S. A. Wang, L. A. Moyer, B. P. Bell, and M. J. Alter. 2005. A comprehensive immunization strategy to eliminate transmission of hepatitis B virus infection in the United States. Recommendations of the Advisory Committee on Immunization Practices (ACIP). Part 1: Immunization of infants, children, and adolescents. *Morbidity and Mortality Weekly Report* 54(RR-16):1-31.

McNeil, D. G., Jr. 2015. Curing hepatitis C, in an experiment the size of Egypt. *New York Times*, December 25. http://www.nytimes.com/2015/12/16/health/hepatitis-c-treatment-egypt.html?_r=0 (accessed October 26, 2016).

Mehta, S. H., J. Astemborski, G. D. Kirk, S. A. Strathdee, K. E. Nelson, D. Vlahov, and D. L. Thomas. 2011. Changes in blood-borne infection risk among injection drug users. *Journal of Infectious Diseases* 203(5):587-594.

Mongolia WHO (World Health Organization) Representative Office. 2010. *WHO country cooperation strategy for Mongolia 2010-2015*. Geneva, Switzerland: WHO, Western Pacific Region.

NASEM (National Academies of Sciences, Engineering, and Medicine). 2016. *Eliminating the public health problem of hepatitis B and C in the United States: Phase one report*. Washington, DC: The National Academies Press.

Nelson, N. P., T. V. Murphy, and D. J. Jamieson. 2014. Prevention of perinatal hepatitis B virus transmission. *Journal of the Pediatric Infectious Diseases Society* 3(Suppl 1):S7-S12.

Ryerson, A. B., C. R. Eheman, S. F. Altekruse, J. W. Ward, A. Jemal, R. L. Sherman, S. J. Henley, D. Holtzman, A. Lake, A. Noone, R. N. Anderson, J. Ma, K. N. Ly, K. A. Cronin, L. Penberthy, and B. A. Kohler. 2016. Annual report to the nation on the status of cancer, 1975-2012, featuring the increasing incidence of liver cancer. *Cancer* 122(9):1312-1337.

Sherman, M., and J. M. Llovet. 2011. Smoking, hepatitis B virus infection, and development of hepatocellular carcinoma. *Journal of the National Cancer Institute* 103(22):1642-1643.

Stanaway, J. D., A. D. Flaxman, M. Naghavi, C. Fitzmaurice, T. Vos, I. Abubakar, L. J. Abu-Raddad, R. Assadi, N. Bhala, B. Cowie, M. H. Forouzanfour, J. Groeger, K. M. Hanafiah, K. H. Jacobsen, S. L. James, J. MacLachlan, R. Malekzadeh, N. K. Martin, A. A. Mokdad, A. H. Mokdad, C. J. L. Murray, D. Plass, S. Rana, D. B. Rein, J. H. Richardus, J. Sanabria, M. Saylan, S. Shahraz, S. So, V. V. Vlassov, E. Weiderpass, S. T. Wiersma, M. Younis, C. Yu, M. El Sayed Zaki, and G. S. Cooke. 2016. The global burden of viral hepatitis from 1990 to 2013: Findings from the Global Burden of Disease Study 2013. *Lancet* 388(10049):1081-1088.

Strickland, G. T. 2006. Liver disease in Egypt: Hepatitis C superseded schistosomiasis as a result of iatrogenic and biological factors. *Hepatology* 43(5):915-922.

Thomas, D. L. 2013. Global control of hepatitis C: Where challenge meets opportunity. *Nature Medicine* 19(7):850-858.

White, D. L., A. P. Thrift, F. Kanwal, J. Davila, and H. B. El-Serag. 2016. Incidence of hepatocellular carcinoma in all 50 United States, from 2000 through 2012. *Gastroenterology* 152(4):812-820.e5.

WHO (World Health Organization). 2015. *Hepatitis B*. http://www.who.int/mediacentre/factsheets/fs204/en (accessed July 22, 2016).

WHO. 2016a. *Global health sector strategy on viral hepatitis, 2016-2021: Towards ending viral hepatitis*. Geneva, Switzerland: WHO. http://apps.who.int/iris/bitstream/10665/246177/1/WHO-HIV-2016.06-eng.pdf (accessed July 19, 2016).

WHO. 2016b. *Schistosomiasis: Fact sheet*. http://www.who.int/mediacentre/factsheets/fs115/en (accessed December 30, 2016).

WHO and Center for Disease Analysis. 2015. *Public health and economic impact of a population based approach to HCV treatment in Mongolia*. WHO, Center for Disease Analysis.

WHO Regional Office for the Western Pacific. 2014. *Meeting report. Technical meeting on raising awareness, surveillance, prevention and management of viral hepatitis in Mongolia.* Manila, Philippines: WHO Regional Office for the Western Pacific.

WHO Regional Office for the Western Pacific. 2015. *Viral hepatitis in Mongolia: Situation and response.* Geneva, Switzerland: WHO.

WHO Regional Office for the Western Pacific. n.d. *Hepatitis: A crisis in Mongolia.* http://www.wpro.who.int/hepatitis/resource/features/mongolia_story/en (accessed June 30, 2016).

Wiktor, S. Z., and Y. J. F. Hutin. 2016. The global burden of viral hepatitis: Better estimates to guide hepatitis elimination efforts. *The Lancet* 388(10049):1030-1031.

Zoulim, F., T. J. Liang, A. L. Gerbes, A. Aghemo, S. Deuffic-Burban, G. Dusheiko, M. W. Fried, S. Pol, J. K. Rockstroh, N. A. Terrault, and S. Wiktor. 2015. Hepatitis C virus treatment in the real world: Optimising treatment and access to therapies. *Gut* 64(11):1824-1833.

2

Targets for Elimination

The World Health Organization's (WHO's) hepatitis strategy document set targets for reducing the world's burden of viral hepatitis (see Table 2-1). The document makes clear, however, that the proposed targets are global and will not necessarily be suitable for any one country. The emphasis on the screening of donor blood and the use of safety-engineered syringes, for example, does not apply to the United States but to countries where such measures are not already required. The proposed reductions in incidence and mortality shown in Table 2-1 are similarly broad. One percent prevalence of hepatitis B surface antigen (HBsAg) among children is an aspirational goal for 2020 in most of the world's hepatitis B endemic countries but considerably higher than 2006 estimates suggest for the United States (Wasley et al., 2010).

Given differences in epidemiology and disease burden, WHO guidance asks every country to identify its most affected populations and tailor its response accordingly (WHO, 2016b). The organization's strategy document directs countries to "develop as soon as practicable ambitious national goals and targets for 2020 and beyond [. . .]. Targets should be feasible and developed based on country realities, the best possible data [. . .], trends and responses, and monitored through a set of standard and measurable indicators" (WHO, 2016b, p. 23). Box 2-1, for example, describes the Republic of Georgia's viral hepatitis strategy in response to the country's high prevalence of hepatitis C.

As a first step to identifying feasible targets for hepatitis B and C elimination in the United States, the committee commissioned modeling analysis to estimate how different interventions might reduce the national burden of

TABLE 2-1 WHO Targets for Reducing the Global Burden of Viral Hepatitis

Target Area	Baseline 2015	2020 Targets	2030 Targets
Impact targets			
Incidence: New cases of chronic viral hepatitis B and C infections	Between 6 and 10 million infections are reduced to 0.9 million infections by 2030 (95% decline in hepatitis B virus infections, 80% decline in hepatitis C virus infections)	30% reduction (equivalent to 1% prevalence of HBsAg among children)	90% reduction (equivalent to 0.1% prevalence of HBsAg among children)
Mortality: Viral hepatitis B and C deaths	1.4 million deaths reduced to less than 500,000 by 2030 (65% for both viral hepatitis B and C)	10% reduction	65% reduction
Service coverage targets			
Hepatitis B virus vaccination: childhood vaccine coverage (third dose coverage)	82% in infants	90%	90%
Prevention of hepatitis B virus mother-to-child transmission: hepatitis B virus birth-dose vaccination coverage or other approach to prevent mother-to-child transmission	38%	50%	90%
Blood safety	39 countries do not routinely test all blood donations for transfusion-transmissible infections 89% of donations screened in a quality-assured manner	95% of donations screened in a quality-assured manner	100% of donations are screened in a quality-assured manner

TABLE 2-1 Continued

Target Area	Baseline 2015	2020 Targets	2030 Targets
Safe injections: percentage of injections administered with safety-engineered devices in and out of health facilities	5%	50%	90%
Harm reduction: number of sterile needles and syringes provided per person who injects drugs per year	20	200	300
Viral hepatitis B and C diagnosis	<5% of chronic hepatitis infections diagnosed	30%	90%
Viral hepatitis B and C treatment	<1% receiving treatment	5 million people will be receiving hepatitis B virus treatment 3 million people have received hepatitis C virus treatment (Both targets are cumulative by 2020)	80% of eligible persons with chronic hepatitis B virus infection treated 80% of eligible persons with chronic hepatitis C virus infection treated

NOTE: HBsAg = hepatitis B surface antigen; WHO = World Health Organization.
SOURCE: WHO, 2016b.

hepatitis B and C, including liver cancer, cirrhosis, and liver-related deaths (see Appendixes A and B). The modelers were chosen on the basis of their prior work in the field; only models that have been extensively validated and peer-reviewed were considered.[1]

Given the inherent differences in the biology, epidemiology, natural history, and treatment options for hepatitis B and C, the models presented in this chapter are not directly comparable. Broadly, the hepatitis B model considers the effects of varying rates of diagnosis, care, and treatment on

---

[1] Staff at Center for Disease Analysis can make the hepatitis C model available upon request to employees of government or academic institutions. The hepatitis B model can be re-created using TreeAge software and the information presented in Appendix A.

BOX 2-1
Hepatitis Control and Elimination in the Republic of Georgia

The Republic of Georgia is a small country with an estimated 6.7 percent prevalence of hepatitis C, one of the highest rates in the world (Stvilia et al., 2006; WHO Regional Office for Europe, 2015). Experience in HIV programming has afforded the country a cadre of technical workers with transferable expertise for hepatitis C elimination (WHO Regional Office for Europe, 2015). Despite the challenges of high disease burden in a middle-income country, the Georgian authorities have made an elimination plan and secured support to implement it from donors.

The highly effective direct-acting antivirals that were first licensed in 2013 are the cornerstone of the effort (Mitruka et al., 2015). Results of a population sero-survey in May 2015 informed the selection of seven clinical sites for the start of the elimination program. The U.S. Centers for Disease Control and Prevention is working with the Georgian ministry to develop the national program, particularly essential pieces such as case management, laboratory quality assurance and control, and provider training (Mitruka et al., 2015). The pharmaceutical company Gilead also views Georgia as a demonstration project in eliminating hepatitis C. In April 2015, Gilead donated 5,000 courses of Sovaldi® and 20,000 courses of Harvoni® for use in patients with hepatitis C and severe liver disease (Mitruka et al., 2015; WHO Regional Office for Europe, 2015).

Advocacy, surveillance, testing and care, harm reduction, and blood safety have all been identified as target areas for the next phase of the Georgian hepatitis C elimination program (WHO Regional Office for Europe, 2015). At the 2015 World Hepatitis Summit, the minister of health cited a goal for 2020 of 95 percent of hepatitis C cases diagnosed, 95 percent of those diagnosed in care, 95 percent of those in care treated, and 95 percent of those treated cured (Sergeenko, 2015). (Though more recent statements have suggested a diagnosis goal of 90 percent of cases [Tsertsvadze, 2016].) By April 2016, 27,392 Georgians registered with the elimination program. Of those enrolled, 8,448 started treatment (Gvinjilia et al., 2016).

---

liver health outcomes. The hepatitis C model, in contrast, considers the absolute number of people treated and diagnosed as inputs, then compares the consequences of different treatment strategies. Both provide useful insight into realistic targets for hepatitis B and C elimination in the United States.

HEPATITIS B MODELS

The author's full report *Population Health Impact and Cost-Effectiveness of Chronic Hepatitis B Diagnosis, Care, and Treatment in the United States* is shown in Appendix A. Briefly, the author adapted a Markov model originally developed to study hepatitis B interventions in Shanghai, China

(Toy et al., 2014). Updated data from recent cohort studies and a meta-analysis of mostly North American research were used to estimate disease progression (Campsen et al., 2013; Chen et al., 2010; Chu and Liaw, 2007, 2009; Fattovich et al., 2008; Kanwal et al., 2006; Lin et al., 2005; Raffetti et al., 2016; Thiele et al., 2014) and treatment effectiveness (Heathcote et al., 2011; Lok et al., 2016; Papatheodoridis et al., 2015; Tenney et al., 2009; Wong et al., 2013). The model's assumptions regarding the likelihood of developing cirrhosis and liver cancer during antiviral treatment are based on recent data (Arends et al., 2015; Marcellin et al., 2013). Background mortality by age and probability of receiving a liver transplant were drawn from the Organ Procurement and Transplant Network (HRSA, 2016).

The model then compared different rates of diagnosis, care, treatment (among the subset of chronic hepatitis B patients for whom treatment is appropriate), and patient adherence to serological monitoring, as shown in Table 2-2. The estimates for current practice are based on peer-reviewed studies (Chotiyaputta et al., 2011; Hu et al., 2013; Juday et al., 2011; Kim et al., 2014; Lin et al., 2007). The next scenario (HHS 2020 Target) showed the effect of meeting the Department of Health and Human Services (HHS) goal of increasing diagnosis from one-third to two-thirds of all patients with chronic hepatitis B (HHS, 2015). A third scenario (HHS 2020 Target + Improved Treatment) added improvements in rates of care and treatment to the stated HHS target. For additional comparison, the modeler then included a scenario of 80 percent diagnosed, 80 percent of those in care, with 80 percent treatment among those eligible, and 80 and 95 percent patient adherence to monitoring and treatment. This scenario is slightly lower coverage than the next scenario, modeling the WHO's proposed global targets of 90 percent of chronic hepatitis B cases diagnosed, and 80 percent of treatment among those eligible, assuming that 90 percent of diagnosed patients are in care, with (for comparison's sake) perfect patient adherence (WHO, 2016a). Finally, the analysis considered an ideal scenario where everyone with chronic hepatitis B is diagnosed and adheres perfectly to treatment and monitoring.

The modeled prevalence of chronic hepatitis B in the United States in 2015 was 1.29 million people (95 percent confidence interval [CI]: 855,000 to 2.02 million), similar to the Center for Disease Control and Prevention's (CDC's) current estimate of 850,000 to 2.2 million people (CDC, 2016a). This prevalence amounts to 0.4 percent (95 percent CI: 0.27 to 0.63 percent) of the total U.S. population, compared to the most recent NHANES[2] estimate of 0.3 percent (95 percent CI: 0.2 to 0.4 percent) (Roberts et al., 2016). Foreign-born blacks and people born in Asia account for 72.6 percent of cases. Appendix A gives more detail on the age breakdown of

---

[2] Officially, National Health and Nutrition Examination Survey.

TABLE 2-2 Scenario Analysis Rates

Scenario	Diagnosed	Received HBV Care	Treatment Rate Among Treatment Eligible Patients	Adherence to Monitoring	Adherence to Treatment
Natural History	—	—	—	—	—
Current Practice	34.6%[a]	33.3%[b]	45%[c]	35.1%[d]	85%[e]
HHS 2020 Target	66%	33.3%	45%	35.1%	85%
HHS 2020 Target + Improved Rx	66%	80%	80%	35.1%	85%
Hypothetical Scenario	80%	80%	80%	80%	95%
WHO 2030 Target	90%	90%	80%	100%	100%
Idealistic (Utopian)	100%	100%	100%	100%	100%

NOTE: HBV = hepatitis B virus; HHS = Department of Health and Human Services; WHO = World Health Organization.

[a] Lin et al., 2007.
[b] Hu et al., 2013.
[c] Kim et al., 2014.
[d] Juday et al., 2011.
[e] Chotiyaputta et al., 2011.

this cohort, about 25 percent of whom are eligible for antiviral treatment because of chronic active hepatitis or cirrhosis.

Table 2-3 shows the cumulative risks in 2030 of hepatocellular carcinoma, cirrhosis, and HBV-related death among chronic hepatitis B patients in the United States, based on the current practice for diagnosis, care, and treatment. Table 2-4 shows cumulative reductions in these outcomes relative to 2015 practice. Improving the rate of diagnosis to the two-thirds level cited in the HHS strategy document would reduce deaths related to hepatitis B by only about 4 percent by 2030 (HHS, 2015). Table 2-4 makes it clear that higher levels of diagnosis, care, and treatment will be necessary to meaningfully reduce morbidity and mortality from chronic hepatitis B. If the United States were to meet the WHO target of 90 percent of chronic hepatitis B patients diagnosed, 90 percent of those in care, and 80 percent treatment among those eligible (hereafter the 90/90/80 scenario), there would be about 50 percent fewer cumulative deaths related to hepatitis B in the United States over the next 15 years. Meeting the same targets would reduce new cases of cirrhosis by about 45 percent and new cases of hepatocellular carcinoma by about one-third.

Under the current practice, about 9.4 percent of HBV-infected people would die by 2030, only 4.7 percent would die if the WHO target levels of diagnosis, testing, and treatment were met. Given the size of the infected population, this would translate into about 60,630 deaths averted by 2030. (Working off the lower bound of the estimate of HBV-infected people in the United States, 40,185 deaths averted; given the higher bound, 94,940 deaths averted.)

At the same time, the model's analysis of the WHO 2030 target scenario assumed almost perfect adherence to serological monitoring and treatment. This would be a significant improvement over current practice and will require changing the system for delivering hepatitis B care; such changes are discussed more in Chapter 5. Sensitivity analysis shown in Appendix A indicates that increasing care has the strongest effect on the outcomes, followed by increasing diagnosis. Increasing treatment had the least effect on the model's outcomes.

As with all such analyses, this model has several important limitations. First, it works with a hypothetical cohort of chronic hepatitis B patients in the United States in 2015. This cohort does not include the estimated 23,370 new chronic hepatitis B cases (95 percent CI: 17,800 to 31,660 cases) entering the United States every year from immigration, or the relatively small number (fewer than 2,000 a year) of chronic infections acquired domestically.[3] When considering new cases from immigration, the preva-

---

[3] The CDC estimates about 19,200 acute infections every year, including roughly 900 newborns a year acquiring the infection from their mothers (95 percent CI: 800 to 1,000) (CDC, 2016b; Ko et al., 2014).

TABLE 2-3 Cumulative Risks of Hepatocellular Carcinoma, Cirrhosis, and HBV-Related Deaths by 2030 in the 2015 Cohort of Chronic HBV-Infected Persons in the United States

Cumulative Risk	Scenario					
	Current Practice D35/C33/T45	HHS 2020 Target D66/C33/T45	HHS + Improved Rx D66/C80/T80	Hypothetical Scenario D80/C80/T80	WHO 2030 Target D90/C90/T80	Idealistic D100/C100/T100
Hepatocellular carcinoma risk	6.00%	5.84%	5.27%	4.46%	3.91%	3.14%
Cirrhosis risk	10.31%	10.15%	9.01%	6.84%	5.70%	3.79%
HBV-related deaths	9.40%	8.98%	7.60%	5.98%	4.66%	2.84%

NOTE: HBV = hepatitis B virus; HHS = Department of Health and Human Services; WHO = World Health Organization.

TABLE 2-4 Cumulative Reduction in Hepatocellular Carcinoma, Cirrhosis, and HBV-Related Deaths in the 2015 Cohort of Chronic HBV-Infected Persons with Various Improved Diagnosis, Care, and Treatment Scenarios Compared with the Base Scenario (D35/C33/T45) in 15 Years

Cumulative Reduction	Scenario				
	HHS 2020 Target D66/C33/T45	HHS + Improved Rx D66/C80/T80	Hypothetical Scenario D80/C80/T80	WHO 2030 Target D90/C90/T80	Idealistic D100/C100/T100
Hepatocellular carcinoma cases	2.66%	12.16%	25.66%	34.83%	47.66%
Cirrhosis cases	1.55%	12.60%	33.65%	44.71%	63.23%
HBV-related deaths	4.46%	19.14%	36.38%	50.42%	69.78%

NOTE: HBV = hepatitis B virus; HHS = Department of Health and Human Services; WHO = World Health Organization.

lence of chronic hepatitis B increases to about 1.64 million by 2030. (These additional cases would not, however, affect the estimated percent reduction in cumulative risk if they follow the same diagnosis, care, and treatment patterns.) NHANES estimates put the prevalence of chronic hepatitis B around 730,000 from 1999 to 2006 (Wasley et al., 2010). After 2007, when more attention was given to identifying participants of Asian descent, the estimate rose to 850,000 (Roberts et al., 2016). But since people born in HBV endemic countries are still not well-represented in NHANES this figure is likely an underestimate (Cohen et al., 2008; Kim, 2009). If the foreign-born populations in the United States have the same prevalence rates as in their birth countries, as many as 2.2 million additional people may have hepatitis B (Kowdley et al., 2012). At the same time, immigrants are not entirely representative of their native country; the hepatitis B prevalence in an immigrant's birth country may not apply to the people living in the United States (Uddin et al., 2010). With this is mind, the modeler used age-specific U.S. prevalence rates, reported in studies of various racial and ethnic groups, including people born in the United States and abroad. To accommodate the range in prevalence estimates, the committee based its conclusions on percentage reductions in morbidity and mortality rather than absolute numbers.

Furthermore, the work presented in Appendix A does not model strategies to end mother-to-child transmission of hepatitis B or horizontal transmission, as this is not a question for which the modeler has developed peer-reviewed analytic tools. Both are now rare in the United States. Only about 900 infants a year contract HBV infection at birth (Ko et al., 2014); less than 5 percent of the roughly 19,200 adults and children over five who acquire HBV every year develop chronic hepatitis B (CDC, 2016b; Mast et al., 2006). Therefore, new cases entering the population from horizontal transmission would not substantively change the estimates.

Work in Alaska has shown that it is possible to fully eliminate mother-to-child transmission of HBV. Despite HBV infection being endemic among Alaska Natives and 70 percent of chronic hepatitis B patients living in remote areas without road connection, there has not been a single case of acute hepatitis B in an Alaska Native child since 1992[4] (FitzSimons et al., 2013; McMahon et al., 2014). This work, coupled with an assessment of the relative rarity of vertical transmission of HBV, may have inspired the support for elimination of mother-to-child transmission of viral hepatitis expressed in the U.S. government's *Viral Hepatitis Action Plan, 2017-2020* (HHS, 2017b). Chapter 4 discusses management of HBsAg+ pregnant women and steps that may be taken to replicate the Alaskan success nation-

---

[4] Barring one or two international adoptions (McMahon, 2015).

ally. This chapter also describes measures to bring hepatitis B vaccination to more adults, thereby preventing horizontal transmission of HBV.

**The Committee's Conclusions Regarding
Targets for Hepatitis B Elimination**

- A 50 percent reduction in mortality from chronic hepatitis B, averting over 60,000 deaths, is possible in the United States by 2030. Meeting this goal will require diagnosing 90 percent of chronic hepatitis B cases, bringing 90 percent of those to care, and treating 80 percent of those for whom treatment is indicated.
- The same level of diagnosis, care, and treatment will reduce new cases of HBV-related hepatocellular carcinoma by about a third and new cases of HBV-related cirrhosis by about 45 percent.
- Prevalence of chronic hepatitis B in the United States will continue to increase because of in-migration of infected people.
- The elimination of hepatitis B virus infection in neonates and children under 5 is possible, as demonstrated in Alaska Natives.

HEPATITIS C MODELS

The author's full report, *Modeling the Elimination of Hepatitis C in the United States*, is shown in Appendix B. The author used a Markov model developed to estimate how morbidity, mortality, and total number of viremic HCV infections would change between 2015 and 2030 (Razavi et al., 2013, 2014). The model has been used previously to project disease burden in 100 countries; results have been validated with a panel of local experts in 59 of these countries (Blach et al., 2016). The model estimates the number of incident cases of hepatitis C, accounting for spontaneous clearance (Razavi et al., 2014). An older version of the model (predating direct-acting antiviral treatment for chronic hepatitis C) was validated with U.S. data (Kershenobich et al., 2011).

The model drew on published data from multiple sources. Estimates of the current U.S. population, including mortality by gender and age, came from United Nations (UN) data (Razavi et al., 2014; UN, 2015). Estimates of the percentage of the population who are HCV antibody positive and HCV RNA positive, the age and sex distribution of this prevalence, and the total number of cases diagnosed in a given year were drawn from peer-reviewed literature (Denniston et al., 2014; Edlin et al., 2015; Seeff, 2002; Volk et al., 2009). CDC data informed estimates of the distribution of HCV genotypes in the population and across newly diagnosed cases, while national reports and drug sale data were used to estimate the number of patients treated each year (Klevens et al., 2009, 2014; NCHS, 2015).

Information on the number of liver transplants, incidence of hepatocellular carcinoma, and deaths from hepatitis C came from published sources (Altekruse et al., 2014; CDC, 2016a; HRSA, 2016; NCI, 2015; Yang et al., 2012). The model's results were validated against incident cases of hepatocellular carcinoma attributable to chronic hepatitis C as reported to the Surveillance, Epidemiology, and End Results program.

The model compared four scenarios with different assumptions about screening and treatment on hepatitis C incidence and deaths, hepatocellular carcinoma, and decompensated cirrhosis due to hepatitis C. Table 2-5 describes the four scenarios. Briefly, the first scenario (labeled "Base 2013") reflects historical treatment data before the 2014 introduction of direct-acting antivirals. This scenario assumes 110,000 new patients diagnosed every year between 2013 and 2017. This number is shown to decline after 2017, both because of the preventive effect of removing infectious cases from the population and because over time the treatment-eligible patients remaining will be harder to find. This scenario allows for about 30,000 patients treated a year, and a rate of sustained virologic response[5] of 58 percent. The second scenario (labeled "Base 2015") assumes relatively little change in the number of new infections annually, but the use of current drug therapy, with its vastly better rates of sustained virologic response and far more people eligible for treatment. The model also assumes annual treatment of 260,000 people (about what has been reported since direct-acting agents came on the market) gradually declining to 130,000 between 2020 and 2030, but with current restrictions limiting treatment to patients with fibrosis grade 2 or worse. This model makes the same assumptions as the base scenario regarding the number of cases diagnosed and new infections each year. The third scenario (labeled "Aggressive ≥F0") assumes no fibrosis restrictions on treatment after 2017, with aggressive efforts made to diagnose new cases, but allows that the annual number diagnosed will begin to decrease around 2020 because there will be fewer infected cases in the population and the cases left will be harder to find. The final scenario (labeled "Aggressive ≥F2") also assumes 260,000 people will be treated every year and that aggressive measures will be taken to diagnose new cases, but limits treatment only to people with hepatitis fibrosis stage 2 or higher. The drop-off in the number of newly diagnosed cases is less pronounced in this model because HCV transmission will not decline much in a situation where only people with more advanced fibrosis are treated.

Estimates of the percentage change in total viremic HCV infections (meaning cases with detectable HCV RNA) and the percentage change in

---

[5] Sustained virologic response refers to eradication of HCV from the body, indicated by no detectable viral RNA 24 weeks after therapy. Relapse after sustained virologic response occurs in less than 1 percent of cases (NASEM, 2016a).

TABLE 2-5 Model Assumptions Regarding Numbers of People Treated, Diagnosed, and Newly Infected with HCV, as well as Their Ages and the Effectiveness of Treatment Over Time

Scenario	Assumption	Wave 1	Wave 2	Wave 3	Wave 4	Wave 5
Base 2013	Years	2013-2015	2016-2017	2018-2019	2020-2024	2025-2030
	Annual Treated	32,000	32,000	32,000	32,000	32,000
	Annual Newly Diagnosed	110,000	110,000	77,780	55,000	55,000
	Fibrosis Stage	≥F0	≥F0	≥F0	≥F0	≥F0
	Annual New Infections	29,690	30,270	30,100	29,980	29,800
	Treated Age	15-64	15-64	15-64	15-64	15-64
	SVR	58%	58%	58%	58%	58%
Base 2015	Years	2013-2014	2015-2016	2017-2019	2020-2024	2025-2030
	Annual Treated	32,000	260,000	183,800	130,000	130,000
	Annual Newly Diagnosed	110,000	110,000	77,780	55,000	55,000
	Fibrosis Stage	≥F0	≥F2	≥F2	≥F2	≥F2
	Annual New Infections	29,690	30,340	30,160	29,980	29,830
	Treated Age	15-64	15-64	15-74	15-74	15-74
	SVR	58%	90%	95%	95%	95%

Aggressive ≥F0	Years	2013-2014	2015-2016	2017-2019	2020-2024	2025-2030
	Annual Treated	32,000	260,000	260,000	260,000	260,000
	Annual Newly Diagnosed	110,000	110,000	110,000	88,790	71,660
	Fibrosis Stage	≥F0	≥F1	≥F0	≥F0	≥F0
	Annual New Infections	29,690	30,340	22,620	11,150	2,730
	Treated Age	15-64	15-64	15-74	15-74	15-74
	SVR	58%	90%	95%	95%	95%
Aggressive ≥F2	Years	2013-2014	2015-2016	2017-2019	2020-2024	2025-2030
	Annual Treated	32,000	260,000	260,000	260,000	260,000
	Annual Newly Diagnosed	110,000	110,000	110,000	95,940	83,670
	Fibrosis Stage	≥F0	≥F2	≥F2	≥F2	≥F2
	Annual New Infections	29,690	30,330	30,150	29,960	29,800
	Treated Age	15-64	15-64	15-74	15-74	15-74
	SVR	58%	90%	95%	95%	95%

NOTE: HCV = hepatitis C virus; SVR = sustained virologic response.

cumulative incident hepatocellular carcinoma, decompensated cirrhosis, and liver-related deaths relative to the 2015 baseline scenario are shown in Figure 2-1. As with the hepatitis B models, the value of the models lies in comparing the different scenarios and identifying important influences on the outcomes.

Removing all disease severity restrictions and taking aggressive efforts to diagnose new cases would reduce cumulative liver deaths between 2015 and 2030 by 10 percent (relative to 2015). As Figure 2-1 shows, the scenario combining aggressive diagnosis and treatment with restriction to only patients with advanced fibrosis results in a 35 percent reduction in deaths over the same time period. This counterintuitive result is partly a function of the model that holds constant the annual number of treated patients. The treatment restriction scenario modeled therefore includes some relatively healthy people in the 260,000 treated each year. Given that chronic hepatitis C infection is usually asymptomatic for decades, many of the people cured in this scenario would not have died by 2030, but they are more likely to transmit the infection (Hagan et al., 2004; Zeiler et al., 2010). For this reason, unrestricted treatment has a pronounced influence on incidence of chronic hepatitis C.

The model indicates considerable public health benefit to unrestricted treatment. Figure 2-1 shows that the total number of infected cases would drop 75 percent by 2030 (relative to the 2015 base scenario) if treatment were allocated without regard for disease stage. The trade-off between a sharp reduction in disease prevalence and a marginally larger reduction in deaths implied by these models is a function of holding the number of patients treated as an input parameter. Data from recent drug sales and national reports inform the model estimate of 260,000 patients treated every year. There is no reason why this number could not increase, especially if the recommendations made in Chapter 5 are implemented. Increasing the number of patients treated annually, so as to treat those with minimal fibrosis *and* those with more advanced disease at the same time, would allow for larger reductions in both chronic hepatitis C incidence and prevalence and liver-related mortality.

As Appendix B discusses, there were an estimated 21,600 deaths from chronic hepatitis C in the United States in 2015 (95 percent CI: 10,300 to 36,700 deaths). With no change to current practice, about 13,500 deaths related to hepatitis C would be expected in 2030, or 37.5 percent fewer than in 2015. The scenario combining unrestricted treatment with aggressive diagnosis (labeled "Aggressive ≥F0") would result in 7,100 hepatitis C-related deaths in 2030, about a two-thirds reduction from the 2015 level. The same scenario would reduce the incidence of chronic hepatitis C by 90 percent. Table 2-6 presents this information as well as the reduction in prevalence relative to the 2015 scenario.

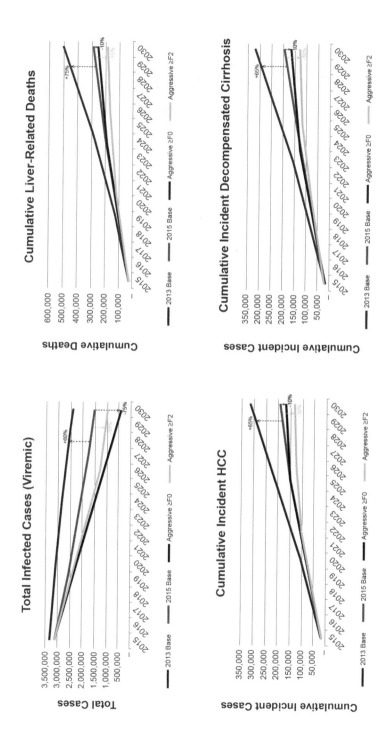

FIGURE 2-1 Cumulative disease burden by scenario with percentage reduction relative to 2015 Base, United States, 2015-2030.

NOTE: HCC = hepatocellular carcinoma.

TABLE 2-6 Reduction in Number of Deaths, Prevalence, and Incidence of Hepatitis C in 2030 Relative to 2015

	No Change from 2015	Aggressive ≥F0	Aggressive ≥F2
Number of deaths in 2030	13,500	7,100	4,100
Reduction in mortality relative 2015	38%	65%	80%
Total viremic cases in 2030	1,495,000	390,000	980,000
Reduction in prevalence relative 2015	50%	85%	70%
Total incident cases in 2030	29,830	2,730	29,800
Reduction in incidence relative 2015	2%	90%	2%
Cumulative HCV deaths	289,200	260,400	190,700
Deaths averted by 2030	—	28,800	98,500

NOTE: HCV = hepatitis C virus.

The committee's first report discussed a theoretical trade-off in eliminating hepatitis C: ending HCV transmission and ending deaths from hepatitis C are both possible with treatment, but meeting those goals requires attention to different populations (NASEM, 2016a). This model makes the same point. As Table 2-6 shows, more deaths would be averted by 2030 under the scenario where only patients with advanced fibrosis were treated, but unrestricted treatment reduces incident infections by 90 percent. Given that this committee was charged with identifying a strategy for the elimination of viral hepatitis, it favors the scenario that would elicit a sharp reduction in incidence. This incidence reduction, in turn, results in 85 percent fewer viremic cases in the population by 2030.

Replicating the success of this scenario, however, depends on aggressive diagnosis of new infections. As shown in Table 2-5, this scenario depends on diagnosing 110,000 cases a year until 2020, dropping to almost 89,000 from 2020 to 2024 and nearly 72,000 from 2025 to 2030. Diagnosis of 110,000 new infections a year was possible in the past partly because transmission was still so high. Over time, undiagnosed cases will be harder to find. People in contact with the health system will be cured of their HCV infection, and meeting the ambitious elimination target will depend on finding and curing individuals who have so far remained largely hidden.

People who inject drugs account for most HCV transmission in the United States; depending on the setting, hepatitis C prevalence in this group ranges from a third to over 80 percent, and these estimates, for the most part, predate the opioid epidemic (Alter, 1997; Hagan et al., 2008). Prisoners account for a (somewhat overlapping) third of national hepatitis C cases (Varan et al., 2014). One way to ensure sufficient case finding and treatment to allow for a 90 percent reduction in incidence and 65 percent reduction in mortality is to actively test and treat in these populations. The comprehensive harm reduction and prison health services described in Chapters 4 and 5 will be crucial to meeting these targets.

The main limitations of this model stem from its structure; it considers the number of patients treated every year as a model input. As Appendix B explains, the estimate of the number of patients treated every year comes from published data combined with expert consultation. This number is a bottleneck in the model, and it stands to reason that increasing the capacity of the health system to treat hepatitis C patients would allow a greater reduction in deaths, without compromising the reduction in total viremic cases or incident infections.

The model is also not designed to account for the effects of enhanced harm reduction on disease incidence, or how efforts to diagnose and treat in high-risk populations might have varying effects on morbidity and mortality. (That is, efforts to diagnose and treat clusters of people who inject drugs may elicit a sharper decrease in incidence than the same work spread among the general population.)

As with the hepatitis B models, underestimating the prevalence of hepatitis C in the population may also affect the results. The sensitivity analysis presented in Appendix B cites disease incidence as the variable with the largest effect on the results. It also explains that incidence of HCV infection is mostly driven by injection drug use, and that the opiate epidemic is not distributed evenly across the country. If the HCV incidence rates reported in Massachusetts were applied to the national model there would be considerably more incident infections and a greater prevalence of hepatitis C. At the same time, a greater prevalence of hepatitis C in the population would make it easier to diagnose a sufficient number of new cases every year to provide candidates for treatment.

**The Committee's Conclusions Regarding
Targets for Hepatitis C Elimination**

- A 90 percent reduction in incidence of hepatitis C (relative to the 2015 incidence carried forward) is possible in the United States by 2030. Meeting this goal will require treatment without restrictions on severity of disease and a consistent ability to diagnose new cases, even as prevalence decreases.
- The same levels of diagnosis and treatment would reduce mortality from hepatitis C in 2030 to 65 percent relative to 2015, and avert 28,800 deaths by 2030.
- Meeting these targets depends on diagnosing at least 110,000 cases a year until 2020, almost 89,000 a year between 2020 and 2024, and over 70,000 each year between 2025 and 2030.

A CENTRAL COORDINATING OFFICE

The targets suggested in this report are appropriately ambitious for the United States. The committee chose them in consideration of the country's resources and its responsibility to the global hepatitis elimination program. These targets have motivational value, but caution should be taken to prevent them from becoming purely aspirational. Overly ambitious targets, after all, can have discouraging consequences, as did the WHO's 2003 pledge to enroll 3 million HIV patients in poor countries on antiretrovirals in 2 years (Rice, 2016). When the goal was not met, Jim Kim, then head of the WHO's HIV and AIDS program, apologized for the failure, acknowledging the chosen timeline had not been realistic (Morris, 2005). Nevertheless, Kim ventured that the ambition of the pledge drove its eventual realization in 2007 (Rice, 2016).

The indicators and timelines given in this chapter represent the committee's best effort to balance a compelling public health target against practical constraints. The previous sections make clear, however, that meeting the targets will depend on aggressive testing, diagnosis, and treatment, as well as considerably increased attention to primary prevention methods such as needle exchange. In short, eliminating hepatitis B and C will require a significant departure from the status quo.

The next four chapters of this report discuss the committee's proposed strategy for viral hepatitis elimination. Recommendations are directed to various federal and state government agencies, as well as to legislators and different private sector organizations. With work spread among so many players, the opportunity for distraction is high. The leadership of a single office would help avoid diffusion of responsibility and ensure efficient and harmonious work.

President Clinton established the Office of National AIDS policy to make AIDS programming more cohesive (ONAP, n.d.). The office coordinates national and global HIV and AIDS programming to ensure that the national program is smoothly integrated at different levels of government and with foreign programs (ONAP, n.d.). Similar leadership would be a boon to the viral hepatitis strategy described in this report.

Recommendation 2-1: The highest level of the federal government should oversee a coordinated effort to manage viral hepatitis elimination.

Successful public health programs are characterized by high political commitment, financial support, and coordination. During the polio epidemics of the mid-20th century, for example, leaders understood that advances in science were necessary to stop children from becoming paralyzed. Pressure from the White House hastened the development of the Salk vaccine necessary for the eventual elimination of polio from the western hemisphere (Juskewitch et al., 2010). Similar cooperation at the highest levels of government has been characteristic of the guinea worm eradication campaign, one of the most successful disease eradication programs to date, and measles elimination (Orenstein, 2006; The Carter Center, n.d.).

History also provides examples of times when failure of high-level coordination prevented success. In the early years of the smallpox eradication campaign, the vaccine, though effective, was not reaching the public in the quantities necessary to stop the spread of infection. Immunizing vulnerable people became the responsibility of a relatively small team at the WHO that managed fieldwork (WHO, 1980).

The importance of central leadership, particularly at the White House level, would be invaluable to the fight against viral hepatitis. Leadership from the White House conveys a certain authority and indicates commitment to the effort across the executive branch; no department would be likely to command the same convening power. If HHS or one of its agencies were to lead the initiative, its ability to direct the Department of Justice or the Department of Veterans Affairs would be hard to establish. Such coordination is of particular concern for viral hepatitis response. The most recent nation action plan for viral hepatitis involved 23 different agencies and offices from 4 departments (HHS, 2017a).

If the president prefers not to create a new office, the coordinating role might also be filled by White House Office of National AIDS Policy mentioned above. This office has experience working across federal and state government agencies to implement the national strategy on HIV and AIDS (ONAP, 2015). Its staff hosted regional HIV forums around the country to encourage open discussion about how to reduce new infections and disparities and increase access to care (Brooks, 2015). Something similar may be appropriate as part of the viral hepatitis elimination strategy.

At the same time, the new administration might prefer that an office in HHS manage viral hepatitis elimination. In this case, the best choice would be the Office of HIV/AIDS and Infectious Disease Policy under the Office of the Assistant Secretary for Health. As the convener for the national viral hepatitis action plan this office already has experience working with the relevant federal agencies on viral hepatitis. Its staff also have technical depth on the topic (HHS, 2015, 2017b). Another viable candidate within HHS would be the Office of the Surgeon General, charged with managing public health practice (HHS, n.d.).

There is also room for active state support of viral hepatitis programming. Ideally, the states would be fully supported by a national office, but motivated state health commissioners may be able to adjust their state's priorities to make viral hepatitis programming more prominent.

The Problem of Stigma

As this committee's earlier report made clear, there are aspects of the viral hepatitis epidemic that resist easy remedy (NASEM, 2016a). Stigma is one such problem. Viral hepatitis patients often feel deeply ashamed of their condition, partly because HBV and HCV are commonly acquired through sexual contact or drug use and because liver disease in general is associated with substance use (Butt, 2008; Cotler et al., 2012; Golden et al., 2006; Moore et al., 2008; Wu et al., 2009; Yoo et al., 2012). Both HBV and HCV are infectious, so patients may fear social rejection if their diagnosis is widely known (Marinho and Barreira, 2013). In the face of such stigma, people may avoid testing, preferring not to know if they are infected, and people with chronic infection may avoid situations that force them to think about their condition (namely, medical care) (Vaughn-Sandler et al., 2014). In short, stigma encourages silence and inaction. It could undo the best viral hepatitis elimination campaign.

Stigma alleviation, while challenging, is possible. A recent National Academies of Sciences, Engineering, and Medicine report found mixed evidence on the effectiveness of education programs to change public attitudes toward mental illness, for example (NASEM, 2016b). In reviewing large campaigns, the report promoted legislative and policy change as valuable goals for anti-stigma efforts. These so-called hard goal campaigns may have particular promise for improving quality of life for people with substance use disorders and other mental health problems (NASEM, 2016b). A large central office at the level of the White House might be in the best position to manage such efforts to reduce stigma.

Other aspects of elimination described later in this report will also require a central coordinating office. The models presented in this chapter make it clear that elimination will depend on considerable improvements to diagnosis and treatment of infected patients. Many such patients were born abroad, and others may have a history of substance use disorders or incarceration. Outreach to such groups can be sensitive and could benefit from a unified plan for communication and service provision with an emphasis on bringing services to the target populations.

Finally, this report discusses key gaps in the research on viral hepatitis and suggests research priorities for different federal agencies. The oversight of a single office could help ensure that various research agendas are balanced efficiently among funding agencies and devoid of unnecessary redundancy.

REFERENCES

Altekruse, S. F., S. J. Henley, J. E. Cucinelli, and K. A. McGlynn. 2014. Changing hepatocellular carcinoma incidence and liver cancer mortality rates in the United States. *American Journal of Gastroenterology* 109(4):542-553.

Alter, M. J. 1997. Epidemiology of hepatitis C. *Hepatology* 26(3 Suppl 1):62S-65S.

Arends, P., M. J. Sonneveld, R. Zoutendijk, I. Carey, A. Brown, M. Fasano, D. Mutimer, K. Deterding, J. G. Reijnders, Y. Oo, J. Petersen, F. van Bommel, R. J. De Knegt, T. Santantonio, T. Berg, T. M. Welzel, H. Wedemeyer, M. Buti, P. Pradat, F. Zoulim, B. Hansen, and H. L. Janssen. 2015. Entecavir treatment does not eliminate the risk of hepatocellular carcinoma in chronic hepatitis B: Limited role for risk scores in Caucasians. *Gut* 64(8):1289-1295.

Blach, S., S. Zeuzem, M. Manns, I. Altraif, A.-S. Duberg, D. H. Muljono, I. Waked, S. M. Alavian, M.-H. Lee, F. Negro, F. Abaalkhail, A. Abdou, M. Abdulla, A. A. Rached, I. Aho, U. Akarca, I. Al Ghazzawi, S. Al Kaabi, F. Al Lawati, K. Al Namaani, Y. Al Serkal, S. A. Al-Busafi, L. Al-Dabal, S. Aleman, A. S. Alghamdi, A. A. Aljumah, H. E. Al-Romaihi, M. I. Andersson, V. Arendt, P. Arkkila, A. M. Assiri, O. Baatarkhuu, A. Bane, Z. Ben-Ari, C. Bergin, F. Bessone, F. Bihl, A. R. Bizri, M. Blachier, A. J. Blasco, C. E. B. Mello, P. Bruggmann, C. R. Brunton, F. Calinas, H. L. Y. Chan, A. Chaudhry, H. Cheinquer, C.-J. Chen, R.-N. Chien, M. S. Choi, P. B. Christensen, W.-L. Chuang, V. Chulanov, L. Cisneros, M. R. Clausen, M. E. Cramp, A. Craxi, E. A. Croes, O. Dalgard, J. R. Daruich, V. de Ledinghen, G. J. Dore, M. H. El-Sayed, G. Ergör, G. Esmat, C. Estes, K. Falconer, E. Farag, M. L. G. Ferraz, P. R. Ferreira, R. Flisiak, S. Frankova, I. Gamkrelidze, E. Gane, J. García-Samaniego, A. G. Khan, I. Gountas, A. Goldis, M. Gottfredsson, J. Grebely, M. Gschwantler, M. G. Pessôa, J. Gunter, B. Hajarizadeh, O. Hajelssedig, S. Hamid, W. Hamoudi, A. Hatzakis, S. M. Himatt, H. Hofer, I. Hrstic, Y.-T. Hui, B. Hunyady, R. Idilman, W. Jafri, R. Jahis, N. Z. Janjua, P. Jarčuška, A. Jeruma, J. G. Jonasson, Y. Kamel, J.-H. Kao, S. Kaymakoglu, D. Kershenobich, J. Khamis, Y. S. Kim, L. Kondili, Z. Koutoubi, M. Krajden, H. Krarup, M.-s. Lai, W. Laleman, W.-c. Lao, D. Lavanchy, P. Lázaro, H. Leleu, O. Lesi, L. A. Lesmana, M. Li, V. Liakina, Y.-S. Lim, B. Luksic, A. Mahomed, M. Maimets, M. Makara, A. O. Malu, R. T. Marinho, P. Marotta, S. Mauss, M. S. Memon, M. C. M. Correa, N. Mendez-Sanchez, S. Merat, A. M. Metwally, R. Mohamed, C. Moreno, F. H. Mourad, B. Müllhaupt, K. Murphy, H. Nde, R. Njouom, D. Nonkovic, S. Norris, S. Obekpa, S. Oguche, S. Olafsson, M. Oltman, O. Omede, C. Omuemu, O. Opare-Sem, A. L. H. Øvrehus, S. Owusu-Ofori, T. S. Oyunsuren, G. Papatheodoridis, K. Pasini, K. M. Peltekian, R. O. Phillips, N. Pimenov, H. Poustchi, N. Prabdial-Sing, H. Qureshi, A. Ramji, D. Razavi-Shearer, K. Razavi-Shearer, B. Redae, H. W. Reesink, E. Ridruejo, S. Robbins, L. R. Roberts, S. K.

Roberts, W. M. Rosenberg, F. Roudot-Thoraval, S. D. Ryder, R. Safadi, O. Sagalova, R. Salupere, F. M. Sanai, J. F. S. Avila, V. Saraswat, R. Sarmento-Castro, C. Sarrazin, J. D. Schmelzer, I. Schréter, C. Seguin-Devaux, S. R. Shah, A. I. Sharara, M. Sharma, A. Shevaldin, G. E. Shiha, W. Sievert, M. Sonderup, K. Souliotis, D. Speiciene, J. Sperl, P. Stärkel, R. E. Stauber, C. Stedman, D. Struck, T.-H. Su, V. Sypsa, S.-S. Tan, J. Tanaka, A. J. Thompson, I. Tolmane, K. Tomasiewicz, J. Valantinas, P. Van Damme, A. J. van der Meer, I. van Thiel, H. Van Vlierberghe, A. Vince, W. Vogel, H. Wedemeyer, N. Weis, V. W. S. Wong, C. Yaghi, A. Yosry, M.-f. Yuen, E. Yunihastuti, A. Yusuf, E. Zuckerman, and H. Razavi. 2016. Global prevalence and genotype distribution of hepatitis C virus infection in 2015: A modelling study. *The Lancet Gastroenterology & Hepatology* 2(3):161-176.

Brooks, D. M. 2015. *Office of National AIDS Policy to host national HIV/AIDS strategy regional forums.* https://obamawhitehouse.archives.gov/blog/2015/03/27/office-national-aids-policy-host-national-hivaids-strategy-regional-forums (accessed February 24, 2017).

Butt, G. 2008. Stigma in the context of hepatitis C: Concept analysis. *Journal of Advanced Nursing* 62(6):712-724.

Campsen, J., M. Zimmerman, J. Trotter, J. Hong, C. Freise, R. Brown, A. Cameron, M. Ghobrial, I. Kam, R. Busuttil, S. Saab, C. Holt, J. Emond, J. Stiles, T. Lukose, M. Chang, and G. Klintmalm. 2013. Liver transplantation for hepatitis B liver disease and concomitant hepatocellular carcinoma in the United States with hepatitis B immunoglobulin and nucleoside/nucleotide analogues. *Liver Transplantation* 19(9):1020-1029.

CDC (Centers for Disease Control and Prevention). 2016a. *Viral hepatitis–Statistics and surveillance.* https://www.cdc.gov/hepatitis/statistics (accessed December 20, 2016).

CDC. 2016b. *What is viral hepatitis?* https://www.cdc.gov/hepatitis/abc/index.htm (accessed December 27, 2016).

Chen, Y. C., C. M. Chu, and Y. F. Liaw. 2010. Age-specific prognosis following spontaneous hepatitis B e antigen seroconversion in chronic hepatitis B. *Hepatology* 51(2):435-444.

Chotiyaputta, W., C. Peterson, F. A. Ditah, D. Goodwin, and A. S. Lok. 2011. Persistence and adherence to nucleos(t)ide analogue treatment for chronic hepatitis B. *Journal of Hepatology* 54(1):12-18.

Chu, C. M., and Y. F. Liaw. 2007. HBsAg seroclearance in asymptomatic carriers of high endemic areas: Appreciably high rates during a long-term follow-up. *Hepatology* 45(5): 1187-1192.

Chu, C. M., and Y. F. Liaw. 2009. Incidence and risk factors of progression to cirrhosis in inactive carriers of hepatitis B virus. *American Journal of Gastroenterology* 104(7): 1693-1699.

Cohen, C., A. A. Evans, W. T. London, J. Block, M. Conti, and T. Block. 2008. Underestimation of chronic hepatitis B virus infection in the United States of America. *Journal of Viral Hepatitis* 15(1):12-13.

Cotler, S., S. Cotler, H. Xie, B. Luc, T. Layden, and S. Wong. 2012. Characterizing hepatitis B stigma in Chinese immigrants. *Journal of Viral Hepatitis* 19(2):147-152.

Denniston, M. M., R. B. Jiles, J. Drobeniuc, R. M. Klevens, J. W. Ward, G. M. McQuillan, and S. D. Holmberg. 2014. Chronic hepatitis C virus infection in the United States, National Health and Nutrition Examination Survey 2003 to 2010. *Annals of Internal Medicine* 160(5):293-300.

Edlin, B. R., B. J. Eckhardt, M. A. Shu, S. D. Holmberg, and T. Swan. 2015. Toward a more accurate estimate of the prevalence of hepatitis C in the United States. *Hepatology* 62(5):1353-1363.

Fattovich, G., F. Bortolotti, and F. Donato. 2008. Natural history of chronic hepatitis B: Special emphasis on disease progression and prognostic factors. *Journal of Hepatology* 48(2):335-352.

FitzSimons, D., B. McMahon, G. Hendrickx, A. Vorsters, and P. Van Damme. 2013. Burden and prevention of viral hepatitis in the Arctic region, Copenhagen, Denmark, 22-23 March 2012. *International Journal of Circumpolar Health* 72(10).

Golden, J., R. M. Conroy, A. M. O'Dwyer, D. Golden, and J.-B. Hardouin. 2006. Illness-related stigma, mood and adjustment to illness in persons with hepatitis C. *Social Science & Medicine* 63(12):3188-3198.

Gvinjilia, L., M. Nasrullah, D. Sergeenko, T. Tsertsvadze, G. Kamkamidze, M. Butsashvili, A. Gamkrelidze, P. Imnadze, V. Kvaratskhelia, N. Chkhartishvili, L. Sharvadze, J. Drobeniuc, L. Hagan, J. W. Ward, J. Morgan, and F. Averhoff. 2016. National progress toward hepatitis C elimination—Georgia, 2015-2016. *Morbidity and Mortality Weekly Report* 65(41):1132-1135.

Hagan, H., H. Thiede, and D. C. Des Jarlais. 2004. Hepatitis C virus infection among injection drug users: Survival analysis of time to seroconversion. *Epidemiology* 15(5):543-549.

Hagan, H., E. R. Pouget, D. C. Des Jarlais, and C. Lelutiu-Weinberger. 2008. Meta-regression of hepatitis C virus infection in relation to time since onset of illicit drug injection: The influence of time and place. *American Journal of Epidemiology* 168(10):1099-1109.

Heathcote, E. J., P. Marcellin, M. Buti, E. Gane, A. Robert, Z. Krastev, G. Germanidis, S. S. Lee, R. Flisiak, and K. Kaita. 2011. Three-year efficacy and safety of tenofovir disoproxil fumarate treatment for chronic hepatitis B. *Gastroenterology* 140(1):132-143.

HHS (Department of Health and Human Services). 2015. *Action plan for the prevention, care, and treatment of viral hepatitis: 2014-2016.* HHS, Office of the Assistant Secretary for Health, Office of HIV/AIDS and Infectious Disease Policy. https://www.aids.gov/pdf/viral-hepatitis-action-plan.pdf (accessed October 26, 2016).

HHS. 2017a. *Federal agencies & offices engaged in the viral hepatitis action plan 2017-2020.* https://www.hhs.gov/hepatitis/action-plan/federal-agencies-engaged/index.html (accessed February 24, 2017).

HHS. 2017b. *National viral hepatitis action plan 2017-2020.* HHS, Office of the Assistant Secretary for Health, Office of HIV/AIDS and Infectious Disease Policy. https://www.hhs.gov/sites/default/files/National%20Viral%20Hepatitis%20Action%20Plan%202017-2020.pdf (February 24, 2017).

HHS. n.d. *Duties of the Surgeon General.* https://www.surgeongeneral.gov/about/duties/index.html (accessed February 24, 2017).

HRSA (Health Resources and Services Administration). 2016. *OPTN (Organ Procurement and Transplant Network). Data.* https://optn.transplant.hrsa.gov/data (accessed December 22, 2016).

Hu, D. J., J. Xing, R. A. Tohme, Y. Liao, H. Pollack, J. W. Ward, and S. D. Holmberg. 2013. Hepatitis B testing and access to care among racial and ethnic minorities in selected communities across the United States, 2009-2010. *Hepatology* 58(3):856-862.

Juday, T., H. Tang, M. Harris, A. Z. Powers, E. Kim, and G. J. Hanna. 2011. Adherence to chronic hepatitis B treatment guideline recommendations for laboratory monitoring of patients who are not receiving antiviral treatment. *Journal of General Internal Medicine* 26(3):239-244.

Juskewitch, J. E., C. J. Tapia, and A. J. Windebank. 2010. Lessons from the Salk polio vaccine: Methods for and risks of rapid translation. *Clinical and Translational Science* 3(4):182-185.

Kanwal, F., M. Farid, P. Martin, G. Chen, I. M. Gralnek, G. S. Dulai, and B. M. Spiegel. 2006. Treatment alternatives for hepatitis B cirrhosis: A cost-effectiveness analysis. *American Journal of Gastroenterology* 101(9):2076-2089.

Kershenobich, D., H. A. Razavi, C. L. Cooper, A. Alberti, G. M. Dusheiko, S. Pol, E. Zuckerman, K. Koike, K. Han, C. M. Wallace, S. Zeuzem, and F. Negro. 2011. Applying a system approach to forecast the total hepatitis C virus-infected population size: Model validation using US data. *Liver International* 31(Suppl 2):4-17.

Kim, W. R. 2009. Epidemiology of hepatitis B in the United States. *Hepatology* 49(5 Suppl): S28-S34.

Kim, L. H., V. G. Nguyen, H. N. Trinh, J. Li, J. Q. Zhang, and M. H. Nguyen. 2014. Low treatment rates in patients meeting guideline criteria in diverse practice settings. *Digestive Diseases and Sciences* 59(9):2091-2099.

Klevens, R. M., J. Miller, C. Vonderwahl, S. Speers, K. Alelis, K. Sweet, E. Rocchio, T. Poissant, T. M. Vogt, and K. Gallagher. 2009. Population-based surveillance for hepatitis C virus, United States, 2006-2007. *Emerging Infectious Diseases* 15(9):1499-1502.

Klevens, R. M., S. Liu, H. Roberts, R. B. Jiles, and S. D. Holmberg. 2014. Estimating acute viral hepatitis infections from nationally reported cases. *American Journal of Public Health* 104(3):482-487.

Ko, S. C., L. Fan, E. A. Smith, N. Fenlon, A. K. Koneru, and T. V. Murphy. 2014. Estimated annual perinatal hepatitis B virus infections in the United States, 2000–2009. *Journal of the Pediatric Infectious Diseases Society* 5(2):114-121.

Kowdley, K. V., C. C. Wang, S. Welch, H. Roberts, and C. L. Brosgart. 2012. Prevalence of chronic hepatitis B among foreign-born persons living in the United States by country of origin. *Hepatology* 56(2):422-433.

Lin, X., N. J. Robinson, M. Thursz, D. M. Rosenberg, A. Weild, J. M. Pimenta, and A. J. Hall. 2005. Chronic hepatitis B virus infection in the Asia-Pacific region and Africa: Review of disease progression. *Journal of Gastroenterology and Hepatology* 20(6):833-843.

Lin, S. Y., E. T. Chang, and S. K. So. 2007. Why we should routinely screen Asian American adults for hepatitis B: A cross-sectional study of Asians in California. *Hepatology* 46(4):1034-1040.

Lok, A. S. F., B. J. McMahon, R. S. Brown, J. B. Wong, A. T. Ahmed, W. Farah, J. Almasri, F. Alahdab, K. Benkhadra, M. A. Mouchli, S. Singh, E. A. Mohamed, A. M. Abu Dabrh, L. J. Prokop, Z. Wang, M. H. Murad, and K. Mohammed. 2016. Antiviral therapy for chronic hepatitis B viral infection in adults: A systematic review and meta-analysis. *Hepatology* 63(1):284-306.

Marcellin, P., E. Gane, M. Buti, N. Afdhal, W. Sievert, I. M. Jacobson, M. K. Washington, G. Germanidis, J. F. Flaherty, R. Aguilar Schall, J. D. Bornstein, K. M. Kitrinos, G. M. Subramanian, J. G. McHutchison, and E. J. Heathcote. 2013. Regression of cirrhosis during treatment with tenofovir disoproxil fumarate for chronic hepatitis B: A 5-year open-label follow-up study. *Lancet* 381(9865):468-475.

Marinho, R. T., and D. P. Barreira. 2013. Hepatitis C, stigma and cure. *World Journal of Gastroenterology* 19(40):6703-6709.

Mast, E. E., C. Weinbaum, A. E. Fiore, M. J. Alter, B. Bell, L. Finelli, L. Rodewald, J. M. Douglas, Jr., R. S. Janssen, and J. W. Ward. 2006. A comprehensive immunization strategy to eliminate transmission of hepatitis B virus infection in the United States. Recommendations of the Advisory Committee on Immunization Practices (ACIP). Part II: Immunization of adults. *Morbidity and Mortality Weekly Report* 55(RR16):1-25.

McMahon, B. J. 2015. *Management of patients with chronic hepatitis B: The Alaska experience.* PowerPoint presentation to the Committee on a National Strategy for the Elimination of Hepatitis B and C, Washington, DC, November 30, 2015. http://www.nationalacademies. org/hmd/~/media/Files/Activity%20Files/PublicHealth/HepatitisBandC/1-November2015/8%20-%20Brian%20McMahon.pdf (accessed January 10, 2017).

McMahon, B. J., L. Bulkow, B. Simons, Y. Zhang, S. Negus, C. Homan, P. Spradling, E. Teshale, D. Lau, and M. Snowball. 2014. Population-based longitudinal study of hepatitis B "e" antigen negative persons with chronic hepatitis B: Level of HBV DNA and liver disease. *Clinical Gastroenterology and Hepatology* 12(4):701.

Mitruka, K., T. Tsertsvadze, M. Butsashvili, A. Gamkrelidze, P. Sabelashvili, E. Adamia, M. Chokheli, J. Drobeniuc, L. Hagan, A. M. Harris, T. Jiqia, A. Kasradze, S. Ko, V. Qerashvili, L. Sharvadze, I. Tskhomelidze, V. Kvaratskhelia, J. Morgan, J. W. Ward, and F. Averhoff. 2015. Launch of a nationwide hepatitis C elimination program—Georgia, April 2015. *Morbidity and Mortality Weekly Report* 64(28):753-757.

Moore, G. A., D. A. Hawley, and P. Bradley. 2008. Hepatitis C: Studying stigma. *Gastroenterology Nursing* 31(5):346-352.

Morris, M. 2005. Apology over missed AIDS target. *BBC*, November 28.

NASEM (National Academies of Sciences, Engineering, and Medicine). 2016a. *Eliminating the public health problem of hepatitis B and C in the United States: Phase one report.* Washington, DC: The National Academies Press.

NASEM. 2016b. *Ending discrimination against people with mental and substance use disorders: The evidence for stigma change.* Washington, DC: The National Academies Press.

NCHS (National Center for Health Statistics). 2015. *National Health and Nutrition Examination Survey data, 2003-2014.* Hyattsville, MD: Department of Health and Human Services, Centers for Disease Control and Prevention.

NCI (National Cancer Institute). 2015. SEER*Stat Database: Incidence - SEER 9 Regs Research Data, Nov 2015 Sub (1973-2013). Surveillance, Epidemiology, and End Results (SEER) Program.

ONAP (Office of National AIDS Policy). 2015. *National HIV/AIDS strategy for the United States: Updated to 2020. Federal action plan.* Washington, DC: White House Office of National AIDS Policy.

ONAP. n.d. *Office of National AIDS Policy.* https://clinton2.nara.gov/ONAP/accomp.html (accessed February 24, 2017).

Orenstein, W. A. 2006. The role of measles elimination in development of a national immunization program. *The Pediatric Infectious Disease Journal* 25(12):1093-1101.

Papatheodoridis, G. V., H. L.-Y. Chan, B. E. Hansen, H. L. Janssen, and P. Lampertico. 2015. Risk of hepatocellular carcinoma in chronic hepatitis B: Assessment and modification with current antiviral therapy. *Journal of Hepatology* 62(4):956-967.

Raffetti, E., G. Fattovich, and F. Donato. 2016. Incidence of hepatocellular carcinoma in untreated subjects with chronic hepatitis B: A systematic review and meta-analysis. *Liver International* 36(9):1239-1251.

Razavi, H., C. Estes, K. Pasini, E. Gower, and S. Hindman. 2013. HCV treatment rate in select European countries in 2004–2010. *Journal of Hepatology* 58(Suppl 1):S22-S23.

Razavi, H., I. Waked, C. Sarrazin, R. Myers, R. Idilman, F. Calinas, W. Vogel, M. Correa, C. Hézode, and P. Lázaro. 2014. The present and future disease burden of hepatitis C virus (HCV) infection with today's treatment paradigm. *Journal of Viral Hepatitis* 21(S1):34-59.

Rice, A. 2016. How the World Bank's biggest critic became its president. *Guardian*, August 11. https://www.theguardian.com/news/2016/aug/11/world-bank-jim-yong-kim (accessed September 22, 2016).

Roberts, H., D. Kruszon-Moran, K. N. Ly, E. Hughes, K. Iqbal, R. B. Jiles, and S. D. Holmberg. 2016. Prevalence of chronic hepatitis B virus (HBV) infection in U.S. households: National Health and Nutrition Examination Survey (NHANES), 1988-2012. *Hepatology* 63(2):388-397.

Seeff, L. B. 2002. Natural history of chronic hepatitis C. *Hepatology* 36(5B):S35-S46.

Sergeenko, D. 2015. *Progress towards hepatitis C elimination in Georgia.* World Hepatitis Summit 2015. http://www.worldhepatitissummit.org/docs/default-source/default-document-library/2015/resources/hepatitis-at-a-national-level.pdf?sfvrsn=4 (accessed October 26, 2016).

Stvilia, K., T. Tsertsvadze, L. Sharvadze, M. Aladashvili, C. del Rio, M. H. Kuniholm, and K. E. Nelson. 2006. Prevalence of hepatitis C, HIV, and risk behaviors for blood-borne infections: A population-based survey of the adult population of T'bilisi, Republic of Georgia. *Journal of Urban Health* 83(2):289-298.

Tenney, D. J., R. E. Rose, C. J. Baldick, K. A. Pokornowski, B. J. Eggers, J. Fang, M. J. Wichroski, D. Xu, J. Yang, and R. B. Wilber. 2009. Long-term monitoring shows hepatitis B virus resistance to entecavir in nucleoside-naïve patients is rare through 5 years of therapy. *Hepatology* 49(5):1503-1514.

The Carter Center. n.d. *Guinea worm eradication program.* https://www.cartercenter.org/health/guinea_worm (accessed September 22, 2016).

Thiele, M., L. L. Gluud, A. D. Fialla, E. K. Dahl, and A. Krag. 2014. Large variations in risk of hepatocellular carcinoma and mortality in treatment naïve hepatitis B patients: Systematic review with meta-analyses. *PLoS One* 9(9):e107177.

Toy, M., J. A. Salomon, H. Jiang, H. Gui, H. Wang, J. Wang, J. H. Richardus, and Q. Xie. 2014. Population health impact and cost-effectiveness of monitoring inactive chronic hepatitis B and treating eligible patients in Shanghai, China. *Hepatology* 60(1):46-55.

Tsertsvadze, T. 2016. *National hepatitis C elimination program in Georgia.* Ninth Paris Hepatitis Conference, Paris, France, January 11.

Uddin, G., D. Shoeb, S. Solaiman, R. Marley, C. Gore, M. Ramsay, R. Harris, I. Ushiro-Lumb, S. Moreea, S. Alam, H. C. Thomas, S. Khan, B. Watt, R. N. Pugh, S. Ramaiah, R. Jervis, A. Hughes, S. Singhal, S. Cameron, W. F. Carman, and G. R. Foster. 2010. Prevalence of chronic viral hepatitis in people of South Asian ethnicity living in England: The prevalence cannot necessarily be predicted from the prevalence in the country of origin. *Journal of Viral Hepatitis* 17(5):327-335.

UN (United Nations). 2015. *World population prospects: The 2015 revision, key findings and advance tables.* New York: Department of Economic and Social Affairs, Population Division.

Varan, A. K., D. W. Mercer, M. S. Stein, and A. C. Spaulding. 2014. Hepatitis C seroprevalence among prison inmates since 2001: Still high but declining. *Public Health Reports* 129(2):187-195.

Vaughn-Sandler, V., C. Sherman, A. Aronsohn, and M. L. Volk. 2014. Consequences of perceived stigma among patients with cirrhosis. *Digestive Diseases and Sciences* 59(3):681-686.

Volk, M. L., R. Tocco, S. Saini, and A. S. Lok. 2009. Public health impact of antiviral therapy for hepatitis C in the United States. *Hepatology* 50(6):1750-1755.

Wasley, A., D. Kruszon-Moran, W. Kuhnert, E. P. Simard, L. Finelli, G. McQuillan, and B. Bell. 2010. The prevalence of hepatitis B virus infection in the United States in the era of vaccination. *Journal of Infectious Diseases* 202(2):192-201.

WHO (World Health Organization). 1980. *The global eradication of smallpox: Final report of the Global Commission for the Certification of Smallpox Eradication, Geneva, December 1979.* Geneva, Switzerland: WHO.

WHO. 2016a. *Combating hepatitis B and C to reach elimination by 2030.* Geneva, Switzerland: WHO.

WHO. 2016b. *Global health sector strategy on viral hepatitis, 2016-2021: Towards ending viral hepatitis.* Geneva, Switzerland: WHO. http://apps.who.int/iris/bitstream/10665/246177/1/WHO-HIV-2016.06-eng.pdf (July 19, 2016).

WHO Regional Office for Europe. 2015. *Georgia sets sights on eliminating hepatitis C.* http://www.euro.who.int/en/countries/georgia/news/news/2015/07/georgia-sets-sights-on-eliminating-hepatitis-c (accessed July 11, 2016).

Wong, G. L. H., H. L. Y. Chan, C. W. H. Mak, S. K. Y. Lee, Z. M. Y. Ip, A. T. H. Lam, H. W. H. Iu, J. M. S. Leung, J. W. Y. Lai, and A. O. S. Lo. 2013. Entecavir treatment reduces hepatic events and deaths in chronic hepatitis B patients with liver cirrhosis. *Hepatology* 58(5):1537-1547.

Wu, H., C. Yim, A. Chan, M. Ho, and J. Heathcote. 2009. Sociocultural factors that potentially affect the institution of prevention and treatment strategies for hepatitis B in Chinese Canadians. *Canadian Journal of Gastroenterology* 23(1):31-36.

Yang, J. D., B. Kim, S. O. Sanderson, J. L. S. Sauver, B. P. Yawn, R. A. Pedersen, J. J. Larson, T. M. Therneau, L. R. Roberts, and W. R. Kim. 2012. Hepatocellular carcinoma in Olmsted County, Minnesota, 1976-2008. *Mayo Clinic Proceedings* 87(1):9-16.

Yoo, G. J., T. Fang, J. Zola, and W. M. Dariotis. 2012. Destigmatizing hepatitis B in the Asian American community: Lessons learned from the San Francisco Hep B Free campaign. *Journal of Cancer Education* 27(1):138-144.

Zeiler, I., T. Langlands, J. M. Murray, and A. Ritter. 2010. Optimal targeting of hepatitis C virus treatment among injecting drug users to those not enrolled in methadone maintenance programs. *Drug and Alcohol Dependence* 110(3):228-233.

3

Public Health Information

The recent *Lancet* Global Burden of Disease analysis found viral hepatitis to account for almost 1.5 million deaths (1.45 million, 95 percent confidence interval [CI]: 1.38 to 1.54 million) and 41.6 million years of life lost to society every year (95 percent CI: 39.1 to 44.7 years) (Stanaway et al., 2016). An editorial in the same issue of *Lancet* pointed out that despite causing more deaths than HIV, tuberculosis, and malaria, viral hepatitis gets relatively little funding or attention from policy makers (Wiktor and Hutin, 2016). "One reason for this," the authors propose, "is the difficulty in accurately quantifying and explaining the morbidity and mortality related to viral hepatitis" (Wiktor and Hutin, 2016, p. 1). Hepatitis B virus (HBV) and hepatitis C virus (HCV) infections are clinically silent in most patients for decades, and when symptoms do emerge they are often non-specific or mild. Serious clinical consequences of infection may occur decades later, with the root infection often not recorded on death certificates (Mahajan et al., 2014; Wiktor and Hutin, 2016).

In forming a national hepatitis strategy, the World Health Organization (WHO) advises each country to "know your epidemic," and respond accordingly (WHO, 2016). Reliable data on new infections, morbidity, and mortality from hepatitis B and C are a fundamental part of tailoring an effective response strategy. This is not to say that collecting such data is an end in itself. The WHO guidance emphasizes the importance of a system that "translates up-to-date data on viral hepatitis into usable information" to drive political commitment (WHO, 2016, p. 26). Such data also have immediate practical value. When, for example, surveillance identifies a spike in HBV infections associated with a medical or dental practice, the health department can respond with suitable counter-measures.

In the United States, measuring the burden of disease is the primary responsibility of state and local health departments that collect data and send the de-identified information to the Centers for Disease Control and Prevention (CDC). The CDC defines public health surveillance as "the ongoing, systematic collection, analysis, interpretation, and dissemination of data regarding a health-related event for use in public health action to reduce morbidity and mortality and to improve health" (German et al., 2001; Rutherford, 2001; Thacker and Berkelman, 1988). A 2010 Institute of Medicine committee further discussed the role of surveillance for HBV and HCV (IOM, 2010). In its report, the committee cited a role for the health department in identifying and responding to outbreaks, developing well-targeted estimates of disease burden, and evaluating ongoing prevention programs (IOM, 2010).

State and local health departments are legally required to conduct surveillance on reportable conditions, including hepatitis B and C, though privacy laws prevent them from sharing identifiable information outside their jurisdictions. In order to keep the data consistent across states, the CDC has developed a standardized case reporting format, though states often collect additional data that are not shared with the CDC. Increased surveillance for viral hepatitis would surely bring more cases to light. Case finding with proper follow-up could ensure patients access to medical care. Using such data, state and local health authorities can describe the HBV- and HCV-infected populations, calculate what proportion of them receive care, and set targets for improved use of services. Understanding the incidence and prevalence of viral hepatitis is complementary to surveillance activities. Such research, combined with surveillance, will provide needed information about viral hepatitis in the United States. This chapter describes ways through which both could be improved.

As discussed in this committee's phase one report, not all state or local health departments are in a position to measure morbidity and mortality attributable to viral hepatitis (NASEM, 2016). Meeting the goals set in the previous chapter will require this and more: well-placed preventive services, efficient screening and testing, and care that reaches all patients, especially the poor and people who inject drugs. The full range of services for viral hepatitis elimination is sometimes presented as a cascade, as shown in the next chapter, with the preventive measures intended for the whole population at one end and progressively more specific services reaching the patients who need them. Information about every step on this cascade will be essential in elimination. This chapter discusses improvements to the national viral hepatitis information system that would advance this goal.

DESCRIBING THE VIRAL HEPATITIS EPIDEMIC

Routine surveillance at the state and local levels will be essential to meet the goals discussed in the previous chapter. The same was true for smallpox eradication and for all disease elimination programs (Broekmans et al., 2002; Cattand et al., 2001; de Quadros et al., 1996; Nesheim et al., 2012; WHO, 1980; Zhou et al., 2013). In the United States, the same state and local health authorities that coordinate control efforts also conduct surveillance. Every week, health departments around the country send the CDC electronic data on nationally notifiable diseases, usually communicable diseases of public health significance (Smith et al., 2013). Both acute and chronic hepatitis B and C are notifiable conditions, but because of the chronic and frequently asymptomatic nature of the infections, surveillance for viral hepatitis is different from that for many other infectious diseases. Viral hepatitis surveillance requires tracking individual patients over time and processing a large amount of information for every case. In some ways, the best transferable examples for hepatitis surveillance systems come from HIV, also a communicable, chronic infection. HIV surveillance data are increasingly used to measure patients' progress from diagnosis to care to suppression of viral load (Medland et al., 2015).

Data gleaned from routine surveillance can give insight into patterns of access to care; help estimate disease burden in a particular region; and tailor prevention and response activities (Barton et al., 2014; Cocoros et al., 2014; HHS, 2015; Kinnard et al., 2014; Klevens et al., 2009; Viner et al., 2015). But in 2014, the most recent year for which data are available, 11 states did not report any newly detected cases of chronic HBV infection; another 11 states did not report any cases of acute HCV infection; and 17 states did not report any past or present cases of HCV infection (CDC, 2016b). These limitations raise concerns about the fitness of the hepatitis surveillance system. Elimination will depend on a more accurate picture of disease burden, as described in Box 3-1.

Integrated, highly automated, electronic surveillance systems could go far toward improving our understanding of the national disease burden (Troppy et al., 2014). To be effective, informatics tools need to be paired with human expertise, ongoing maintenance and technological support. CDC investment in both would advance viral hepatitis elimination in the United States.

Recommendation 3-1: The Centers for Disease Control and Prevention (CDC), in partnership with state and local health departments, should support standard hepatitis case finding measures, and the follow-up, monitoring, and linkage to care of all viral hepatitis cases reported through public health surveillance. The CDC should work with the

National Cancer Institute to attach viral etiology to reports of liver cancer in its periodic national reports on cancer.

The widespread use of electronic medical records holds promise for better understanding of the viral hepatitis epidemic, but this promise has not yet been realized. Traditionally, health departments rely on providers

---

BOX 3-1
Australia's Hepatitis B Mapping Project

In Australia, as in the United States, liver cancer is the fastest growing cause of cancer death. In response to this problem, the government has a hepatitis B strategy that aims to reduce hepatitis B virus transmission, morbidity, and mortality. Increasing the diagnosis of hepatitis B is a major part of the strategy, as is the appropriate management and care for chronic hepatitis B.

In order to better understand the geographic distribution of hepatitis B, the Australasian Society for HIV Medicine and the Victorian Infectious Diseases Reference Laboratory at the Peter Doherty Institute for Infection and Immunity began the Hepatitis B Mapping Project in 2012. Starting with census data, researchers mapped the burden of hepatitis B across Australia. Their first report, published in 2013, presents estimates of infection prevalence as well as information on the proportion of patients who speak little or no English or who are of Aboriginal or Torres Strait Islander descent. Estimates are presented at the national, state or territorial, and local levels. The second and third project reports, published in 2015 and 2016, estimate hepatitis B diagnosis, monitoring, treatment, and immunization coverage across the country, as well as rates of liver cancer. These data are used to measure progress toward the government's national elimination targets. For example, about 239,000 Australians, or 1 percent of the population, had chronic hepatitis B in 2015, and about 38 percent of these cases were not diagnosed. The national goal is to diagnose 80 percent of chronic hepatitis B patients, so the mapping project gave a helpful benchmark. Similarly, the government's national strategy is to treat about 15 percent of chronically infected patients with antivirals, but in 2015 only about 6 percent were prescribed treatment.

The mapping exercise identified 22 areas and populations disproportionately affected by hepatitis B, many of whom are already marginalized, such as people born overseas, Australians of Aboriginal or Torres Strait Islander descent, people who inject drugs, and men who have sex with men. Immigrants from east and southeast Asia account for most chronic hepatitis B infections in Australia, suggesting that the pediatric vaccination program needs to be supplemented with secondary prevention measures. The project also provides useful data about the areas and groups most affected by hepatitis B, allowing for a better tailored prevention program, possibly one that presents important health messages in Asian languages.

SOURCES: ASHM, n.d.; Australia Government Department of Health, 2014; MacLachlan and Cowie, 2012, 2013, 2015, 2016; MacLachlan et al., 2013.

and laboratories to report cases of viral hepatitis and other notifiable conditions (CDC, 2015). Such reporting obligations compete for providers' limited time and attention and are often late or incomplete (CDC, 2013, 2014; Dixon et al., 2013; Jajosky and Groseclose, 2004; Lazarus et al., 2009). Automated, electronic reporting from diagnostic laboratories has improved the speed and efficiency of reporting, but the reports typically lack important clinical details (Birkhead et al., 2015; Heisey-Grove et al., 2011; Klompas et al., 2012; Lazarus et al., 2009; Overhage et al., 2008). Electronic health records contain comprehensive information and may help improve viral hepatitis surveillance. Box 3-2 describes how such a system has been used in Massachusetts.

The informatics tools developed in Massachusetts and described in Box 3-2 can improve health departments' ability to find viral hepatitis patients, but such improvement depends on the ability of staff epidemiologists to evaluate the electronic reports and integrate them into daily work. Massachusetts is one of seven jurisdictions that the CDC chose for enhanced viral hepatitis surveillance (CDC, 2016b). These seven sites provide insight into the changing nature of viral hepatitis in the United States, such as the increase in HCV infection among young people who inject drugs (Altarum Institute, 2013; CDC, 2011). Data from the enhanced sites also help illuminate the true burden of disease. Research in Europe suggests that health departments' notification of viral hepatitis infection is more a function of local testing practices than full burden of disease (Duffell et al., 2015). As the enhanced surveillance sites tend to find more cases of viral hepatitis, their data can be used to model the difference between reported and unreported infections (Klevens et al., 2014).

The use of electronic medical records in surveillance would provide health departments with a wealth of information about viral hepatitis. A patient's history of prior negative antibody tests before a positive test could allow for precise identification of a new infection, for example. Analysis of claims data could also supplement hepatitis surveillance, as it has with zoonotic diseases (Jones et al., 2013; Tseng et al., 2015). The Robert Wood Johnson Foundation's Digital Bridge Project aims to develop systems to make such information available to public health authorities (Digital Bridge, n.d.). With input from the CDC, various state and local health departments, and industry, the goal is creating a computing platform capable of using clinical data for public health (Digital Bridge, n.d.). It is possible that such a system might eventually be able to run algorithms for viral hepatitis outcomes of public health interest.

Automated, electronic systems cannot replace traditional public health surveillance, however. The work of tracking cases through the care cascade, identifying pregnant women with HBV infection and counseling them on neonatal prophylaxis, and describing the demographic characteristics of

---

BOX 3-2
Using Electronic Health Record Data
in Public Health Surveillance

In 2007, the Harvard Center of Excellence in Public Health Informatics and the Massachusetts Department of Health launched an automatic disease detection and reporting system that draws on the information in electronic patient records. The program aims to automate disease reporting, thereby reducing human errors and burden on providers. The program extracts data from patients' electronic records and applies case detection algorithms to find events of public health interest. It then electronically sends these data to health departments for further assessment and investigation. Code for the program is publicly available and compatible with different electronic medical record packages. The program server can also be kept in the same place as a practice's electronic medical records server, making it easier to secure patient data.

The use of algorithms based on multiple criteria increases the likelihood of detecting cases of notifiable diseases. The algorithm can also help avoid problems with incomplete data or an inaccurate diagnosis. In identifying acute hepatitis C, for example, the system looks for one of three different patterns of clinical or laboratory test results, integrating the two data streams. This method gives a more complete picture than either the laboratory or clinical data alone. New tests, clinical codes, and revised epidemiological case definitions can be easily incorporated.

The system has been shown to have good sensitivity and positive predictive value; it is faster and more accurate than other surveillance methods. The acute

---

and risk factors for viral hepatitis in a community will continue to fall on health department staff working in partnership with providers.

The CDC's Epidemiology and Laboratory Capacity for Infectious Disease funds, through cooperative agreements to support basic surveillance, epidemiology, laboratory, and information systems, health departments in all 50 states, as well as 8 territories and 6 cities (CDC, 2016a). This cooperative agreement might be a valuable way to continue funding enhanced viral hepatitis surveillance as part of an elimination program. As the cooperatives already fund capacity building for other infectious diseases, using this funding tool might allow for better integration of viral hepatitis surveillance with other infectious diseases on a national scale. Funding could be used to improve informatics, giving other jurisdictions access to tools like those used in Massachusetts to mine electronic records, to improve electronic laboratory reporting for all viral hepatitis laboratory results, and to support increased staff capacity. Each health department should have suf-

hepatitis B algorithm is 97 percent sensitive, has a 97 percent positive predictive value, and was found to be superior to the alternative surveillance methods of hepatitis B core antigen and immunoglobulin M testing and diagnosis coding. When applied to electronic patient data from Massachusetts, the acute hepatitis B algorithm missed no cases, identified four additional cases not previously reported to the health department, and was even able to distinguish between acute and chronic infections.

To take advantage of the software, health care providers must use an electronic medical record system in their routine practice. Clearly, people who are not in care or not tested for viral hepatitis will never be identified. Health department staff need to assess reported cases and maintain the proper technology to integrate the program's reports into their existing workflow. Some data require follow-up investigation, especially determination of a case's risk history, which is not always consistently documented. But the adoption of the system is growing. It is now used at five sites in Massachusetts and one site each in Ohio and Texas for surveillance of tuberculosis, influenza-like illness, Lyme disease, sexually transmitted infections, and diabetes mellitus as well as viral hepatitis. Health departments around the country could, in theory, make use of this software, though such changes require technical and informatics support on both the providers' and health departments' sides, as well as epidemiological support for additional case investigation. While electronic health records are used around the country, the systems are different, and code would have to be customized for each one.

SOURCES: Allen-Dicker and Klompas, 2012; Birkhead et al., 2015; Klompas, 2016; Klompas et al., 2008, 2012; Lazarus et al., 2009.

ficient staff to manage the electronic system, follow reported cases, confirm their enrollment in care, and conduct outbreak investigations.

Enhancement of viral hepatitis surveillance will require changes to regulations in some states. As it is now, states have different regulations for the reporting of hepatitis B and C cases (CDC, 2015). Understanding the hepatitis care continuum in a given jurisdiction means having data on care and treatment, as well as a series of test results over time. For example, a negative HCV RNA test on a hepatitis C case after treatment provides health departments with valuable evidence of sustained virologic response. In New York, reporting of negative HCV RNA has been required since 2014, allowing the New York City health department staff to determine that about 40 percent of HCV infections reported in 2015 were cleared, either spontaneously or through treatment (Flanigan, 2017; New York City Department of Health and Mental Hygiene, 2016). Similarly, improvement in how chronic hepatitis B cases are captured would not only inform a better estimate of local prevalence, it would also help ensure that all HBsAg+

pregnant women are provided case management to prevent mother-to-child transmission of HBV.

In its guidance to member states, the WHO advises that "the hepatitis information system should be fully integrated into the broader national health information system to ensure standardized and coordinated reporting and to maximize efficiencies" (WHO, 2016, p. 27). In the United States, one important area where the information system might be improved is cancer registries. These registries are usually run by state health departments and can be used to calculate cancer incidence and monitor disease burden over time (American Cancer Society, 2014; Parkin et al., 2001). The National Cancer Institute's SEER[1] program is another major cancer resource that draws data from some of the best cancer registries around the country to calculate national statistics on cancer incidence and mortality (American Cancer Society, 2014).

Cancer registries generally report information on primary liver cancer (cancer that begins in the liver) by combining data on the two main types: hepatocellular carcinoma and intrahepatic bile duct cancer. These two types of disease have different etiologies, however. Intrahepatic bile duct cancer is rarer in the United States and occurs more frequently in patients with ulcerative colitis and primary sclerosing cholangitis (NCI, 2016b). Hepatocellular carcinoma, on the other hand, accounts for 90 percent of primary liver cancers in the United States; hepatitis B and C are its most common causes (Altekruse et al., 2009; London and McGlynn, 2006; NCI, 2016a).

Hepatitis B and C cause hepatocellular carcinoma through different mechanisms (Barazani et al., 2007). HBV acts by disrupting the host's genomic stability when inserting its genetic material into the host's DNA and through the expression of certain proteins that may affect normal cell function and cause cancer in non-cirrhotic patients (Chisari et al., 2010; Xu et al., 2014). Chronic HBV infection can cause cirrhosis, leading to multiple cycles of cellular injury and regeneration, also a pathway to cancer (El-Serag, 2012; Fernandez-Rodriguez and Gutierrez-Garcia, 2014). The process of chronic inflammation and cirrhosis is also the mechanism through which HCV causes cancer (Hoshida et al., 2014). The different etiologies can affect clinical presentation and tumor burden, which influence patients' treatment options, outcomes, and long-term survival (Barazani et al., 2007). It is therefore important to be able to estimate the burden of hepatocellular carcinoma *by cause* across different demographic groups in the United States (Altekruse et al., 2009; Barazani et al., 2007; Yu et al., 2006). But the classification system used in cancer registries does not allow for reporting of etiology. Collecting this information could help measure the cancer burden attributable to chronic HBV and HCV infection, as well

---

[1] Officially, the Surveillance, Epidemiology, and End Results program.

as identify disparities and study trends in cancer burden over time. Cross-referencing cases of liver cancer with state viral hepatitis registries would be one way to determine a viral hepatitis etiology of liver cancer. It would also help to have the cancer registry request and include viral serology in patient charts and electronic records when they collect information about new cases.

In the same way, surveillance for viral hepatitis would be improved by linking health department data to other vital records. Linking to death registries would allow for better understanding of mortality among HBV- and HCV-infected people, and matching with birth registries could help women at risk of mother-to-child transmission of HBV (Kuncio et al., 2016; Moore et al., 2016; Pinchoff et al., 2014). The sharing of data among states could also be helpful, but it would require an automated system to identify duplicate cases in multiple state registries. Tracking cases across states is a complicated and time-consuming process, currently done only for HIV and AIDS cases, a smaller number than for HBV and HCV infections (Glynn et al., 2008).

A Better Understanding of Incidence and Prevalence

Public health surveillance can be an invaluable tool in disease elimination and one that is crucial if local estimates of disease burden are to be compared to national data. While surveillance can support improved local estimates of incidence and prevalence, data are typically derived from cases that are already in care. A more complete understanding of the epidemiology of viral hepatitis and associated complications comes from epidemiological research, especially in select populations with known risk factors. Such research is challenging, as much of the burden of disease is borne by people on society's margins: the imprisoned, people who inject drugs, and people born in endemic countries.

The seven jurisdictions that are doing enhanced viral hepatitis surveillance are finding higher burden and more cases among young people than CDC estimates would suggest (CDC, 2016b; Flanigan, 2017; Hart-Malloy et al., 2013; Massachusetts Department of Public Health, 2016; Michigan DHHS, 2015). Their findings point to a higher true incidence and prevalence of HBV and HCV infections than previously thought, a hypothesis that could be best explored with a population sero-survey of people thought to be most at risk for viral hepatitis.

The National Health and Nutrition Examination Survey

In some ways, the most efficient strategy for conducting sero-surveys would be to work through an existing national study, such as NHANES[2]. For over 50 years, NHANES has provided invaluable data on the health and nutritional status of Americans. The surveys are population-based and combine interviews, clinical examination, and collection of biological specimens. NHANES is repeated every year in adults and children; its results form the evidence base for numerous health policy decisions (NCHS, n.d.-b).

The relevance of the NHANES model to understanding viral hepatitis is questionable, however (Edlin et al., 2015). Though the survey has been used to estimate the prevalence of chronic HBV and HCV infections in the United States, the study design excludes or undersamples some groups known to be at high risk of viral hepatitis (Denniston et al., 2014; Edlin et al., 2015; Roberts et al., 2016). NHANES participants are chosen from households; they cannot be institutionalized or homeless (Edlin et al., 2015; NCHS, n.d.-a). For these reasons, NHANES likely underestimates the prevalence of chronic hepatitis C infection by about 30 percent (Edlin et al., 2015).

Furthermore, participation in population-based studies like NHANES is declining, and even when the overall refusal rate is low, there is a risk of systematic differences between the participants and those who decline or ignore the invitation (Galea and Tracy, 2007). In the past, the National Center for Health Statistics has responded to concerns about NHANES participants by oversampling key populations (NCHS, 2015). The oversampling of Asian Americans in the 2011-2012 survey indicated a prevalence of hepatitis B 10 times higher than the rest of the population (Roberts et al., 2016).

The Chronic Hepatitis Cohort Study

Another ongoing epidemiological study of viral hepatitis in the United States, the Chronic Hepatitis Cohort Study (CHeCS), has improved our understanding of the characteristics of and prognosis of chronic hepatitis B and C patients (Moorman et al., 2013; Niederau et al., 1998). CHeCS works through health systems in Hawaii, Michigan, Oregon, and Pennsylvania (Moorman et al., 2013). Patients' electronic and billing records are analyzed for evidence of chronic HBV and HCV infection (Moorman et al., 2013). Research in this cohort has helped determine that chronic hepatitis C infection is incorrectly omitted from tens of thousands of death certificates

---

[2] Officially, the National Health and Nutrition Examination Survey.

a year and that fewer than half of patients with liver enzyme elevation were tested for HBV or HCV (Mahajan et al., 2014; Spradling et al., 2012).

CHeCS is not a sero-study, however, and, because data are drawn from patient records, about 97 percent of participants have some form of health insurance (Moorman et al., 2013). Key populations for viral hepatitis, including prisoners and people who inject drugs, are not captured in claims studies, limiting generalizability. CHeCS is, therefore, not the most promising framework in which to ask broader questions about viral hepatitis in the at-risk population. This is not to say that CHeCS and other claims databases could not be used to create a more accurate picture of the burden of viral hepatitis. The Agency for Healthcare Research and Quality's Healthcare Cost and Utilization Project databases contain information on cost, medical practice, and quality of services that could also be used for hepatitis research (AHRQ, 2016).

There is no ongoing cross-sectional or cohort study of sufficient reach, especially in high-risk populations, from which to form reliable estimates of the prevalence and incidence of viral hepatitis and liver-related outcomes such as cirrhosis. A cohort study that tracked high-risk patients in multiple, representative settings would inform a better understanding of disease incidence. Periodic cross-sectional surveys that include similar populations would form the basis for an accurate estimate of disease prevalence. These studies would complement data about viral hepatitis coming from NHANES.

Recommendation 3-2: The Centers for Disease Control and Prevention should support cross-sectional and cohort studies to measure HBV and HCV infection incidence and prevalence in high-risk populations.

The Bureau of Justice Statistics' *Survey of Inmates in Federal Correctional Facilities, Survey of Inmates in State Correctional Facilities,* and *Survey of Inmates in Local Jails* are promising vehicles for reaching a key population. The survey in federal facilities has been conducted three times since 1991, the survey in state facilities seven times since 1974, and the survey in jails six times since 1972 (BJS, 2002, 2004a,b). Participants are chosen in a two-stage process, with the facility selected first, then the inmate (BJS, 2002, 2004a,b). The questions have changed slightly in different survey iterations; questions about health, medical problems, and drug use are already part of the process (BJS, 2002, 2004a,b). At the same time, epidemiological research is not within the purview of the Department of Justice; such questions and expertise would have to come from partners at the CDC. It is also possible that imprisoned people would be reluctant to participate in a physical exam that includes a blood draw. Employing public health nurses for the medical portion of the exam may help overcome these concerns and has been an effective strategy in other correctional settings (Ruiz et al., 1999).

The blood draw component of the proposed viral hepatitis cohort and cross-sectional studies is crucial. In its efforts to develop these studies, the CDC should promote a basic panel of hepatitis B serum biomarkers, including HBsAg (to check for chronic infection), total hepatitis B core antibody (anti-HBc) (to check for prior infection), and hepatitis B surface antibody (anti-HBs) (to check for immunity). This would not be a departure from standard practice. As for hepatitis C tests, HCV RNA should be reported in addition to HCV antibody. About 25 percent of people infected with HCV clear the infection spontaneously (Micallef et al., 2006). These patients will continue to test positive for HCV antibody, as will people who have been cured medically. As the CDC tracks progress toward the elimination targets proposed in Chapter 2, accurate information about current, viremic infections, as indicated by HCV RNA, will be essential (since chronic hepatitis B infection is not curable currently, there is no parallel requirement for hepatitis B reporting).

Traditionally, the relatively crude measure of hepatitis C disease burden afforded by HCV antibody was accepted because there was no good biomarker to estimate incidence. The recent development of an HCV immunoglobulin antibody avidity assay could change this (Patel et al., 2016). By measuring biomarkers that change with the duration of infection, the assay can identify recent infections in a cross-section of the population (Patel et al., 2016). The test is still being validated and has been shown to precisely estimate incidence of HCV infection if it is considered along with a measure of HCV RNA (Patel et al., 2016). The test is most accurate in populations with a high incidence of HCV infection, such as for use among people who inject drugs, but it can be used in any population, provided the sample size is large enough.

There is a need for better information about disease burden and the care cascade of viral hepatitis in the United States, including likelihood of linkage to care, sustained virologic response, and risk of reinfection. Research on key populations could provide such information, especially if conducted as a complement to comprehensive public health surveillance. Such studies should be repeated periodically to monitor the situation. Viral hepatitis elimination will depend on an accurate understanding of the epidemic, including who is most affected and where. Identifying these people will become more difficult over time, as there will be fewer cases left to find. It is therefore essential to set up a sensitive surveillance system and to invest in a better understanding of viral hepatitis incidence and prevalence now, allowing for better targeted public health programs and an accurate baseline measure. Investments in measuring disease burden will pay off more over time, when the success of the elimination program depends on finding an ever smaller group of patients.

REFERENCES

AHRQ (Agency for Healthcare Reseach and Quality). 2016. HCUP overview. Healthcare Cost and Utilization Oroject (HCUP). https://www.hcup-us.ahrq.gov/overview.jsp (accessed January 25, 2017).

Allen-Dicker, J., and M. Klompas. 2012. Comparison of electronic laboratory reports, administrative claims, and electronic health record data for acute viral hepatitis surveillance. *Journal of Public Health Management and Practice* 18(3):209-214.

Altarum Institute. 2013. *Technical consultation: Hepatitis C virus infection in young persons who inject drugs. February 26-27, 2013. Consultation report.* Altarum Institute. https://www.aids.gov/pdf/hcv-and-young-pwid-consultation-report.pdf (accessed December 29, 2016).

Altekruse, S. F., K. A. McGlynn, and M. E. Reichman. 2009. Hepatocellular carcinoma incidence, mortality, and survival trends in the United States from 1975 to 2005. *Journal of Clinical Oncology* 27(9):1485-1491.

American Cancer Society. 2014. *Cancer surveillance programs in the United States.* http://www.cancer.org/cancer/cancerbasics/cancer-surveillance-programs-and-registries-in-the-united-states (accessed October 26, 2016).

ASHM (Australasian Society for HIV, Viral Hepatitis and Sexual Health Medicine). n.d. *Hepatitis B mapping project.* http://www.ashm.org.au/HBV/more-about/hepatitis-b-mapping-project (accessed July 20, 2016).

Australia Government Department of Health. 2014. *Second national hepatitis B strategy, 2014-2017.* http://www.health.gov.au/internet/main/publishing.nsf/Content/C353814FE3255962CA257BF0001DE841/$File/Hep-B-Strategy2014-v3.pdf (accessed July 25, 2016).

Barazani, Y., J. R. Hiatt, M. J. Tong, and R. W. Busuttil. 2007. Chronic viral hepatitis and hepatocellular carcinoma. *World Journal of Surgery* 31(6):1243-1248.

Barton, K., D. Church, S. Onofrey, N. Cocoros, and A. DeMaria, Jr. 2014. Follow-up testing for hepatitis C virus infection: An analysis of Massachusetts surveillance data, 2007-2010. *Public Health Reports* 129(5):403-407.

Birkhead, G. S., M. Klompas, and N. R. Shah. 2015. Uses of electronic health records for public health surveillance to advance public health. *Annual Review of Public Health* 36:345-359.

BJS (Bureau of Justice Statistics). 2002. *Data collection: Survey of Inmates in Local Jails (SILJ).* https://www.bjs.gov/index.cfm?ty=dcdetail&iid=274 (accessed December 30, 2016).

BJS. 2004a. *Data collection: Survey of Inmates in Federal Correctional Facilities (SIFCF).* https://www.bjs.gov/index.cfm?ty=dcdetail&iid=273 (accessed December 30, 2016).

BJS. 2004b. *Data collection: Survey of Inmates in State Correctional Facilities (SISCF).* https://www.bjs.gov/index.cfm?ty=dcdetail&iid=275#Methodology;%20https://www.bjs.gov/index.cfm?ty=dcdetail&iid=274#Methodology (accessed December 29, 2016).

Broekmans, J. F., G. B. Migliori, H. L. Rieder, J. Lees, P. Ruutu, R. Loddenkemper, and M. C. Raviglione. 2002. European framework for tuberculosis control and elimination in countries with a low incidence. Recommendations of the World Health Organization (WHO), International Union Against Tuberculosis and Lung Disease (IUATLD) and Royal Netherlands Tuberculosis Association (KNCV) working group. *European Respiratory Journal* 19(4):765-775.

Cattand, P., J. Jannin, and P. Lucas. 2001. Sleeping sickness surveillance: An essential step towards elimination. *Tropical Medicine & International Health* 6(5):348-361.

CDC (Centers for Disease Control and Prevention). 2011. Hepatitis C virus infection among adolescents and young adults: Massachusetts, 2002-2009. *Morbidity and Mortality Weekly Report* 60(17):537-541.

CDC. 2013. Completeness of reporting of chronic hepatitis B and C virus infections—Michigan, 1995-2008. *Morbidity and Mortality Weekly Report* 62(6):99-102.

CDC. 2014. *Manual for the surveillance of vaccine-preventable diseases.* https://www.cdc.gov/vaccines/pubs/surv-manual/chpt04-hepb.html (accessed January 10, 2016).

CDC. 2015. *State reporting requirements for viral hepatitis.* https://www.cdc.gov/hepatitis/featuredtopics/statereportingrequirements.htm (accessed December 29, 2016).

CDC. 2016a. *Epidemiology and laboratory capacity for infectious diseases (ELC) cooperative agreement.* https://www.cdc.gov/ncezid/dpei/epidemiology-laboratory-capacity.html (accessed April 27, 2017).

CDC. 2016b. *Viral hepatitis surveillance: United States, 2014.* http://www.cdc.gov/hepatitis/statistics/2014surveillance/pdfs/2014hepsurveillancerpt.pdf (accessed September 22, 2016).

Chisari, F. V., M. Isogawa, and S. F. Wieland. 2010. Pathogenesis of hepatitis B virus infection. *Pathologie Biologie* 58(4):258-266.

Cocoros, N., E. Nettle, D. Church, L. Bourassa, V. Sherwin, K. Cranston, R. Carr, H. D. Fukuda, and A. DeMaria, Jr. 2014. Screening for Hepatitis C as a Prevention Enhancement (SHAPE) for HIV: An integration pilot initiative in a Massachusetts County correctional facility. *Public Health Reports* 129(Suppl 1):5-11.

de Quadros, C. A., J. M. Olive, B. S. Hersh, M. A. Strassburg, D. A. Henderson, D. Brandling-Bennett, and G. A. Alleyne. 1996. Measles elimination in the Americas: Evolving strategies. *JAMA* 275(3):224-229.

Denniston, M. M., R. B. Jiles, J. Drobeniuc, R. M. Klevens, J. W. Ward, G. M. McQuillan, and S. D. Holmberg. 2014. Chronic hepatitis C virus infection in the United States, National Health and Nutrition Examination Survey, 2003 to 2010. *Annals of Internal Medicine* 160(5):293-300.

Digital Bridge. n.d. *About.* http://www.digitalbridge.us/about (accessed February 23, 2017).

Dixon, B. E., J. A. Siegel, T. V. Oemig, and S. J. Grannis. 2013. Electronic health information quality challenges and interventions to improve public health surveillance data and practice. *Public Health Reports* 128(6):546-553.

Duffell, E. F., M. J. van de Laar, and A. J. Amato-Gauci. 2015. Enhanced surveillance of hepatitis C in the EU, 2006–2012. *Journal of Viral Hepatitis* 22(7):590-595.

Edlin, B. R., B. J. Eckhardt, M. A. Shu, S. D. Holmberg, and T. Swan. 2015. Toward a more accurate estimate of the prevalence of hepatitis C in the United States. *Hepatology* 62(5):1353-1363.

El-Serag, H. B. 2012. Epidemiology of viral hepatitis and hepatocellular carcinoma. *Gastroenterology* 142(6):1264-1273.

Fernandez-Rodriguez, C. M., and M. L. Gutierrez-Garcia. 2014. Prevention of hepatocellular carcinoma in patients with chronic hepatitis B. *World Journal of Gastrointestinal Pharmacology and Therapeutics* 5(3):175-182.

Flanigan, C. 2017. Burden of hepatitis C in NYS. PowerPoint presentation at NYS Hepatitis C Elimination Summit in Albany, NY, February 7, 2017. Received February 8, 2017. Available by request from the National Academies of Sciences, Engineering, and Medicine Public Access Records Office. For more information, email PARO@nas.edu.

Galea, S., and M. Tracy. 2007. Participation rates in epidemiologic studies. *Annals of Epidemiology* 17(9):643-653.

German, R. R., L. M. Lee, J. M. Horan, R. L. Milstein, C. A. Pertowski, and M. N. Waller. 2001. Updated guidelines for evaluating public health surveillance systems: Recommendations from the guidelines working group. *Morbidity and Mortality Weekly Report* 50(RR-13):1-35; quiz CE31-CE37.

Glynn, M. K., Q. Ling, R. Phelps, J. Li, and L. M. Lee. 2008. Accurate monitoring of the HIV epidemic in the United States: Case duplication in the national HIV/AIDS surveillance system. *Journal of Acquired Immune Deficiency Syndromes* 47(3):391-396.

Hart-Malloy, R., A. Carrascal, A. G. Dirienzo, C. Flanigan, K. McClamroch, and L. Smith. 2013. Estimating HCV prevalence at the state level: A call to increase and strengthen current surveillance systems. *American Journal of Public Health* 103(8):1402-1405.

Heisey-Grove, D. M., D. R. Church, G. A. Haney, and A. Demaria, Jr. 2011. Enhancing surveillance for hepatitis C through public health informatics. *Public Health Reports* 126(1):13-18.

HHS (Department of Health and Human Services). 2015. *Action plan for the prevention, care, and treatment of viral hepatitis: 2014-2016.* HHS, Office of the Assistant Secretary for Health, Office of HIV/AIDS and Infectious Disease Policy. https://www.aids.gov/pdf/viral-hepatitis-action-plan.pdf (accessed October 26, 2016).

Hoshida, Y., B. C. Fuchs, N. Bardeesy, T. F. Baumert, and R. T. Chung. 2014. Pathogenesis and prevention of hepatitis C virus-induced hepatocellular carcinoma. *Journal of Hepatology* 61(1 Suppl):S79-S90.

IOM (Institute of Medicine). 2010. *Hepatitis and liver cancer: A national strategy for prevention and control of hepatitis B and C.* Washington, DC: The National Academies Press.

Jajosky, R. A., and S. L. Groseclose. 2004. Evaluation of reporting timeliness of public health surveillance systems for infectious diseases. *BMC Public Health* 4:29.

Jones, S. G., S. Coulter, and W. Conner. 2013. Using administrative medical claims data to supplement state disease registry systems for reporting zoonotic infections. *Journal of the American Medical Informatics Association* 20(1):193-198.

Kinnard, E. N., L. E. Taylor, O. Galarraga, and B. D. Marshall. 2014. Estimating the true prevalence of hepatitis C in Rhode Island. *Rhode Island Medical Journal* 97(7):19-24.

Klevens, R. M., J. Miller, C. Vonderwahl, S. Speers, K. Alelis, K. Sweet, E. Rocchio, T. Poissant, T. M. Vogt, and K. Gallagher. 2009. Population-based surveillance for hepatitis C virus, United States, 2006-2007. *Emerging Infectious Diseases* 15(9):1499-1502.

Klevens, R. M., S. Liu, H. Roberts, R. B. Jiles, and S. D. Holmberg. 2014. Estimating acute viral hepatitis infections from nationally reported cases. *American Journal of Public Health* 104(3):482-487.

Klompas, M. 2016. *Enhancing hepatitis C surveillance using electronic health record data.* Presentation to the Committee on a National Strategy for the Elimination of Hepatitis B and C, Washington, DC, June 9, 2016. http://www.nationalacademies.org/hmd/~/media/Files/Activity%20Files/PublicHealth/HepatitisBandC/8-June2016/Klompas.pdf (accessed December 29, 2016).

Klompas, M., G. Haney, D. Church, R. Lazarus, X. Hou, and R. Platt. 2008. Automated identification of acute hepatitis B using electronic medical record data to facilitate public health surveillance. *PLoS One* 3(7):e2626.

Klompas, M., J. McVetta, R. Lazarus, E. Eggleston, G. Haney, B. A. Kruskal, W. K. Yih, P. Daly, P. Oppedisano, B. Beagan, M. Lee, C. Kirby, D. Heisey-Grove, A. DeMaria, Jr., and R. Platt. 2012. Integrating clinical practice and public health surveillance using electronic medical record systems. *American Journal of Public Health* 102(Suppl 3):S325-S332.

Kuncio, D. E., E. C. Newbern, C. C. Johnson, and K. M. Viner. 2016. Failure to test and identify perinatally infected children born to hepatitis C virus-infected women. *Clinical Infectious Diseases* 62(8):980-985.

Lazarus, R., M. Klompas, F. X. Campion, S. J. McNabb, X. Hou, J. Daniel, G. Haney, A. DeMaria, L. Lenert, and R. Platt. 2009. Electronic support for public health: Validated case finding and reporting for notifiable diseases using electronic medical data. *Journal of the American Medical Informatics Association* 16(1):18-24.

London, W. T., and K. A. McGlynn. 2006. Liver cancer. In *Cancer epidemiology and prevention*. 3rd ed, edited by D. Schottenfeld and J. F. Fraumeni. New York: Oxford University Press. Pp. 763-786.

MacLachlan, J. H., and B. C. Cowie. 2012. Liver cancer is the fastest increasing cause of cancer death in Australians. *Medical Journal of Australia* 197(9):492-493.

MacLachlan, J., and B. Cowie. 2013. *Hepatitis B mapping project: Estimates of chronic hepatitis B prevalence and cultural and linguistic diversity by Medicare local, 2011—National report*. Darlinghurst, NSW, Australia: Australasian Society for HIV, Viral Hepatitis and Sexual Health Medicine.

MacLachlan, J., and B. Cowie. 2015. *Hepatitis B mapping project: Estimates of chronic hepatitis B infection diagnosis, monitoring and treatment by Medicare local, 2012/13—National report*. Darlinghurst, NSW, Australia: Australasian Society for HIV, Viral Hepatitis and Sexual Health Medicine.

MacLachlan, J., and B. Cowie. 2016. *Hepatitis B mapping project: Estimates of chronic hepatitis B prevalence, diagnosis, monitoring, and treatment by primary health network, 2014/15—National report*. Darlinghurst, NSW, Australia: Australasian Society for HIV, Viral Hepatitis and Sexual Health Medicine.

MacLachlan, J. H., N. Allard, V. Towell, and B. C. Cowie. 2013. The burden of chronic hepatitis B virus infection in Australia, 2011. *Australian and New Zealand Journal of Public Health* 37(5):416-422.

Mahajan, R., J. Xing, S. J. Liu, K. N. Ly, A. C. Moorman, L. Rupp, F. Xu, and S. D. Holmberg. 2014. Mortality among persons in care with hepatitis C virus infection: The Chronic Hepatitis Cohort Study (CHeCS), 2006-2010. *Clinical Infectious Diseases* 58(8):1055-1061.

Massachusetts Department of Public Health. 2016. *Hepatitis C virus infection 2015 surveillance report*. Massachusetts Department of Public Health, Bureau of Infectious Disease and Laboratory Sciences.

Medland, N. A., J. H. McMahon, E. P. Chow, J. H. Elliott, J. F. Hoy, and C. K. Fairley. 2015. The HIV care cascade: A systematic review of data sources, methodology and comparability. *Journal of the International AIDS Society* 18:20634.

Micallef, J. M., J. M. Kaldor, and G. J. Dore. 2006. Spontaneous viral clearance following acute hepatitis C infection: A systematic review of longitudinal studies. *Journal of Viral Hepatitis* 13(1):34-41.

Michigan DHHS (Department of Health and Human Services). 2015. *2015 hepatitis B and C surveillance report*. Michigan DHHS.

Moore, M. S., E. Ivanina, K. Bornschlegel, B. Qiao, M. J. Schymura, and F. Laraque. 2016. Hepatocellular carcinoma and viral hepatitis in New York City. *Clinical Infectious Diseases* 63(12):1577-1583.

Moorman, A. C., S. C. Gordon, L. B. Rupp, P. R. Spradling, E. H. Teshale, M. Lu, D. R. Nerenz, C. C. Nakasato, J. A. Boscarino, E. M. Henkle, N. J. Oja-Tebbe, J. Xing, J. W. Ward, and S. D. Holmberg. 2013. Baseline characteristics and mortality among people in care for chronic viral hepatitis: The Chronic Hepatitis Cohort Study. *Clinical Infectious Diseases* 56(1):40-50.

NASEM (National Academies of Sciences, Engineering, and Medicine). 2016. *Eliminating the public health problem of hepatitis B and C in the United States: Phase one report*. Washington, DC: The National Academies Press.

NCHS (National Center for Health Statistics). 2015. *National Health and Nutrition Examination Survey. NHANES 2011-2012 overview.* https://wwwn.cdc.gov/nchs/nhanes/continuousnhanes/overview.aspx?BeginYear=2011 (accessed January 26, 2017).

NCHS. n.d.-a. *Key concepts about NHANES survey design.* http://www.cdc.gov/Nchs/tutorials/Nhanes/SurveyDesign/SampleDesign/Info1.htm (accessed October 21, 2016).

NCHS. n.d.-b. *National Health and Nutrition Examination Survey, 2013-2014: Overview.* Hyattsville, MD: NCHS.

NCI (National Cancer Institute). 2016a. *Adult primary liver cancer treatment (PDQ®)–Health professional version.* https://www.cancer.gov/types/liver/hp/adult-liver-treatment-pdq (accessed October 28, 2016).

NCI. 2016b. *Bile duct cancer treatment (PDQ®)–Patient version.* https://www.cancer.gov/types/liver/patient/bile-duct-treatment-pdq (accessed October 28, 2016).

Nesheim, S., A. Taylor, M. A. Lampe, P. H. Kilmarx, L. Fitz Harris, S. Whitmore, J. Griffith, M. Thomas-Proctor, K. Fenton, and J. Mermin. 2012. A framework for elimination of perinatal transmission of HIV in the United States. *Pediatrics* 130(4):738-744.

New York City Department of Health and Mental Hygiene. 2016. Hepatitis B and C in New York City 2015. https://www1.nyc.gov/assets/doh/downloads/pdf/cd/hepatitis-b-and-c-annual-report-2015.pdf (accessed February 8, 2017).

Niederau, C., S. Lange, T. Heintges, A. Erhardt, M. Buschkamp, D. Hurter, M. Nawrocki, L. Kruska, F. Hensel, W. Petry, and D. Haussinger. 1998. Prognosis of chronic hepatitis C: Results of a large, prospective cohort study. *Hepatology* 28(6):1687-1695.

Overhage, J. M., S. Grannis, and C. J. McDonald. 2008. A comparison of the completeness and timeliness of automated electronic laboratory reporting and spontaneous reporting of notifiable conditions. *American Journal of Public Health* 98(2):344-350.

Parkin, D. M., F. Bray, J. Ferlay, and P. Pisani. 2001. Estimating the world cancer burden: GLOBOCAN 2000. *International Journal of Cancer* 94(2):153-156.

Patel, E. U., A. L. Cox, S. H. Mehta, D. Boon, C. E. Mullis, J. Astemborski, W. O. Osburn, J. Quinn, A. D. Redd, G. D. Kirk, D. L. Thomas, T. C. Quinn, and O. Laeyendecker. 2016. Use of hepatitis C virus (HCV) immunoglobulin G antibody avidity as a biomarker to estimate the population-level incidence of HCV infection. *Journal of Infectious Diseases* 214(3):344-352.

Pinchoff, J., A. Drobnik, K. Bornschlegel, S. Braunstein, C. Chan, J. K. Varma, and J. Fuld. 2014. Deaths among people with hepatitis C in New York City, 2000-2011. *Clinical Infectious Diseases* 58(8):1047-1054.

Roberts, H., D. Kruszon-Moran, K. N. Ly, E. Hughes, K. Iqbal, R. B. Jiles, and S. D. Holmberg. 2016. Prevalence of chronic hepatitis B virus (HBV) infection in U.S. households: National Health and Nutrition Examination Survey (NHANES), 1988-2012. *Hepatology* 63(2):388-397.

Ruiz, J. D., F. Molitor, R. K. Sun, J. Mikanda, M. Facer, J. M. Colford, Jr., G. W. Rutherford, and M. S. Ascher. 1999. Prevalence and correlates of hepatitis C virus infection among inmates entering the California correctional system. *Western Journal of Medicine* 170(3): 156-160.

Rutherford, G. W. 2001. Principles and practices of public health surveillance, 2nd ed. *American Journal of Epidemiology* 154(4):385-386.

Smith, P. F., J. L. Hadler, M. Stanbury, R. T. Rolfs, and R. S. Hopkins. 2013. "Blueprint version 2.0": Updating public health surveillance for the 21st century. *Journal of Public Health Management and Practice* 19(3):231-239.

Spradling, P. R., L. Rupp, A. C. Moorman, M. Lu, E. H. Teshale, S. C. Gordon, C. Nakasato, J. A. Boscarino, E. M. Henkle, D. R. Nerenz, M. M. Denniston, and S. D. Holmberg. 2012. Hepatitis B and C virus infection among 1.2 million persons with access to care: Factors associated with testing and infection prevalence. *Clinical Infectious Diseases* 55(8):1047-1055.

Stanaway, J. D., A. D. Flaxman, M. Naghavi, C. Fitzmaurice, T. Vos, I. Abubakar, L. J. Abu-Raddad, R. Assadi, N. Bhala, B. Cowie, M. H. Forouzanfour, J. Groeger, K. M. Hanafiah, K. H. Jacobsen, S. L. James, J. MacLachlan, R. Malekzadeh, N. K. Martin, A. A. Mokdad, A. H. Mokdad, C. J. L. Murray, D. Plass, S. Rana, D. B. Rein, J. H. Richardus, J. Sanabria, M. Saylan, S. Shahraz, S. So, V. V. Vlassov, E. Weiderpass, S. T. Wiersma, M. Younis, C. Yu, M. El Sayed Zaki, and G. S. Cooke. 2016. The global burden of viral hepatitis from 1990 to 2013: Findings from the Global Burden of Disease Study 2013. *Lancet* 388(10049):1081-1088.

Thacker, S. B., and R. L. Berkelman. 1988. Public health surveillance in the United States. *Epidemiologic Reviews* 10(1):164-190.

Troppy, S., G. Haney, N. Cocoros, K. Cranston, and A. DeMaria, Jr. 2014. Infectious disease surveillance in the 21st century: An integrated web-based surveillance and case management system. *Public Health Reports* 129(2):132-138.

Tseng, Y. J., A. Cami, D. A. Goldmann, A. DeMaria, Jr., and K. D. Mandl. 2015. Using nationwide health insurance claims data to augment Lyme disease surveillance. *Vector Borne and Zoonotic Diseases* 15(10):591-596.

Viner, K., D. Kuncio, E. C. Newbern, and C. C. Johnson. 2015. The continuum of hepatitis C testing and care. *Hepatology* 61(3):783-789.

WHO (World Health Organization). 1980. *The global eradiction of smallpox: Final report of the Global Commission for the Certification of Smallpox Eradication, Geneva, December 1979*. Geneva, Switzerland: WHO.

WHO. 2016. *Global health sector strategy on viral hepatitis, 2016-2021: Towards ending viral hepatitis*. Geneva, Switzerland: WHO. http://apps.who.int/iris/bitstream/10665/246177/1/WHO-HIV-2016.06-eng.pdf (accessed July 19, 2016).

Wiktor, S. Z., and Y. J. F. Hutin. 2016. The global burden of viral hepatitis: Better estimates to guide hepatitis elimination efforts. *Lancet* 388(10049):1030-1031.

Xu, H. Z., Y. P. Liu, B. Guleng, and J. L. Ren. 2014. Hepatitis B virus-related hepatocellular carcinoma: Pathogenic mechanisms and novel therapeutic interventions. *Gastrointestinal Tumors* 1(3):135-145.

Yu, L., D. A. Sloane, C. Guo, and C. D. Howell. 2006. Risk factors for primary hepatocellular carcinoma in black and white Americans in 2000. *Clinical Gastroenterology and Hepatology* 4(3):355-360.

Zhou, X. N., R. Bergquist, and M. Tanner. 2013. Elimination of tropical disease through surveillance and response. *Infectious Diseases of Poverty* 2(1).

4

Essential Interventions

Viral hepatitis elimination is an international effort, but the scope of the problem varies by country. This committee's previous report discussed the epidemiology of hepatitis B virus (HBV) and hepatitis C virus (HCV) infection in the United States (NASEM, 2016). It discussed opportunities for ending transmission of both viruses, as well as steps to prevent the progression of HBV and HCV infection to cirrhosis and liver cancer (NASEM, 2016). With this epidemiological perspective in mind, this chapter discusses some crucial actions that would help reduce the national burden of both infections. In identifying interventions with the greatest potential effect, the committee considered the care cascade across the continuum of services shown in Figure 4-1. As much as possible, this chapter distinguishes between specific interventions against viral hepatitis and the manner in which such interventions are delivered, a topic covered in the next chapter.

PREVENTION AND TESTING

Prevention is the first step to making HBV and HCV infections rare. Hepatitis B is preventable with immunization, so prevention is a matter of ensuring widespread vaccination and taking steps to prevent transmission from mother to child. There is no prophylactic vaccine for HCV, so services to prevent hepatitis C involve controlling the practices known to spread the virus and curing chronic infections. Since both viruses are transmitted primarily through blood contact, risk reduction measures most associated with hepatitis C and HIV are also useful to prevent HBV infection.

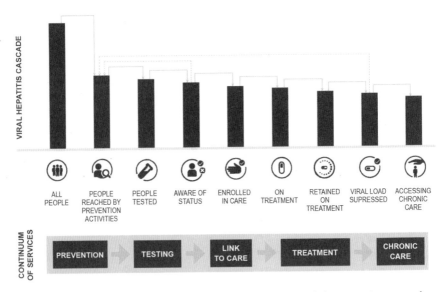

FIGURE 4-1 The continuum of viral hepatitis services and the retention cascade. SOURCE: WHO, 2016a.

Prevention of HBV Infection

Hepatitis B is preventable. The vaccines licensed in the 1980s confer durable immunity to 95 percent of people who receive three doses (CDC, 2016d,f; Mast et al., 2005; Walayat et al., 2015). When the three-dose vaccine series is started at birth, children are protected against acquisition during the vulnerable preschool years; the birth dose also helps prevent vertical transmission of HBV. Among a subset of HBsAg+ pregnant women with high viremia, risk of prophylaxis failure is higher (Chen et al., 2012). About 900 neonates a year contract HBV at birth in the United States (Ko et al., 2014). This number too could be reduced.

Perfect vaccination of children would end HBV transmission in two generations, but the elimination goals set out in Chapter 2 require faster action than that (Forcione et al., 2002). In the United States, better attention to adult vaccination and changes to the management of HBsAg+ pregnant women may be all that stands in the way of ending the transmission of HBV.

Vaccination of Adults

The prevalence of HBV in children decreased markedly after the introduction of hepatitis B vaccine (Wasley et al., 2010). As of 2013, about

90 percent of children under 3 were fully immunized against HBV (Elam-Evans et al., 2014). Vaccine-induced immunity is far less common in adults, however (Wasley et al., 2010). Only about a quarter of adults older than 19 participating in the 2014 National Health Interview Survey reported having had three doses of hepatitis B vaccine (24.5 percent, 95 percent confidence interval [CI]: 23.8 to 25.3), roughly the same percentage as the previous year (Williams et al., 2016). Likelihood of full vaccination is only slightly better among people who travel internationally (30.5 percent, 95 percent CI: 29.2 to 31.8) (Williams et al., 2016).

In 2006, the Centers for Disease Control and Prevention's (CDC's) Advisory Committee on Immunization Practices (ACIP) recommended universal adult hepatitis B vaccination in places where a high proportion of people are likely at risk for HBV infection, such as clinics targeting people who inject drugs or men who have sex with men; it also recommended a standing order to identify adults for whom hepatitis B immunization is recommended in primary care and specialty clinics; it recommended that all diabetes patients be immunized against HBV in 2011 (CDC, 2011b; Mast et al., 2006). Yet adult hepatitis B vaccination coverage remains low, even in high-risk groups (CDC, 2011b; Mast et al., 2005). Only 29.8 percent of patients with chronic liver disease (95 percent CI: 23.9 to 36.5 percent), and 23.5 percent of diabetics aged 19 to 59 (95 percent CI: 20.7 to 26.7 percent) have been immunized (Williams et al., 2016). Studies have found low immunization coverage among people who inject drugs, men who have sex with men at HIV clinics, and clients at sexually transmitted disease clinics (Bowman et al., 2014; Collier et al., 2015; Henkle et al., 2015; Hoover et al., 2012). Hepatitis B infection is also an occupational hazard for health care workers, who can be exposed to infected blood or tissue through needle stick and other sharp injuries, yet many health care workers remain unvaccinated. Only about two-thirds of providers in direct patient care have been immunized—well below the Healthy People 2020 target of 90 percent (Byrd et al., 2013; HHS, n.d.; Talas, 2009; Williams et al., 2016).

Unvaccinated adults remain vulnerable to HBV infection through unprotected sex, unsafe injections and transfusions, and contact with infected blood. Thirty to 50 percent of adults who contract HBV will develop symptoms of acute hepatitis, a condition with a mortality rate of 0.5 to 1 percent (CDC, 2016f; Immunization Action Coalition, n.d.; Mast et al., 2006). About 5 percent will develop chronic hepatitis B (Mast et al., 2006; WHO, 2016b).

From 2009 to 2013, three Appalachian states reported a 114 percent increase in the incidence of acute hepatitis B infection associated with increased injection drug use among white men in their thirties (Harris et al., 2016a). In 2014, adults accounted for about 95 percent of the estimated 19,200 cases of acute hepatitis B in the United States (CDC, 2016i). Rates of acute infection were highest in those aged 30 to 39 years in 2014 (2.23 cases per 100,000 people) and have increased slightly in ages 40 to 59 years from 2010 to 2014 (CDC, 2016i). Non-Hispanic blacks had the highest rate of acute hepatitis B infection in 2014 (CDC, 2016i).

There are many reasons for low adult hepatitis B vaccine coverage. There is not good public awareness about hepatitis B; even health workers can be uninformed of its risk (Ferrante et al., 2008; Patil et al., 2013; Williams et al., 2016). Clinics often fail to stock the hepatitis B vaccine, partly because there is no funding to deliver it to uninsured and underinsured people, and partly because they fear losing clients over the lengthy three-dose schedule (Daley et al., 2009; Williams et al., 2016). Some states require a prescription even for vaccination at a pharmacy (ASTHO, 2014).

Adult immunization does not have to be so complicated. Every year since 2009 about 40 percent of adults in the United States have received seasonal flu vaccine; coverage among those over 65 years is even better, around two-thirds (CDC, 2016b,c). If states supported hepatitis B vaccination to the same level as seasonal influenza vaccine, great improvements could be made in hepatitis B immunization.

Recommendation 4-1: States should expand access to adult hepatitis B vaccination, removing barriers to free immunization in pharmacies and other easily accessible settings.

The relative success of seasonal influenza immunization is partly a matter of making vaccination convenient, especially for hard-to-reach patients, including homeless people and substance users (Vlahov et al., 2007). Offering vaccination in pharmacies is one way to reach a broader cross-section of the population. Many pharmacies are open evenings and weekends, making them convenient to people whose jobs do not allow paid leave. Data from Walgreens pharmacies in 49 states showed that about 30 percent of vaccinations were given during off-clinic hours (meaning weekends, evenings, and holidays) (Goad et al., 2013). The same data showed 40 percent of 18- to 49-year-olds seeking immunizations at Walgreens came during off-hours; 37 percent were uninsured (Goad et al., 2013).

All states now authorize pharmacists to vaccinate, but many restrict the types of vaccines and circumstances under which pharmacists can administer them (American Pharmacists Association, 2015; Bach and Goad, 2015; Immunization Action Coalition, 2016). Pharmacists can administer hepatitis B vaccine in all states except New Hampshire and New York, although Georgia, Hawaii, Indiana, North Carolina, and Puerto Rico require a prescription for the vaccine, and 34 states have age restrictions on hepatitis B vaccination in pharmacies (American Pharmacists Association, 2016).

State laws on the reimbursement of vaccination delivered in pharmacies also vary widely (Bach and Goad, 2015). Payment for vaccination can come from private insurance, Medicare, Medicaid, or out-of-pocket (ASTHO, 2014). Provisions to simplify reimbursement, such as the Medicare mass immunizer program, reduce the administrative barriers to vaccination, but hepatitis B vaccine is not included in the mass immunizer program (ASTHO, 2014; CMS, 2016a,b).

The CDC can fund state and local health departments to buy vaccines through section 317 of the Public Health Service Act, but the vast majority of these funds go to childhood immunizations (Orenstein et al., 2007). Section 317 funding is meant "to fill critical public health needs," and as such would be appropriately spent on viral hepatitis elimination (CDC, 2016h).

The specific actions needed to make hepatitis B vaccine more widely available will vary by state. In Hawaii, which has a large population of Asian Americans and Native Hawaiians, pharmacies can provide the hepatitis B vaccine series; the state's MinuteClinics can also screen for HCV (CVS Health, 2016). Prisons and jails are also an ideal venue for hepatitis B vaccination, a topic discussed in the next chapter.

Reluctance to vaccinate against HBV in nontraditional settings may stem from some confusion over the importance of adherence to the standard dose schedule. Protective immunity to HBV is found in 30 to 55 percent of healthy adults after one dose of the vaccine (Mast et al., 2004, 2006). A two-dose vaccine schedule has been shown to confer immunity in 82.9 percent of healthy adults (95 percent CI 76.1 to 89.7 percent) (Wong et al., 2014). Patients may fear, erroneously, that receiving extra doses of the vaccine is harmful, a point that should be clarified for all vaccine providers. Similarly, when the interval between doses is lengthened there is no need to restart the series (CDC, 2016e). Some research has shown that delaying the last dose for years may even improve antibody response (Jackson et al., 2007; Junewicz et al., 2014).

Prevention of Mother-to-Child Transmission

HBV is far more efficiently transmitted from mother to child than HIV or HCV (Benova et al., 2014; Connor et al., 1994; Dienstag, 2015). Without intervention, about 90 percent of infants born to HBeAg+ women will contract the virus at birth (CDC, 2016d; Ko et al., 2014). Infants infected at birth are prone to chronic hepatitis B infection, which carries a 25 percent risk of premature death from liver cancer or cirrhosis later in life (Beasley and Hwang, 1991; CDC, 2016e; Mast et al., 2005). Timely hepatitis B vaccination and hepatitis B immune globulin after birth are highly effective in preventing most infants born to HBsAg+ mothers from developing chronic hepatitis B infection (Mast et al., 2005). In 1988, ACIP recommended universal screening of all pregnant women for HBsAg and that babies born to HBsAg+ mothers receive hepatitis B immune globulin and the first dose of hepatitis B vaccine within 12 hours of birth (CDC, 1988). In 1990, the CDC established a national perinatal hepatitis B prevention program (CDC, 2011a). The program aims to identify HBsAg+ pregnant women and enroll them in case management to ensure their infants receive timely immunoprophylaxis and serologic testing after completion of the vaccine series (CDC, 2011a). By 2000, 50 percent of the more than 20,000 births to HBsAg+ mothers were enrolled in the program, and new cases of chronic hepatitis B in infants declined from almost 6,000 cases in 1990 to about 1,000 in 2000 (Smith et al., 2012b; Ward, 2015).

Despite the initial good progress, further reduction in perinatal HBV transmission has lagged. Ideally all HBsAg+ pregnant women should be referred to a specialist for perinatal and long-term care, as ACIP recommended in 2005 (Mast et al., 2005). But of the estimated 25,000 to 26,000 HBsAg+ women who give birth in the United States each year, only about half are identified for case management, a proportion unchanged since 2000 (Smith et al., 2012b). In 2015 the CDC and American College of Obstetricians and Gynecologists (ACOG) developed an algorithm showing the tests necessary for HBsAg+ pregnant women and the results which should trigger referral to a specialist (see Figure 4-2). Still, every year an estimated 800 to 1,000 infants (or about 3.8 percent of babies born to HBsAg+ mothers) become chronically infected from vertical transmission (Ko et al., 2014).

By some estimates as many as 96.7 percent of HBsAg+ pregnant women are tested in their first trimester (Ko et al., 2014). It is crucial that their newborns receive a dose of hepatitis B vaccine within 12 to 24 hours of birth to prevent transmission of the virus, but hepatitis B birth dose coverage[1] in the United States was only 63.9 percent in 2015 (CDC, 2016a). ACIP aimed to correct this in 2016 by recommending that all infants receive the initial dose of the hepatitis B vaccine within 24 hours of birth (Chitnis, 2016; Jenco, 2016).

Infants born to highly viremic HBsAg+ mothers have increased risk of immunoprophylaxis failure. A prospective observational study in Australia found that 9 percent of infants born to mothers with HBV DNA greater than 20 million IU/mL ($7.3 \log_{10}$ IU/mL or 100 million copies/mL) developed chronic hepatitis B infection (despite post-exposure prophylaxis with hepatitis B vaccine and immune globulin), but none of the babies born to women with lower HBV DNA did (Wiseman et al., 2009). A recent analysis of cases of hepatitis B immunoprophylaxis failure in California between 2005 and 2011 found 92 percent of cases had HBV DNA greater than 20 million IU/mL (Burgis et al., 2014).

Prophylactic antiviral therapy in the third trimester of pregnancy will

---

[1] Within 24 hours of birth.

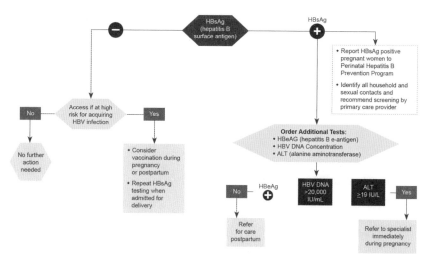

FIGURE 4-2 Screening and referral algorithm for HBV infection among pregnant women.
SOURCE: CDC, 2015.

further reduce perinatal HBV transmission among highly viremic women. A recent randomized trial of prophylactic tenofovir treatment in such patients (median HBV DNA 8.19 $\log_{10}$ IU/mL) prevented transmission of HBV without serious consequences to the newborn or complications to the delivery (Pan et al., 2016). At the same time, women may experience hepatitis flare after stopping treatment postpartum and require long-term antiviral therapy, which carries a risk of unclear potential for drug resistance in subsequent pregnancies (ter Borg et al., 2008).

Current practice guidelines in Australia recommend that pregnant women with HBV DNA greater than 10 million IU/mL (7 $\log_{10}$ IU/mL) be referred to a specialist for consideration for prophylactic tenofovir therapy (ASHM, 2014). The 2015, AASLD[2] guidelines set a lower threshold, recommending pregnant women with an HBV DNA level greater than 200,000 IU/mL be considered for prophylactic antiviral therapy, while acknowledging the need for research to establish a more precise treatment threshold (Terrault et al., 2016).

Hepatitis B flare is common during pregnancy and after delivery and can lead to liver failure (Elefsiniotis et al., 2015; Giles et al., 2015; Nguyen et al., 2009; ter Borg et al., 2008). It is therefore important to monitor

---

[2] Officially, the American Association for the Study of Liver Diseases.

liver enzymes in HBsAg+ pregnant women. A retrospective study of 29 pregnant women with chronic hepatitis B found three women developed severe hepatitis flare or liver failure and required antiviral therapy, and one woman required a liver transplant (Nguyen et al., 2009).

> **Recommendation 4-2: The Centers for Disease Control and Prevention, the American Association for the Study of Liver Diseases, the Infectious Diseases Society of America, and the American College of Obstetricians and Gynecologists should recommend that all HBsAg+ pregnant women have early prenatal HBV DNA and liver enzyme tests to evaluate whether antiviral therapy is indicated for prophylaxis to eliminate mother-to-child transmission or for treatment of chronic active hepatitis.**

Prevention of mother-to-child transmission of HBV is clearly a priority for the CDC, one referenced in the national viral hepatitis action plan (HHS, 2015). Affirmation of the importance of early viremia testing from CDC leadership would help enforce this point. The Infectious Diseases Society of America (IDSA), AASLD, and ACOG also command the attention of important stakeholders on this question: the doctors who manage hepatitis B in pregnant women. Leadership from these societies would help draw attention to this essential service and end the vertical transmission of HBV.

Prevention of HBV and HCV Infections

Until there is a vaccine for HCV, prevention will be mainly a matter of limiting exposure to the virus. One component of prevention (discussed later in this chapter) is curing all infected persons of their chronic infection. Another is preventing the blood contact that spreads HCV, as well as HBV and HIV infections. In some countries this means better screening of donor blood, ending use of reusable syringes, or reducing demand for unnecessary medical injections (WHO, 2016a). In the United States about 75 percent of the roughly 30,500 new HCV infections a year are caused by injection drug use (Klevens et al., 2014; University of Washington, n.d.-a). A key step to ending transmission of HCV in the United States is reducing the risk of infection among people who inject drugs.

Injection Drug Use and HCV Infection

The United States has a drug injection problem of epidemic proportions (Dart et al., 2015; Kolodny et al., 2015). The nonmedical use of prescription opioids has risen sharply since 2000 (Keyes et al., 2014). National survey data suggest that 435,000 Americans use heroin, and another 4.3

million report illicit use of prescription pain medicines (SAMHSA, 2015a). These proportions could shift over time; heroin is often easier to buy and cheaper than prescription opioids, causing people addicted to painkillers to switch (Cicero et al., 2014; Dart et al., 2015). The CDC estimates that death from opioid overdose has increased 200 percent since 2000, a situation described as "an unprecedented epidemic" (HHS, 2013; Rudd et al., 2016).

The opioid problem is not simply a matter of more people using addictive drugs; a different cross-section of society is involved than was a generation ago. In the 1960s, heroin use was mostly confined to cities; users were predominantly young, male, and disproportionately racial and ethnic minorities (Cicero et al., 2014). In contrast, people who have become addicted to opioids in the last decade are male and female, overwhelmingly white, and living in rural areas, suburbs, and small towns (Akyar et al., 2016; Cicero et al., 2014). Nowadays about half of people who inject drugs live outside of cities, often in relative isolation, in areas not well equipped to access medical care or addiction treatment services (Havens et al., 2013; Oster et al., 2015). In rural counties deaths from drug overdose have increased three times faster than in urban ones (Keyes et al., 2014).

HCV infection is a serious health consequence of injection drug use. Studies from the early 2000s suggest an HCV antibody prevalence among people who inject drugs of 70 to 77 percent (Nelson et al., 2011). About a third of people who inject drugs acquire HCV infection in their first year of injecting (Hagan et al., 2008). Controlling HCV among drug injectors is challenging. The syringe exchange programs[3] that have reduced HIV incidence are less effective against hepatitis C (Des Jarlais et al., 2015; Holtzman et al., 2009). HCV transmission by needle stick is 10 times more efficient than for HIV (Bruggmann and Grebely, 2015; Siddharta et al., 2016). HCV is also a relatively hardy virus, able to survive on fomites for hours or even days (Krawczynski et al., 2003; Valdiserri et al., 2014). For these reasons, needle or syringe sharing accounts for only about 63 percent of the risk of HCV infection among people who inject drugs, because the virus can survive on other equipment including cotton filters and rinse water (Hagan et al., 2010).

Opioid Agonist Therapy

The most effective way to prevent hepatitis C among people who inject drugs is to combine strategies that improve the safety of injection with those that treat the underlying addiction (Cox and Thomas, 2013; Hagan et al.,

---

[3] Also called syringe services.

2010). Opioid agonist therapy[4] refers to the use of prescription medicines to bind opiate receptors in the brain, thereby relieving the symptoms of withdrawal (IOM, 1995). Such therapy is part of the tertiary prevention of substance use disorders, meaning that it prevents the worst complications of the disorder, including overdose and transmission of blood-borne infections (Kolodny et al., 2015). Before 2000, opioid agonists could only be prescribed in drug treatment clinics, but now the Substance Abuse and Mental Health Services Administration (SAMHSA) issues waivers to doctors who, after registering with the Drug Enforcement Agency (DEA), can prescribe buprenorphine-based formulations in routine practice (FDA, n.d.; SAMHSA, 2017).[5] Still, the opioid epidemic created more demand for services, and by 2012 demand exceeded capacity by between 1.3 and 1.4 million (Jones et al., 2015). In response to this shortage, SAMHSA increased the maximum patient load per waived provider to 275, and expanded the role of nurse practitioners and physician assistants in managing buprenorphine therapy (HHS, 2016c; SAMHSA, 2015b).

Nevertheless, most of the waivers have been issued to doctors on the coasts (HHS, 2016c; Rosenblatt et al., 2015; SAMHSA, 2015b). A 2012 analysis found that 30 million Americans live in places where not a single provider can prescribe opioid agonists (Rosenblatt et al., 2015). There is a need for wider access to treatment for opioid dependence, especially in rural areas (Rosenblatt et al., 2015; Stein et al., 2015). Recent studies in rural Colorado, North Carolina, Oklahoma, and Pennsylvania are exploring strategies, such as tele-psychiatry, to bring opioid use treatment to rural areas (AHRQ, 2016). Regarding medications, long-acting buprenorphine and naltrexone formulations may be more suitable in such areas (Kjome and Moeller, 2011; Laffont et al., 2016). When naltrexone is administered via a sustained-release implant, for example, it can be active in blood, controlling drug cravings, for up to 6 months (Hulse et al., 2009; Kjome and Moeller, 2011).

Syringe Exchange

Syringe exchange programs in the United States do not have sufficient coverage even in cities; availability is worse in rural areas (Des Jarlais et al.,

---

[4] Including full agonist therapy with methadone and partial agonist therapy with buprenorphine, sometimes complemented with the antagonist treatment naloxone (SAMHSA, 2015c; 2016).

[5] The waiver program only authorized the prescription of buprenorphine, alone or in combination with naloxone. Other opioid agonists are still restricted. For example, the DEA categorizes methadone as Schedule II drug, meaning that it has a high potential for abuse and dependence (DEA, n.d.). Therefore, methadone can only be prescribed in conjunction with drug treatment programs certified by SAMHSA (SAMHSA, 2015c).

2015). Despite serving, in theory, half the people who inject drugs, rural and suburban areas have only 30 percent of the nation's syringe services and distribute almost 29 million fewer syringes (only about 8 percent of the total) (Des Jarlais et al., 2015; Oster et al., 2015). Of every dollar spent on syringe services in the United States, about 17 cents goes to rural or suburban areas (Des Jarlais et al., 2015). With fewer staff and smaller budgets, rural programs have to reach people injecting drugs in remote parts of the country, such as Appalachia, and vast ones, such as the Central Valley. When syringe services are far away, people are less likely to use them (Allen et al., 2015; Cooper et al., 2011). Transportation challenges can pale in comparison to the problem of protecting clients' privacy, something often taken for granted in the relative anonymity of big cities (Benyo, 2012).

Part of the value of both opioid agonist therapy and syringe exchange programs is that they provide clients with an entry point to the health system (MacNeil and Pauly, 2011). Staff at exchanges, especially case managers, can also help interested clients enroll in drug counseling or cessation programs. A randomized, controlled trial in Baltimore syringe exchange programs found that clients working with case managers were 87 percent more likely to enter drug treatment within a week of their referral than clients without such support (Strathdee et al., 2006). Staff can also counsel clients on the use of naloxone to treat overdose and offer testing for viral hepatitis and HIV. Three-quarters of syringe exchange programs responding to a 2013 survey reported offering HCV testing, though the proportion was lower in rural areas (Des Jarlais et al., 2015). Ensuring linkage to care is more challenging; fewer than half of survey respondents (a third in rural areas) reported tracking the referral process for clients who tested positive (Des Jarlais et al., 2015).

Although legally prohibited in the United States, supervised injection facilities, clinics where people can inject under clinical supervision, may be another means of harm reduction (Drug Policy Alliance, 2016). Supervised injection has been shown to reduce death from overdose; in Vancouver, the introduction of such a facility was associated with a 35 percent reduction in the rate of fatal overdose, compared to only a 9 percent reduction in other parts of the city (Marshall et al., 2011). A 2006 review (predating curative treatment for hepatitis C) concluded that "it is plausible that these rooms can contribute to a reduced incidence of HCV" through reducing the sharing of injecting equipment (Wright and Tompkins, 2006). The possibility of curing HCV infection in a crucial population may warrant revisiting the strategy. A supervised injection facility in Vancouver reported an 87.6 percent prevalence of HCV antibody among its clients (Wood et al., 2005). A systematic review of research (mainly from Canada and Australia) found supervised sites to be effective at reaching people with unstable housing and a recent history of incarceration (Potier et al., 2014).

Syringe exchange and opioid agonist treatment are cornerstones of viral hepatitis elimination. But these services are least available in the places that most need them, rural areas with an injection opioid problem (see Box 4-1). It is no coincidence that the same four states (Kentucky, Tennessee, Virginia, and West Virginia) that saw a 364 percent increase in acute HCV infection between 2006 and 2012 have documented unmet needs for syringe services (Des Jarlais et al., 2015; Zibbell et al., 2015). Expanding harm reduction services (both exchanges and opioid agonist therapy) to rural and suburban areas is complicated, as these parts of the country are characterized by fewer resources for health and principled opposition to anything seen to facilitate illicit drug use (Havens et al., 2013; Valdiserri et al., 2014). Such obstacles can be overcome, but only with commitment from states and federal agencies.

Recommendation 4-3: States and federal agencies should expand access to syringe exchange and opioid agonist therapy in accessible venues.

The epidemic of nonmedical opioid use has captured the attention of policy makers and providers, with new emphasis on diagnosing substance use disorder and using opioid agonist therapy to treat it when possible (Tetrault and Butner, 2015). Syringe services and treatment for substance use disorder, essential parts of the response to the opioid epidemic, can also prevent transmission of HCV (HHS, 2013; Volkow et al., 2014). Action against the opioid epidemic complements work on viral hepatitis elimination, with attention to the two goals benefiting both.

UNAIDS[6] reckons that every person who injects drugs needs about 200 syringes a year, something few exchange programs can provide (UNAIDS, 2014). In some states, drug paraphernalia laws and rules regulating the prescription and sale of syringes can present an obstacle to full coverage (Burris et al., 2002) (see Box 4-1). In states without such restrictions, and with public funding available to syringe exchange programs, more equipment is distributed and the programs can offer complementary services, including HCV testing (Bramson et al., 2015). Tracking the number of syringes distributed and the number of people who inject drugs in a program's coverage area could, in theory, afford a measure of progress against the UNAIDS target, though in practice it is difficult to estimate the latter with any precision (Abdul-Quader et al., 2013). Evidence regarding unmet need for syringe services may help persuade legislators to remove restrictions on them, including the restrictions on the number of syringes exchanged per visit or per client.

The North American Syringe Exchange Network periodically surveys

---

[6] Officially, the Joint United Nations Programme on HIV/AIDS.

exchanges regarding services provided, budget, and annual number of syringes exchanged (CDC, 2010; North American Syringe Exchange Network, n.d.). Such surveys will be valuable in charting progress on this recommendation and determining if the reach of the exchanges is expanding. Other valuable indicators will be the number of providers authorized to provide buprenorphine, and the number of people in opioid treatment programs.

Expansion of syringe exchange to rural and suburban areas may require modifications to models developed in cities. Pharmacies are an accessible venue for people who inject drugs across a range of settings (Hammett et al., 2014). Pharmacies in some jurisdictions can sell or distribute syringes, dispose of used ones, dispense naloxone for overdose, and test for HIV (Hammett et al., 2014). When it is legal to buy syringes at pharmacies, more people who inject drugs do so (Siddiqui et al., 2015). Pharmacies are often reasonably equipped to provide confidential space for patient counseling. Research in Rhode Island suggests that pharmacists and other pharmacy staff are willing to counsel clients who inject drugs on prevention and referrals for treatment when appropriate (Zaller et al., 2010). Where pharmacists are not willing to participate, education may help persuade them (Chiarello, 2016; Crawford et al., 2013). It is also essential to have clear laws and an unambiguous store or franchise policy supporting syringe exchange, so that no pharmacist fears retribution from management for dispensing syringes (Chiarello, 2016; Crawford et al., 2013). Some reluctant pharmacists may be reassured by data showing that syringe sales at pharmacies are not associated with any increase in crime in the surrounding area (Stopka et al., 2014).

Mobile syringe exchange has the potential to reach a wide cross-section of people who inject drugs. Mobile exchanges typically operate from a van or bus, allowing them to bring services to their clients and to cover a wide area, conveying advantages in rural areas (WHO, 2007). In cities, mobile programs are often meant to supplement fixed sites (Ivsins et al., 2010). When the only fixed-site syringe exchange in Victoria, British Columbia, closed, syringe distribution in the city fell by a third (Ivsins et al., 2010). Clients familiar with the fixed site complained that the switch to mobile clinics made it more difficult to safely dispose of syringes and to obtain clean ones (Ivsins et al., 2010). On the other hand, mobile programs often face less community opposition than fixed sites (Ivsins et al., 2010; WHO, 2007). Some observational studies suggest that mobile sites may be more acceptable to younger clients and to people engaging in higher risk behavior (Jones et al., 2010). Mobile programs may also be more desirable in places where clients may fear harassment or public shaming (WHO, 2007).

Widening the reach of syringe exchange is ideologically complicated (Rich and Adashi, 2015). Introducing such programs to new places requires

---

BOX 4-1
The Indiana Syringe Exchange Program

Indiana's syringe exchange program was created in 2015 in response to what became the largest HIV outbreak in state history (Harper, 2015). In early 2015 there were 11 confirmed cases of HIV in Scott County, a rural county of about 24,000 people with high unemployment and poverty (Peters et al., 2016; Sun, 2016). After the local Planned Parenthood clinic closed in 2013, no free HIV testing was available in the county (Peters et al., 2016).

All 11 persons identified at the beginning of the epidemic had injected oxymorphone, a prescription opioid (Peters et al., 2016). The Centers for Disease Control and Prevention was notified in February, and on March 26, 2015, the state declared a public health emergency in Scott County (Janowicz, 2016). The ensuing investigation identified 181 HIV cases infected between November 2014 and November 2015, mostly young white men, about 92 percent of whom also had hepatitis C virus infection (Peters et al., 2016). Through contact tracing, the team identified 536 people with whom the infected people had reported having unprotected sex, sharing syringes, or both (Peters et al., 2016). The outbreak was driven by a network of people of different ages who reported injecting mainly oxymorphone but also heroin, methamphetamine, cocaine, and oxycodone (Conrad et al., 2015; Peters et al., 2016). In response to the public health emergency declaration, the county set up a mobile syringe exchange and community outreach center (Harper, 2015). The center offered HIV and hepatitis C testing and treatment, information about substance use disorder, referral to social services, and help with health insurance enrollment (Janowicz, 2016).

Syringe exchange programs were previously illegal in Indiana; they are seen to be inconsistent with laws against drug use (McCarthy, 2015; Sun, 2016).

---

sensitivity to local norms. Although the evidence indicates that exchange programs do not recruit new users or increase drug use among clients, people whose communities are being devastated by drug use may understandably object to actions seen to enable it (Bramson et al., 2015; Vlahov and Junge, 1998). When such programs were starting in response to HIV, cultural opposition to them was particularly strong among police officers and African American and Hispanic community leaders (Anderson, 1991; Barreras and Torruella, 2013; Bramson et al., 2015; Singer et al., 1991). Such attitudes can change, especially if community members are convinced of the exchange programs' effectiveness to reduce disease and keep used needles off the streets (Barreras and Torruella, 2013; Keyl et al., 1998). Police officers in some areas have come to favor exchange programs, citing reduced risk of needle stick injury on the job and benefit to the community

Therefore, the syringe exchange program was originally limited to Scott County (McCarthy, 2015; Sun, 2016). Critics opposed limiting the program to one county, however. The spike in HCV infection and the large number of people in treatment for heroin use suggested a wider problem (McCarthy, 2015). State officials then extended the law allowing syringe exchange programs statewide, provided the county had declared a public health emergency, a declaration valid for 1 year (State of Indiana, n.d.; Sun, 2016). However, the state does not provide funding for the syringe exchange programs currently approved in eight counties, and federal funds cannot be used to purchase sterile syringes (Callahan, 2016; Rural Center for AIDS/STD Prevention, 2016; Sun, 2016). Since the affected counties are rural and poor, many of the syringe exchange programs rely on donations, non-profit organizations, and foundations to support their services (Callahan, 2016).

Scott County's syringe exchange program distributed more than 97,000 sterile syringes in 2015 (Peters et al., 2016). Participants were given sterile syringes to last 1 week, as well as wound kits and information about harm reduction and substance abuse services (Harper, 2015; Patel et al., 2015). Syringe sharing declined by 85 percent (95 percent CI: 82 to 87 percent) and syringe returns increased within its first 2 months (Patel et al., 2015). Scott County's program recently received permission to remain open through May 2017 (Rudavsky, 2016).

The outbreak provides a warning to 220 counties across 26 states with similar risk factors for an HIV or hepatitis C outbreak (Van Handel et al., 2016). Implementing HIV and hepatitis C testing and syringe exchange programs in rural areas experiencing intensifying opioid epidemics could help prevent similar public health emergencies.

(Davis et al., 2014). Project sponsors would do well to encourage local consultation in new exchange programs.

Expansion of opioid agonist therapy will also be essential to preventing viral hepatitis infections. The Surgeon General's 2016 report *Facing Addiction in America* concluded that while medications are effective in treating serious substance use disorders, too few providers are able to prescribe them (HHS, 2016a). The increase in the allowable patient limit on providers managing buprenorphine therapy could help improve the reach of this essential health service. The Surgeon General's report also argued for better integration of opioid agonist therapy into mainstream medical practices (as opposed to separate substance abuse clinics) as a way to improve efficiency and lead to better health outcomes (HHS, 2016b). Consistent with this emerging consensus, the 2016 Comprehensive Addiction and Recovery Act aimed to make evidence-based treatments for opiate addiction more available around the country, including to incarcerated people (Community

Anti-Drug Coalitions of America, n.d.). A better discussion of reaching people who inject drugs and people in prisons with a range of viral hepatitis services follows in the next chapter.

Testing and Screening

Identifying people infected with HBV or HCV will be crucial to elimination, as the models presented in Chapter 2 indicate. The value of screening is already affirmed in the CDC and U.S. Preventive Services Task Force (USPSTF) guidelines, which recommend screening people at high risk of infection for both HBV and HCV (see Table 4-1); Chapter 5 discusses strategies to improve compliance with these guidelines. At the same time, chronic viral hepatitis is often clinically silent until its later stages. Early detection is the first step to preventing the complications of untreated infection. Wider screening for hepatitis C may be warranted in the United States, as it accounts for a considerably larger share of the national burden of viral hepatitis.

HCV Screening

In 1998 the CDC recommended screening for HCV among people with the known risk factors for infection shown in Box 4-2 (CDC, 1998; University of Washington, n.d.-b). By 2014, however, it was evident that at least 20 percent of people with hepatitis C had no discernable risk factor for the infection, and that almost three-quarters were born between 1945 and 1965 (CDC, 2016i). In 2012 the CDC changed its recommendation to encourage one-time HCV testing for everyone born between 1945 and 1965 (CDC, 2012). The following year the USPSTF followed suit, revising its 2004 statement cautioning against widespread screening of asymptomatic adults, but that was a year before direct-acting antivirals came on the market (Moyer, 2013).

Screening for HCV has increased since 2013, with increasing attention given to the best strategies to implement the USPSTF recommendation (Sidlow and Msaouel, 2015; Turner et al., 2015). Recent estimates suggest that about 15 to 20 percent of the 1945 to 1965 birth cohort is screened in primary care (Bourgi et al., 2016; Linas et al., 2014). Insufficient staff time and competing demands on providers' attention, a problem discussed in the next chapter, has been cited as a reason for the uneven implementation of the recommendation, as has providers' unwillingness to inquire about risk factors (Jewett et al., 2015; Southern et al., 2014). It is not clear that provider education can improve this. One 15-week intervention to improve adherence to national guidelines saw adherence to screening decrease from

TABLE 4-1 USPSTF Recommendations and Important Risk Groups for HBV and HCV Screening

	HBV	HCV
USPSTF Recommendation	The USPSTF recommends screening for HBV infection in persons at high risk for infection.	The USPSTF recommends screening for HCV infection in persons at high risk for infection. The USPSTF also recommends offering one-time screening for HCV infection to adults born between 1945 and 1965.
Important Risk Groups for Screening	Important risk groups (in non-pregnant adolescents and adults) for HBV infection that should be screened include • Persons born in countries and regions with a high prevalence of HBV infection (≥2 percent) • U.S.-born persons not vaccinated as infants whose parents were born in regions with a very high prevalence of HBV infection (≥8 percent), such as sub-Saharan Africa and central and Southeast Asia • HIV-positive persons • Injection drug users • Men who have sex with men • Household contacts or sexual partners of persons with HBV infection	Important risk groups for HCV infection that should be screened include • Past or current injection drug users • Persons who received a blood transfusion, organ or tissue transplant before 1992 • Long-term hemodialysis patients • Persons born to an HCV-infected mother • Incarcerated persons • Intranasal drug users • Persons with an unregulated tattoo • Persons with other percutaneous exposures • Adults born between 1945 and 1965 • Recipients of clotting factor concentrates made before 1987 • Persons with HIV infection

NOTE: HBV = hepatitis B virus; HCV = hepatitis C virus; USPSTF = U.S. Preventive Services Task Force.
SOURCES: CDC, 2016g; LeFevre, 2014; Moyer, 2013.

almost 60 percent at the start to about 13 percent in the last week (Southern et al., 2014).

Some settings have actively pursued wider HCV screening, including urban emergency departments, safety net providers for the uninsured. Screening in an Oakland emergency room found an HCV antibody prevalence of almost 14 percent among those in the 1945 to 1965 birth cohort, 38 percent among people who inject drugs, and about 3 percent among

---

BOX 4-2
CDC 1998 Risk-Based HCV Screening Recommendations

Persons who should be tested routinely for HCV infection based on their risk for infection:

- Persons who ever injected illegal drugs, including those who injected once or a few times many years ago and do not consider themselves as drug users.
- Persons with selected medical conditions, including
  o Persons who received clotting factor concentrates produced before 1987;
  o Persons who were ever on chronic (long-term) hemodialysis; and
  o Persons with persistently abnormal alanine aminotransferase levels.
- Prior recipients of transfusions or organ transplants, including
  o Persons who were notified that they received blood from a donor who later tested positive for HCV infection;
  o Persons who received a transfusion of blood or blood components before July 1992; and
  o Persons who received an organ transplant before July 1992.

Persons who should be tested routinely for HCV infection based on a recognized exposure:

- Health care, emergency medical, and public safety workers after needle sticks, sharps, or mucosal exposures to HCV-positive blood.
- Children born to HCV-positive women.

NOTE: CDC = Centers for Disease Control and Prevention; HCV = hepatitis C virus.
SOURCES: CDC, 1998; University of Washington, n.d.-b.

---

people with neither risk factor (White et al., 2016). A similar program at an urban tertiary care hospital in Alabama found that one in every nine emergency department patients born between 1945 and 1965 had HCV antibody, nearly four times higher than the previously reported prevalence for that group (Galbraith et al., 2015; Smith et al., 2012a). Moreover, cases found in urban emergency rooms could be missed under current risk-based and birth cohort screening guidelines. Twenty-five percent of cases found in Baltimore and 28 percent in Cincinnati emergency departments were among people with no reported risk factor for the virus; an ambulatory care center in the Bronx, also a safety net provider, found 3 percent prevalence of HCV antibody in people with no obvious risk factors (Hsieh et al., 2016; Lyons et al., 2016; Southern et al., 2011). For these reasons, some researchers have suggested universal testing at clinics and hospitals that serve high-risk populations (Southern et al., 2011).

Mathematical models indicate that one-time universal adult screening for HCV would identify 446,700 patients who would be missed with birth cohort screening (Kabiri et al., 2014). As the elimination effort continues, expanding testing, especially in settings likely to see high-risk patients, may be the key to continued progress (Edlin, 2011).

> **Recommendation 4-4:** The Centers for Disease Control and Prevention should work with states to identify settings appropriate for enhanced viral hepatitis testing based on expected prevalence.

The decision to make a policy of widespread testing for any disease cannot be taken lightly. The procedure comes at an expense to the health system and puts a burden on providers. It also has the potential to cause distress in patients, especially when the disease screened for carries a social stigma, as viral hepatitis does. On the other hand, society stands to benefit from any measure that sheds light on the subclinical burden of HBV and HCV infections. The ability of direct-acting antivirals to cure infection can also change the risk to benefit calculation over time. The CDC, in cooperation with its state and local partners, has the ability to identify populations that would benefit from heightened screening, especially if state and local health offices make the surveillance improvements described in Chapter 3.

There are core antigen tests for HCV with sensitivity of 90 percent and specificity of 98 percent (Freiman et al., 2016). There are, at present, no Food and Drug Administration-approved point-of-care hepatitis B tests in the United States, partly because the relatively low prevalence of hepatitis B translates into less incentive to manufacturers to seek market authorization. The next chapter of this report discusses measures that could improve adherence to established screening guidelines. Taken together, adherence to existing guidelines and enhanced screening in certain settings might contribute to a greater demand for screening assays, and prompt manufacturers to seek U.S. licensure for these products.

CARE AND TREATMENT

The direct-acting antivirals that cure chronic HCV infection are what make elimination of hepatitis C as a public health problem a feasible goal in the United States; their importance cannot be understated (Palese, 2016). At this time there are no comparable curative therapies for chronic hepatitis B, a problem discussed in Chapter 7. Identification of chronic HBV infections and their appropriate treatment will be crucial to ending transmission of the virus and to preventing death from chronic infection (NASEM, 2016). Entecavir and tenofovir are highly effective at suppressing the virus and cost-effective even over decades (Eckman et al., 2011; Hutton et al., 2007). The management of chronic HBV infection requires wide access to integrated, comprehensive care, a topic discussed in Chapter 5.

Curing Chronic HCV Infection

Hepatitis C treatments are costly, a topic discussed in detail in Chapter 6. The combination of cost and demand for these medicines has strained the budgets of many payers (Brennan and Shrank, 2014; Saag, 2014; Steinbrook and Redberg, 2014; Trooskin et al., 2015). In response, insurers have established criteria for prescription approval, such as evidence of advanced liver fibrosis or consultation with a specialist (Barua et al., 2015; Simon et al., 2015). Many insurers require a period of abstinence from drugs and alcohol; some confirm this with drug testing (Grebely et al., 2015). Restrictions in state Medicaid programs have drawn particular scrutiny; criteria for approval vary widely among states (Barua et al., 2015; Canary et al., 2015). As of 2015, 74 percent of Medicaid programs required evidence of advanced fibrosis or cirrhosis; 69 percent required prescription by or consultation with a specialist, and half required a period of abstinence from drugs and alcohol (Barua et al., 2015). Another six states required patients to undergo liver biopsy prior to treatment (Barua et al., 2015).

Because of the varying restrictions imposed by insurers, the process to obtain approval for direct-acting antiviral prescriptions has become laborious. These drugs are often listed as specialty products, a classification that requires a higher out-of-pocket payment from the patient, so when coverage is approved, the charge to the patient is often unaffordable (Rodriguez and Reynolds, 2016). Among callers to a hepatitis C hotline, about 40 percent were commercial insurance clients asking for help paying for treatment, and a quarter were Medicare beneficiaries in the same position (Rodriguez and Reynolds, 2016).

Another strategy to control costs is to require these prescriptions undergo a pre-approval process (sometimes called prior authorization) to determine if the patient meets the insurer's criteria for treatment, a process that can require considerable effort on the part of providers (Barua et al., 2015; Edlin, 2011; Trooskin et al., 2015). The insurer reviews the prior authorization request and either approves the filling of the prescription or issues a denial. If the prescription is denied, the prescriber can appeal the decision, but the appeals process requires further documentation and review. Prescriptions that ultimately are not filled because of a lack of approval by the insurer are considered absolutely denied. Absolute denial of direct-acting antivirals is not uncommon. The Yale Liver Center reported that a quarter of its patients were denied ledipasvir-sofosbuvir upon first request (Do et al., 2015).

There is evidence of disparities in access to direct-acting antivirals. A cohort study of hepatitis C patients in the mid-Atlantic region analyzed the rate of absolute denial of treatment among Medicare, Medicaid, and commercial insurers (Lo Re et al., 2016). 16.2 percent (95 percent CI: 14.8 to 17.8 percent) of the 2,321 patients were denied the drugs, most commonly on the grounds that the documentation provided was not sufficient information to assess medical need or lack of medical necessity (Lo Re et al., 2016). Absolute denial was significantly more common among Medicaid patients, whose treatment was refused at a rate of 46.3 percent (adjusted risk relative to commercial insurance patients: 4.14; 95 percent CI: 3.38 to 5.08), compared to Medicare (5.0 percent refusal; adjusted risk relative to commercial insurance patients: 0.61; 95 percent CI: 0.43 to 0.86) or commercial insurance patients (10.2 percent refusal) (Lo Re et al., 2016). Among cirrhotics, a quarter of Medicaid beneficiaries were denied treatment, compared to almost none of those with other types of insurance (Lo Re et al., 2016).

Another cohort study evaluated reasons why hepatitis C patients prescribed a sofosbuvir-based regimen never start it (Younossi et al., 2016). Out of 3,841 patients, 315 (8 percent) did not start the prescribed therapy; financial reasons and the insurance companies' process accounted for 81 percent of such cases. As in the Lo Re study, non-start (among patients who did not start therapy for financial or insurance reasons) was highest among Medicaid beneficiaries (35 percent, 95 percent CI: 30 to 40 percent) compared to patients covered with either Medicare (2 percent, 95 percent CI: 1 to 3 percent) or commercial insurance (6 percent, 95 percent CI: 5 to 7 percent) (Younossi et al., 2016).

The disparity in access to direct-acting antivirals has caught public attention, obliging the Centers for Medicare & Medicaid Services to formally remind state Medicaid directors that restricting access as a way to control costs is disallowed (CMS, 2015). In 2016 a class action lawsuit against the Washington state Medicaid agency ended in the ruling that restricting therapy to patients with advanced fibrosis was a violation of the Social Security Act (Aleccia, 2016). The threat of similar legal action caused the Delaware Medicaid program to rescind its access restrictions in June 2016 (Rini, 2016). State programs in Florida, Massachusetts, New York, and Pennsylvania have recently followed the Department of Veterans Affairs (VA) in removing all disease severity restrictions on hepatitis C treatment (Hughes, 2016; Kennedy, 2016; Lynch and McCarthy, 2016; Massachusetts EOHHS, 2016; Sapatkin, 2016). Since 2014, 16 state Medicaid programs have reduced their restrictions on treatment, although some states are not clear about the details of their policies (Hughes, 2016; Kennedy, 2016;

Lynch and McCarthy, 2016; Massachusetts EOHHS, 2016; NVHR and CHLPI, 2016; Sapatkin, 2016).

The committee commends Medicaid programs that have removed fibrosis restrictions on treatment. Patients denied access to hepatitis C treatment can have continued progression of hepatic fibrosis and remain at risk for cirrhosis, end-stage liver disease, and hepatocellular carcinoma. Delaying treatment until hepatic fibrosis is more advanced has been shown to increase the risk of cirrhosis, liver cancer, and death, and the tests used to stage fibrosis cannot do so with great accuracy (Degos et al., 2010; Tsochatzis et al., 2011). Research in the VA system suggests that deferring anti-HCV therapy until the development of advanced hepatic fibrosis or cirrhosis reduces the value of the treatment and increases the risk of liver-related complications and death (McCombs et al., 2015). Denial of direct-acting antiviral treatment allows for ongoing liver inflammation, which can increase the risk of extra-hepatic complications. There are also consequences to society. As Appendix B makes clear, universal treatment of all hepatitis C patients would reduce infections 90 percent by 2030 (relative to 2015 levels). By the same token, failure to treat chronic HCV infection enlarges the reservoir for transmission, while denying treatment can cause anxiety and may provoke distrust of the health system.

> **Recommendation 4-5: Public and private health plans should remove restrictions that are not medically indicated and offer direct-acting antivirals to all chronic hepatitis C patients.**

Curing chronic hepatitis C has immense clinical benefit (Pearlman and Traub, 2011). Cured patients, even cirrhotics, may experience a reversal of hepatic fibrosis over time (Everson et al., 2008; Mallet et al., 2008; Maylin et al., 2008; Shiratori et al., 2000). Reduction in fibrosis and return to normal liver function is associated with a decreased risk of hepatic decompensation, hepatocellular carcinoma, and all-cause mortality (van der Meer et al., 2012). Cure of chronic hepatitis C can also help eliminate HCV transmission (Harris et al., 2016b; Martin et al., 2016). It is plausible that curing chronic hepatitis C will also improve the many complications of infection, including bone, kidney, cardiovascular, and neuropsychiatric problems (Adinolfi et al., 2015; Butt et al., 2011; Freiberg et al., 2011; Lo Re et al., 2012, 2015; Tsui et al., 2007). It also improves overall quality of life for the hepatitis C patient (Smith-Palmer et al., 2015; Younossi and Henry, 2015).

Treating HCV infection is also cost-effective. In a review of both the clinical and financial value of direct-acting antiviral therapy, the California Technology Assessment Forum found that although treating all patients is costly, the benefits are sufficient to make it cost-effective (Tice et al., 2015).

Delaying treatment increases costs; it costs less to cure people who have never been through a course of treatment before and to cure people before they progress to cirrhosis, further evidence for the effectiveness of early action (Chhatwal et al., 2015; Rein et al., 2015; Younossi et al., 2015). Additionally, patients who are cured of chronic HCV infection have significantly lower medical expenses than those who are not (Smith-Palmer et al., 2015; Younossi and Henry, 2014).

Treating everyone with chronic HCV infection, regardless of disease stage, would avert considerable suffering and anxiety. It is also a financially sensible course of action in the long run. IDSA and AASLD issued a joint statement in collaboration with the International Antiviral Society-USA supporting treatment for everyone with chronic HCV infection (AASLD and IDSA, 2015). The ability of these drugs to eradicate HCV infection in nearly all infected people has made the prospect of eliminating viral hepatitis in the United States plausible. Public and private health plans should not interfere with this goal. They should remove restrictions on direct-acting antiviral treatment for hepatitis C patients. The committee recognizes that the cost of the drugs presents an obstacle to implementing this recommendation. A strategy to better manage these costs is discussed in Chapter 6.

REFERENCES

AASLD and IDSA (American Association for the Study of Liver Diseases and Infectious Diseases Society of America). 2015. *Hepatitis C guidance underscores the importance of treating HCV infection: Panel recommends direct-acting drugs for nearly all patients with chronic hepatitis C.* http://hcvguidelines.org/sites/default/files/when-and-in-whom-to-treat-press-release-october-2015.pdf (accessed November 14, 2016).

Abdul-Quader, A. S., J. Feelemyer, S. Modi, E. S. Stein, A. Briceno, S. Semaan, T. Horvath, G. E. Kennedy, and D. C. Des Jarlais. 2013. Effectiveness of structural-level needle/syringe programs to reduce HCV and HIV infection among people who inject drugs: A systematic review. *AIDS and Behavior* 17(9):2878-2892.

Adinolfi, L. E., R. Nevola, G. Lus, L. Restivo, B. Guerrera, C. Romano, R. Zampino, L. Rinaldi, A. Sellitto, M. Giordano, and A. Marrone. 2015. Chronic hepatitis C virus infection and neurological and psychiatric disorders: An overview. *World Journal of Gastroenterology* 21(8):2269-2280.

AHRQ (Agency for Healthcare Research and Quality). 2016. *Increasing access to medication-assisted treatment of opioid abuse in rural primary care practices.* https://www.ahrq.gov/professionals/systems/primary-care/increasing-access-to-opioid-abuse-treatment.html (accessed February 14, 2017).

Akyar, E., K. H. Seneca, S. Akyar, N. Schofield, M. P. Schwartz, and R. G. Nahass. 2016. Linkage to care for suburban heroin users with hepatitis C virus infection, New Jersey, USA. *Emerging Infectious Diseases* 22(5):907-909.

Aleccia, J. 2016. Judge orders Washington Medicaid to provide lifesaving hepatitis C drugs for all. *Seattle Times,* May 28. http://www.seattletimes.com/seattle-news/health/judge-orders-apple-health-to-cover-hepatitis-c-drugs-for-all (November 9, 2016).

Allen, S., M. Ruiz, and A. O'Rourke. 2015. How far will they go? Assessing the travel distance of current and former drug users to access harm reduction services. *Harm Reduction Journal* 12:3.

American Pharmacists Association. 2015. *Pharmacist-administered immunizations: What does your state allow?* https://www.pharmacist.com/pharmacist-administered-immunizations-what-does-your-state-allow (accessed December 6, 2016).

American Pharmacists Association. 2016. *Pharmacist administered vaccines: Types of vaccines authorized to administer.* http://pharmacist.com/sites/default/files/files/Slides%20 on%20Pharmacist%20IZ%20Authority_July_2016%20v2mcr.pdf?dfptag=imz (accessed December 8, 2016).

Anderson, W. 1991. The New York needle trial: The politics of public health in the age of AIDS. *American Journal of Public Health* 81(11):1506-1517.

ASHM (Australasian Society for HIV, Viral Hepatitis and Sexual Health Medicine). 2014. *10.0 Managing hepatitis B virus infection in pregnancy and children.* http://hepatitisb. org.au/10-0-managing-hepatitis-b-virus-infection-in-pregnancy-and-children (accessed November 21, 2016).

ASTHO (Association of State and Territorial Health Officials). 2014. *Pharmacy legal toolkit: Guidance and templates for state and territorial health agencies when establishing effective partnerships with pharmacies during routine and pandemic influenza seasons.* Arlington, VA: ASTHO.

Bach, A. T., and J. A. Goad. 2015. The role of community pharmacy-based vaccination in the USA: Current practice and future directions. *Dove Press* 4:67-77. https://www.dove-press.com/the-role-of-community-pharmacy-based-vaccination-in-the-usa-current-pr-peer-reviewed-article-IPRP (accessed December 6, 2016).

Barreras, R. E., and R. A. Torruella. 2013. New York City's struggle over syringe exchange: A case study of the intersection of science, activism, and political change. *Journal of Social Issues* 69(4):694-712.

Barua, S., R. Greenwald, J. Grebely, G. J. Dore, T. Swan, and L. E. Taylor. 2015. Restrictions for Medicaid reimbursement of sofosbuvir for the treatment of hepatitis C virus infection in the United States. *Annals of Internal Medicine* 163(3):215-223.

Beasley, R., and L. Hwang. 1991. Overview of the epidemiology of hepatocellular carcinoma. In *Viral hepatitis and liver disease. Proceedings of the 1990 international symposium on viral hepatitis and liver disease*, edited by F. B. Hollinger, S. Lemon, and H. S. Margolis. Baltimore, MD: Williams & Wilkins.

Benova, L., Y. A. Mohamoud, C. Calvert, and L. J. Abu-Raddad. 2014. Vertical transmission of hepatitis C virus: Systematic review and meta-analysis. *Clinical Infectious Diseases* 59(6):765-773.

Benyo, A. 2012. *Promoting secondary exchange: Opportunities to advance public health*, edited by J. Curry and D. Raymond. New York: Harm Reduction Coalition.

Bourgi, K., I. Brar, and K. Baker-Genaw. 2016. Health disparities in hepatitis C screening and linkage to care at an integrated health system in southeast Michigan. *PLoS One* 11(8):e0161241.

Bowman, S., L. E. Grau, M. Singer, G. Scott, and R. Heimer. 2014. Factors associated with hepatitis B vaccine series completion in a randomized trial for injection drug users reached through syringe exchange programs in three U.S. cities. *BMC Public Health* 14:820.

Bramson, H., D. C. Des Jarlais, K. Arasteh, A. Nugent, V. Guardino, J. Feelemyer, and D. Hodel. 2015. State laws, syringe exchange, and HIV among persons who inject drugs in the United States: History and effectiveness. *Journal of Public Health Policy* 36(2):212-230.

Brennan, T., and W. Shrank. 2014. New expensive treatments for hepatitis C infection. *JAMA* 312(6):593-594.

Bruggmann, P., and J. Grebely. 2015. Prevention, treatment and care of hepatitis C virus infection among people who inject drugs. *International Journal of Drug Policy* 26(Suppl 1):S22-S26.

Burgis, J., D. Kong, C. Salibay, J. Zipprich, K. Harriman, and S. So. 2014. Tu1129 Risk factors associated with immunoprophylaxis failure in infants born to mothers with chronic hepatitis B infection in California. *Gastroenterology* 146(5):S-762.

Burris, S., S. A. Strathdee, and J. S. Vernick. 2002. *Syringe access law in the United States: A state of the art assessment of law and policy.* Baltimore, MD: Center for Law and the Public's Health at Johns Hopkins and Georgetown Universities.

Butt, A. A., X. Wang, and L. F. Fried. 2011. HCV infection and the incidence of CKD. *American Journal of Kidney Diseases* 57(3):396-402.

Byrd, K. K., P. J. Lu, and T. V. Murphy. 2013. Hepatitis B vaccination coverage among health-care personnel in the United States. *Public Health Reports* 128(6):498-509.

Callahan, R. 2016. *Indiana counties must fund needle exchanges sans state help.* http://www.wcpo.com/news/state/state-indiana/indiana-counties-must-fund-needle-exchanges-sans-state-help (accessed December 1, 2016).

Canary, L. A., R. M. Klevens, and S. D. Holmberg. 2015. Limited access to new hepatitis C virus treatment under state Medicaid programs. *Annals of Internal Medicine* 163(3):226-228.

CDC (Centers for Disease Control and Prevention). 1988. Recommendations of the Immunization Practices Advisory Committee prevention of perinatal transmission of hepatitis B virus: Prenatal screening of all pregnant women for hepatitis B surface antigen. *Morbidity and Mortality Weekly Report* 37(22):341-346, 351. https://www.cdc.gov/mmwr/preview/mmwrhtml/00000036.htm (accessed December 6, 2016).

CDC. 1998. Recommendations for prevention and control of hepatitis c virus (HCV) infection and HCV-related chronic disease. *Morbidity and Mortality Weekly Report* 47(RR19):1-39.

CDC. 2010. Syringe exchange programs—United States, 2008. *Morbidity and Mortality Weekly Report* 59(45):1488-1491. https://www.cdc.gov/mmwr/preview/mmwrhtml/mm5945a4.htm#tab2 (accessed February 23, 2017).

CDC. 2011a. Assessing completeness of perinatal hepatitis B virus infection reporting through comparison of immunization program and surveillance data—United States. *Morbidity and Mortality Weekly Report* 60(13):410-413.

CDC. 2011b. Use of hepatitis B vaccination for adults with diabetes mellitus: Recommendations of the Advisory Committee on Immunization Practices (ACIP). *Morbidity and Mortality Weekly Report* 60(50):1709-1711.

CDC. 2012. *CDC now recommends all baby boomers receive one-time hepatitis C test.* http://www.cdc.gov/nchhstp/newsroom/2012/hcv-testing-recs-pressrelease.html (accessed November 15, 2016).

CDC. 2015. *Screening and referral algorithm for hepatitis B virus (HBV) infection among pregnant women.* https://www.cdc.gov/hepatitis/hbv/pdfs/prenatalhbsagtesting.pdf (accessed February 6, 2017).

CDC. 2016a. *ChildVaxView. 2015 hepatitis B (HepB) vaccination coverage among children 19-35 months by state, HHS region, and the United States, National Immunization Survey (NIS), 2015.* https://www.cdc.gov/vaccines/imz-managers/coverage/childvaxview/data-reports/hepb/reports/2015.html (accessed January 11, 2017).

CDC. 2016b. *Flu vaccination coverage, United States, 2014-15 influenza season.* http://www.cdc.gov/flu/fluvaxview/coverage-1415estimates.htm (accessed December 6, 2016).

CDC. 2016c. *Flu vaccination coverage, United States, 2015-16 influenza season.* http://www.cdc.gov/flu/fluvaxview/coverage-1516estimates.htm (accessed December 6, 2016).

CDC. 2016d. *Hepatitis B.* http://www.cdc.gov/vaccines/pubs/pinkbook/hepb.html (accessed 2016, November 3).

CDC. 2016e. *Hepatitis B FAQs for health professionals.* http://www.cdc.gov/hepatitis/hbv/hbvfaq.htm#overview (accessed November 7, 2016).

CDC. 2016f. *Hepatitis B FAQs for the public.* https://www.cdc.gov/hepatitis/hbv/bfaq.htm#bFAQ15 (accessed January 24, 2017).

CDC. 2016g. *Hepatitis C FAQs for health professionals.* http://www.cdc.gov/hepatitis/hcv/hcvfaq.htm#section1 (accessed October 25, 2016).

CDC. 2016h. *Questions answered on vaccines purchased with 317 funds.* https://www.cdc.gov/vaccines/imz-managers/guides-pubs/qa-317-funds.html (accessed February 23, 2017).

CDC. 2016i. *Surveillance for viral hepatitis—United States, 2014.* https://www.cdc.gov/hepatitis/statistics/2014surveillance/commentary.htm (accessed December 6, 2016).

Chen, H. L., L. H. Lin, F. C. Hu, J. T. Lee, W. T. Lin, Y. J. Yang, F. C. Huang, S. F. Wu, S. C. Chen, W. H. Wen, C. H. Chu, Y. H. Ni, H. Y. Hsu, P. L. Tsai, C. L. Chiang, M. K. Shyu, P. I. Lee, F. Y. Chang, and M. H. Chang. 2012. Effects of maternal screening and universal immunization to prevent mother-to-infant transmission of HBV. *Gastroenterology* 142(4):773-781.

Chhatwal, J., F. Kanwal, M. S. Roberts, and M. A. Dunn. 2015. Cost-effectiveness and budget impact of hepatitis C virus treatment with sofosbuvir and ledipasvir in the United States. *Annals of Internal Medicine* 162(6):397-406.

Chiarello, E. 2016. Nonprescription syringe sales: Resistant pharmacists' attitudes and practices. *Drug and Alcohol Dependence* 166:45-50.

Chitnis, D. 2016. ACIP approves change to hepatitis B vaccination guidelines. *Pediatric News, MDedge.* http://www.mdedge.com/pediatricnews/article/116025/vaccines/acip-approves-change-hepatitis-b-vaccination-guidelines (accessed November 21, 2016).

Cicero, T. J., M. S. Ellis, H. L. Surratt, and S. P. Kurtz. 2014. The changing face of heroin use in the United States: A retrospective analysis of the past 50 years. *JAMA Psychiatry* 71(7):821-826.

CMS (Centers for Medicare & Medicaid Services). 2015. *Medicaid drug rebate notice: Assuring Medicaid beneficiaries access to hepatitis C (HCV) drugs.* https://www.medicaid.gov/medicaid-chip-program-information/by-topics/prescription-drugs/downloads/rx-releases/state-releases/state-rel-172.pdf (accessed November 14, 2016).

CMS. 2016a. *Mass immunizers and roster billing: Simplified billing for influenza virus and pneumococcal vaccinations.* CMS, HHS, and the Medicare Learning Network.

CMS. 2016b. *Provider resources.* https://www.cms.gov/Medicare/Prevention/Immunizations/Providerresources.html (accessed December 6, 2016).

Collier, M. G., J. Drobeniuc, J. Cuevas-Mota, R. S. Garfein, S. Kamili, and E. H. Teshale. 2015. Hepatitis A and B among young persons who inject drugs—Vaccination, past, and present infection. *Vaccine* 33(24):2808-2812.

Community Anti-Drug Coalitions of America. n.d. *The Comprehensive Addiction and Recovery Act (CARA).* http://www.cadca.org/comprehensive-addiction-and-recovery-act-cara (accessed February 23, 2017).

Connor, E. M., R. S. Sperling, R. Gelber, P. Kiselev, G. Scott, M. J. O'Sullivan, R. VanDyke, M. Bey, W. Shearer, R. L. Jacobson, and et al. 1994. Reduction of maternal-infant transmission of human immunodeficiency virus type 1 with zidovudine treatment. Pediatric AIDS Clinical Trials Group Protocol 076 Study Group. *New England Journal of Medicine* 331(18):1173-1180.

Conrad, C., H. M. Bradley, D. Broz, S. Buddha, E. L. Chapman, R. R. Galang, D. Hillman, J. Hon, K. W. Hoover, M. R. Patel, A. Perez, P. J. Peters, P. Pontones, J. C. Roseberry, M. Sandoval, J. Shields, J. Walthall, D. Waterhouse, P. J. Weidle, H. Wu, and J. M. Duwve. 2015. Community outbreak of HIV infection linked to injection drug use of oxymorphone—Indiana, 2015. *Morbidity and Mortality Weekly Report* 64(16):443-444.

Cooper, H. L., D. C. Des Jarlais, Z. Ross, B. Tempalski, B. Bossak, and S. R. Friedman. 2011. Spatial access to syringe exchange programs and pharmacies selling over-the-counter syringes as predictors of drug injectors' use of sterile syringes. *American Journal of Public Health* 101(6):1118-1125.

Cox, A. L., and D. L. Thomas. 2013. Hepatitis C virus vaccines among people who inject drugs. *Clinical Infectious Diseases* 57(Suppl 2):S46-S50.

Crawford, N. D., S. Amesty, A. V. Rivera, K. Harripersaud, A. Turner, and C. M. Fuller. 2013. Randomized, community-based pharmacy intervention to expand services beyond sale of sterile syringes to injection drug users in pharmacies in New York City. *American Journal of Public Health* 103(9):1579-1582.

CVS Health. 2016. *CVS Health offering expanded hepatitis care options in Hawaii.* https://cvshealth.com/newsroom/press-releases/cvs-health-offering-expanded-hepatitis-care-options-hawaii (accessed December 6, 2016).

Daley, M. F., K. A. Hennessey, C. M. Weinbaum, S. Stokley, L. P. Hurley, L. A. Crane, B. L. Beaty, J. C. Barrow, C. I. Babbel, L. M. Dickinson, and A. Kempe. 2009. Physician practices regarding adult hepatitis B vaccination: A national survey. *American Journal of Preventive Medicine* 36(6):491-496.

Dart, R. C., H. L. Surratt, T. J. Cicero, M. W. Parrino, S. G. Severtson, B. Bucher-Bartelson, and J. L. Green. 2015. Trends in opioid analgesic abuse and mortality in the United States. *New England Journal of Medicine* 372(3):241-248.

Davis, C. S., J. Johnston, L. de Saxe Zerden, K. Clark, T. Castillo, and R. Childs. 2014. Attitudes of North Carolina law enforcement officers toward syringe decriminalization. *Drug and Alcohol Dependence* 144:265-269.

DEA (Drug Enforcement Administration). n.d. *Drug scheduling.* https://www.dea.gov/druginfo/ds.shtml (accessed February 23, 2017).

Degos, F., P. Perez, B. Roche, A. Mahmoudi, J. Asselineau, H. Voitot, and P. Bedossa. 2010. Diagnostic accuracy of FibroScan and comparison to liver fibrosis biomarkers in chronic viral hepatitis: A multicenter prospective study (the FIBROSTIC study). *Journal of Hepatology* 53(6):1013-1021.

Des Jarlais, D. C., A. Nugent, A. Solberg, J. Feelemyer, J. Mermin, and D. Holtzman. 2015. Syringe service programs for persons who inject drugs in urban, suburban, and rural areas—United States, 2013. *Morbidity and Mortality Weekly Report* 64(48):1337-1341.

Dienstag, J. L. 2015. *Overview of the epidemiology and natural history of hepatitis B.* PowerPoint presentation to the Committee on a National Strategy on the Elimination of Hepatitis B and C, Washington, DC, November 30, 2015. http://nationalacademies.org/hmd/~/media/Files/Activity%20Files/PublicHealth/HepatitisBandC/1-November2015/4-%20Jules%20Dienstag.pdf (accessed January 10, 2017).

Do, A., Y. Mittal, A. Liapakis, E. Cohen, H. Chau, C. Bertuccio, D. Sapir, J. Wright, C. Eggers, K. Drozd, M. Ciarleglio, Y. Deng, and J. K. Lim. 2015. Drug authorization for sofosbuvir/ledipasvir (Harvoni) for chronic HCV infection in a real-world cohort: A new barrier in the HCV care cascade. *PLoS One* 10(8):e0135645.

Drug Policy Alliance. 2016. *Supervised injection facilities.* http://www.drugpolicy.org/sites/default/files/DPA%20Fact%20Sheet_Supervised%20Injection%20Facilities%20(Feb.%202016).pdf (accessed December 6, 2016).

Eckman, M. H., T. E. Kaiser, and K. E. Sherman. 2011. The cost-effectiveness of screening for chronic hepatitis B infection in the United States. *Clinical Infectious Diseases* 52(11):1294-1306.

Edlin, B. R. 2011. Perspective: Test and treat this silent killer. *Nature* 474:S18-S19.

Elam-Evans, L. D., D. Yankey, J. A. Singleton, and M. Kolasa. 2014. National, state, and selected local area vaccination coverage among children aged 19-35 months—United States, 2013. *Morbidity and Mortality Weekly Report* 63(34):741-748.

Elefsiniotis, I., E. Vezali, D. Vrachatis, S. Hatzianastasiou, S. Pappas, G. Farmakidis, G. Vrioni, and A. Tsakris. 2015. Post-partum reactivation of chronic hepatitis B virus infection among hepatitis B e-antigen-negative women. *World Journal of Gastroenterology* 21(4):1261-1267.

Everson, G. T., L. Balart, S. S. Lee, R. W. Reindollar, M. L. Shiffman, G. Y. Minuk, P. J. Pockros, S. Govindarajan, E. Lentz, and E. J. Heathcote. 2008. Histological benefits of virological response to peginterferon alfa-2a monotherapy in patients with hepatitis C and advanced fibrosis or compensated cirrhosis. *Alimentary Pharmacology & Therapeutics* 27(7):542-551.

FDA (Food and Drug Administration). n.d. *Information for phamacists. NDA 20-732. NDA 20-733.* http://www.fda.gov/downloads/drugs/drugsafety/postmarketdrugsafetyinformationforpatientsandproviders/ucm191533.pdf (accessed November 15, 2016).

Ferrante, J. M., D. G. Winston, P. H. Chen, and A. N. de la Torre. 2008. Family physicians' knowledge and screening of chronic hepatitis and liver cancer. *Family Medicine* 40(5):345-351.

Forcione, D. G., R. T. Chung, and J. L. Dienstag. 2002. Natural history of hepatitis B virus infection. In *Chronic viral hepatitis: Diagnosis and therapeutics*, edited by R. S. Koff and G. Y. Wu. Totowa, NJ: Humana Press. Pp. 41-58.

Freiberg, M. S., C. C. Chang, M. Skanderson, K. McGinnis, L. H. Kuller, K. L. Kraemer, D. Rimland, M. B. Goetz, A. A. Butt, M. C. Rodriguez Barradas, C. Gibert, D. Leaf, S. T. Brown, J. Samet, L. Kazis, K. Bryant, and A. C. Justice. 2011. The risk of incident coronary heart disease among veterans with and without HIV and hepatitis C. *Circulation: Cardiovascular Quality and Outcomes* 4(4):425-432.

Freiman, J. M., T. M. Tran, S. G. Schumacher, L. F. White, S. Ongarello, J. Cohn, P. J. Easterbrook, B. P. Linas, and C. M. Denkinger. 2016. Hepatitis C core antigen testing for diagnosis of hepatitis C virus infection: A systematic review and meta-analysis. *Annals of Internal Medicine* 165(5):345-355.

Galbraith, J. W., R. A. Franco, J. P. Donnelly, J. B. Rodgers, J. M. Morgan, A. F. Viles, E. T. Overton, M. S. Saag, and H. E. Wang. 2015. Unrecognized chronic hepatitis C virus infection among baby boomers in the emergency department. *Hepatology* 61(3):776-782.

Giles, M., K. Visvanathan, S. Lewin, S. Bowden, S. Locarnini, T. Spelman, and J. Sasadeusz. 2015. Clinical and virological predictors of hepatic flares in pregnant women with chronic hepatitis C. *Gut* 64(11):1810-1815.

Goad, J. A., M. S. Taitel, L. E. Fensterheim, and A. E. Cannon. 2013. Vaccinations administered during off-clinic hours at a national community pharmacy: Implications for increasing patient access and convenience. *Annals of Family Medicine* 11(5):429-436.

Grebely, J., B. Haire, L. E. Taylor, P. Macneill, A. H. Litwin, T. Swan, J. Byrne, J. Levin, P. Bruggmann, and G. J. Dore. 2015. Excluding people who use drugs or alcohol from access to hepatitis C treatments—Is this fair, given the available data? *Journal of Hepatology* 63(4):779-782.

Hagan, H., E. R. Pouget, D. C. Des Jarlais, and C. Lelutiu-Weinberger. 2008. Meta-regression of hepatitis C virus infection in relation to time since onset of illicit drug injection: The influence of time and place. *American Journal of Epidemiology* 168(10):1099-1109.

Hagan, H., E. R. Pouget, I. T. Williams, R. L. Garfein, S. A. Strathdee, S. M. Hudson, M. H. Latka, and L. J. Ouellet. 2010. Attribution of hepatitis C virus seroconversion risk in young injection drug users in 5 U.S. cities. *Journal of Infectious Diseases* 201(3):378-385.

Hammett, T. M., S. Phan, J. Gaggin, P. Case, N. Zaller, A. Lutnick, A. H. Kral, E. V. Fedorova, R. Heimer, W. Small, R. Pollini, L. Beletsky, C. Latkin, and D. C. Des Jarlais. 2014. Pharmacies as providers of expanded health services for people who inject drugs: A review of laws, policies, and barriers in six countries. *BMC Health Services Research* 14:261.

Harper, J. 2015. Indiana's HIV outbreak leads to reversal on needle exchanges. *NPR* (National Public Radio), June 2. http://www.npr.org/sections/health-shots/2015/06/02/411231157/indianas-hiv-outbreak-leads-to-reversal-on-needle-exchanges (accessed December 1, 2016).

Harris, A. M., K. Iqbal, S. Schillie, J. Britton, M. A. Kainer, S. Tressler, and C. Vellozzi. 2016a. Increases in acute hepatitis B virus infections—Kentucky, Tennessee, and West Virginia, 2006-2013. *Morbidity and Mortality Weekly Report* 65(3):47-50.

Harris, R. J., N. K. Martin, E. Rand, S. Mandal, D. Mutimer, P. Vickerman, M. E. Ramsay, D. De Angelis, M. Hickman, and H. E. Harris. 2016b. New treatments for hepatitis C virus (HCV): Scope for preventing liver disease and HCV transmission in England. *Journal of Viral Hepatitis* 23(8):631-643.

Havens, J. R., M. R. Lofwall, S. D. Frost, C. B. Oser, C. G. Leukefeld, and R. A. Crosby. 2013. Individual and network factors associated with prevalent hepatitis C infection among rural Appalachian injection drug users. *American Journal of Public Health* 103(1):e44-e52.

Henkle, E., M. Lu, L. B. Rupp, J. A. Boscarino, V. Vijayadeva, M. A. Schmidt, and S. C. Gordon. 2015. Hepatitis A and B immunity and vaccination in chronic hepatitis B and C patients in a large United States cohort. *Clinical Infectious Diseases* 60(4):514-522.

HHS (Department of Health and Human Services). 2013. *Addressing prescription drug abuse in the United States: Current activities and future opportunities.* Washington, DC: HHS, Behavioral Health Coordinating Committee, Prescription Drug Abuse Subcommittee.

HHS. 2015. *Action plan for the prevention, care, and treatment of viral hepatitis: 2014-2016.* HHS, Office of the Assistant Secretary for Health, Office of HIV/AIDS and Infectious Disease Policy. https://www.aids.gov/pdf/viral-hepatitis-action-plan.pdf (accessed October 26, 2016).

HHS. 2016a. Chapter 4. Early intervention, treatment, and management of substance use disorders. *Facing addiction in America: The Surgeon General's report on alcohol, drugs, and health.* Washington, DC: HHS, Office of the Surgeon General.

HHS. 2016b. Chapter 6. Health care systems and substance use disorders. *Facing addiction in America: The Surgeon General's report on alcohol, drugs, and health.* Washington, DC: HHS, Office of the Surgeon General.

HHS. 2016c. Medication assisted treatment for opioid use disorders. 81 FR 44711. *Federal Register* 81(131):44711-44739. https://www.federalregister.gov/documents/2016/07/08/2016-16120/medication-assisted-treatment-for-opioid-use-disorders (accessed February 23, 2017).

HHS. n.d. *IID-15.3: Increase hepatitis B vaccine coverage among health care personnel* https://www.healthypeople.gov/2020/topics-objectives/topic/immunization-and-infectious-diseases/objectives (accessed March 1, 2017).

Holtzman, D., V. Barry, L. J. Ouellet, D. C. Des Jarlais, D. Vlahov, E. T. Golub, S. M. Hudson, and R. S. Garfein. 2009. The influence of needle exchange programs on injection risk behaviors and infection with hepatitis C virus among young injection drug users in select cities in the United States, 1994-2004. *Preventive Medicine* 49(1):68-73.

Hoover, K. W., M. Butler, K. A. Workowski, S. Follansbee, B. Gratzer, C. B. Hare, B. Johnston, J. L. Theodore, G. Tao, B. D. Smith, T. Chorba, and C. K. Kent. 2012. Low rates of hepatitis screening and vaccination of HIV-infected MSM in HIV clinics. *Sexually Transmitted Diseases* 39(5):349-353.

Hsieh, Y. H., R. E. Rothman, O. B. Laeyendecker, G. D. Kelen, A. Avornu, E. U. Patel, J. Kim, R. Irvin, D. L. Thomas, and T. C. Quinn. 2016. Evaluation of the Centers for Disease Control and Prevention recommendations for hepatitis C virus testing in an urban emergency department. *Clinical Infectious Diseases* 62(9):1059-1065.

Hughes, C. 2016. New York Medicaid to cover hepatitis C treatment. *Times Union*, April 27. http://www.timesunion.com/local/article/Patient-group-presses-state-for-increased-7378967.php (accessed November 1, 2016).

Hulse, G. K., N. Morris, D. Arnold-Reed, and R. J. Tait. 2009. Improving clinical outcomes in treating heroin dependence: Randomized, controlled trial of oral or implant naltrexone. *Archives of General Psychiatry* 66(10):1108-1115.

Hutton, D. W., D. Tan, S. K. So, and M. L. Brandeau. 2007. Cost-effectiveness of screening and vaccinating Asian and Pacific Islander adults for hepatitis B. *Annals of Internal Medicine* 147(7):460-469.

Immunization Action Coalition. 2016. *State information: States authorizing pharmacists to vaccinate.* http://www.immunize.org/laws/pharm.asp (accessed December 6, 2016).

Immunization Action Coalition. n.d. *Hepatitis B: Questions and answers: Information about the disease and vaccines.* http://www.immunize.org/catg.d/p4205.pdf (accessed December 7, 2016).

IOM (Institute of Medicine). 1995. Treatment standards and optimal treatment. In *Federal regulation of methadone treatment*, edited by R. A. Rettig and A. Yarmolinsky. Washington, DC: National Academy Press.

Ivsins, A., C. Chow, D. Marsh, S. Macdonald, T. Stockwell, and K. Vallance. 2010. *Drug use trends in Victoria and Vancouver, and changes in injection drug use after the closure of Victoria's fixed site needle exchange. (CARBCstatistical bulletin).* Victoria, British Columbia, Canada: University of Victoria.

Jackson, Y., F. Chappuis, N. Mezger, K. Kanappa, and L. Loutan. 2007. High immunogenicity of delayed third dose of hepatitis B vaccine in travellers. *Vaccine* 25(17):3482-3484.

Janowicz, D. M. 2016. HIV transmission and injection drug use: Lessons from the Indiana outbreak. *Topics in Antiviral Medicine* 24(2):90-92.

Jenco, M. 2016. ACIP updates recommendations on HPV, HepB, MenB vaccines. *American Academy of Pediatrics (AAP) News.* http://www.aappublications.org/news/2016/10/20/ACIP102016 (accessed November 21, 2016).

Jewett, A., A. Garg, K. Meyer, L. D. Wagner, K. Krauskopf, K. A. Brown, J. J. Pan, O. Massoud, B. D. Smith, and D. B. Rein. 2015. Hepatitis C virus testing perspectives among primary care physicians in four large primary care settings. *Health Promotion Practice* 16(2):256-263.

Jones, L., L. Pickering, H. Sumnall, J. McVeigh, and M. A. Bellis. 2010. Optimal provision of needle and syringe programmes for injecting drug users: A systematic review. *International Journal on Drug Policy* 21(5):335-342.

Jones, C. M., M. Campopiano, G. Baldwin, and E. McCance-Katz. 2015. National and state treatment need and capacity for opioid agonist medication-assisted treatment. *American Journal of Public Health* 105(8):e55-e63.

Junewicz, A., A. Brateanu, and C. Nielsen. 2014. Q: Do patients who received only two doses of hepatitis B vaccine need a booster? *Cleveland Clinic Journal of Medicine* 81(6):346-348.

Kabiri, M., A. B. Jazwinski, M. S. Roberts, A. J. Schaefer, and J. Chhatwal. 2014. The changing burden of hepatitis C virus infection in the United States: Model-based predictions. *Annals of Internal Medicine* 161(3):170-180.

Kennedy, K. 2016. Florida changes hep C drug policy for Medicaid. *Washington Times*, June 1. http://www.washingtontimes.com/news/2016/jun/1/florida-changes-hep-c-drug-policy-for-medicaid-aft/ (accessed November 4, 2016).

Keyes, K. M., M. Cerda, J. E. Brady, J. R. Havens, and S. Galea. 2014. Understanding the rural–urban differences in nonmedical prescription opioid use and abuse in the United States. *American Journal of Public Health* 104(2):e52-e59.

Keyl, P. M., L. Gruskin, K. Casano, H. Montag, B. Junge, and D. Vlahov. 1998. Community support for needle exchange programs and pharmacy sale of syringes: A household survey in Baltimore, Maryland. *Journal of Acquired Immune Deficiency Syndromes and Human Retrovirology* 18(Suppl 1):S82-S88.

Kjome, K. L., and F. G. Moeller. 2011. Long-acting injectable naltrexone for the management of patients with opioid dependence. *Substance Abuse* 5:1-9.

Klevens, R. M., S. Liu, H. Roberts, R. B. Jiles, and S. D. Holmberg. 2014. Estimating acute viral hepatitis infections from nationally reported cases. *American Journal of Public Health* 104(3):482-487.

Ko, S. C., L. Fan, E. A. Smith, N. Fenlon, A. K. Koneru, and T. V. Murphy. 2014. Estimated annual perinatal hepatitis B virus infections in the United States, 2000-2009. *Journal of the Pediatric Infectious Diseases Society* 5(2):114-121.

Kolodny, A., D. T. Courtwright, C. S. Hwang, P. Kreiner, J. L. Eadie, T. W. Clark, and G. C. Alexander. 2015. The prescription opioid and heroin crisis: A public health approach to an epidemic of addiction. *Annual Review of Public Health* 36:559-574.

Krawczynski, K., M. J. Alter, B. H. Robertson, L. Lu, J. E. Spelbring, and K. A. McCaustland. 2003. Environmental stability of hepatitis C virus (HCV): Viability of dried/stored HCV in chimpanzee infectivity studies. *Hepatology* 38(S4):428A.

Laffont, C. M., R. Gomeni, C. Heidbreder, J. P. Jones, and A. F. Nasser. 2016. Population pharmacokinetic modeling after repeated administrations of RBP-6000, a new, subcutaneously injectable, long-acting, sustained-release formulation of buprenorphine, for the treatment of opioid use disorder. *Journal of Clinical Pharmacology* 56(7):806-815.

LeFevre, M. L. 2014. Screening for hepatitis B virus infection in nonpregnant adolescents and adults: U.S. Preventive Services Task Force recommendation statement. *Annals of Internal Medicine* 161(1):58-66.

Linas, B. P., H. Hu, D. M. Barter, and M. Horberg. 2014. Hepatitis C screening trends in a large integrated health system. *American Journal of Medicine* 127(5):398-405.

Lo Re, V. III, J. Volk, C. W. Newcomb, Y. X. Yang, C. P. Freeman, S. Hennessy, J. R. Kostman, P. Tebas, M. B. Leonard, and A. R. Localio. 2012. Risk of hip fracture associated with hepatitis C virus infection and hepatitis C/human immunodeficiency virus coinfection. *Hepatology* 56(5):1688-1698.

Lo Re, V. III, K. Lynn, E. R. Stumm, J. Long, M. S. Nezamzadeh, J. F. Baker, A. N. Hoofnagle, A. J. Kapalko, K. Mounzer, B. S. Zemel, P. Tebas, J. R. Kostman, and M. B. Leonard. 2015. Structural bone deficits in HIV/HCV-coinfected, HCV-monoinfected, and HIV-monoinfected women. *Journal of Infectious Diseases* 212(6):924-933.

Lo Re, V. III, C. Gowda, P. N. Urick, J. T. Halladay, A. Binkley, D. M. Carbonari, K. Battista, C. Peleckis, J. Gilmore, J. A. Roy, J. A. Doshi, P. P. Reese, K. R. Reddy, and J. R. Kostman. 2016. Disparities in absolute denial of modern hepatitis C therapy by type of insurance. *Clinical Gastroenterology and Hepatology* 14(7):1035-1043.

Lynch, T. G., and M. F. McCarthy. 2016. *Hepatitis C virus funding and prioritization status update.* http://www.hepatitis.va.gov/pdf/choice-prioritization-update.pdf (accessed October 26, 2016).

Lyons, M. S., V. A. Kunnathur, S. D. Rouster, K. W. Hart, M. I. Sperling, C. J. Fichtenbaum, and K. E. Sherman. 2016. Prevalence of diagnosed and undiagnosed hepatitis C in a midwestern urban emergency department. *Clinical Infectious Diseases* 62(9):1066-1071.

MacNeil, J., and B. Pauly. 2011. Needle exchange as a safe haven in an unsafe world. *Drug and Alcohol Review* 30(1):26-32.

Mallet, V., H. Gilgenkrantz, J. Serpaggi, V. Verkarre, A. Vallet-Pichard, H. Fontaine, and S. Pol. 2008. Brief communication: The relationship of regression of cirrhosis to outcome in chronic hepatitis C. *Annals of Internal Medicine* 149(6):399-403.

Marshall, B. D., M. J. Milloy, E. Wood, J. S. Montaner, and T. Kerr. 2011. Reduction in overdose mortality after the opening of North America's first medically supervised safer injecting facility: A retrospective population-based study. *Lancet* 377(9775):1429-1437.

Martin, N. K., A. Thornton, M. Hickman, C. Sabin, M. Nelson, G. S. Cooke, T. C. Martin, V. Delpech, M. Ruf, H. Price, Y. Azad, E. C. Thomson, and P. Vickerman. 2016. Can hepatitis C virus (HCV) direct-acting antiviral treatment as prevention reverse the HCV epidemic among men who have sex with men in the United Kingdom? Epidemiological and modeling insights. *Clinical Infectious Diseases* 62(9):1072-1080.

Massachusetts EOHHS (Executive Office of Health and Human Services). 2016. *MassHealth implements new drug rebate program, extends access to hep C treatment.* http://www.mass.gov/eohhs/gov/newsroom/press-releases/eohhs/masshealth-implements-new-drug-rebate-program.html (accessed November 9, 2016).

Mast, E., F. Mahoney, and M. Kane. 2004. Hepatitis B vaccine. In *Vaccines*, 4th ed, edited by S. A. Plotkin and W. A. Orenstein. Philadelphia: W.B. Saunders.

Mast, E. E., H. S. Margolis, A. E. Fiore, E. W. Brink, S. T. Goldstein, S. A. Wang, L. A. Moyer, B. P. Bell, and M. J. Alter. 2005. A comprehensive immunization strategy to eliminate transmission of hepatitis B virus infection in the United States. Recommendations of the Advisory Committee on Immunization Practices (ACIP). Part 1: Immunization of infants, children, and adolescents. *Morbidity and Mortality Weekly* 54(RR-16):1-31.

Mast, E. E., C. Weinbaum, A. E. Fiore, M. J. Alter, B. Bell, L. Finelli, L. Rodewald, J. M. Douglas, Jr., R. S. Janssen, and J. W. Ward. 2006. A comprehensive immunization strategy to eliminate transmission of hepatitis B virus infection in the United States. Recommendations of the Advisory Committee on Immunization Practices (ACIP). Part 2: Immunization of adults. *Morbidity and Mortality Weekly* 55(RR16):1-25.

Maylin, S., M. Martinot-Peignoux, R. Moucari, N. Boyer, M. P. Ripault, D. Cazals-Hatem, N. Giuily, C. Castelnau, A. C. Cardoso, T. Asselah, C. Feray, M. H. Nicolas-Chanoine, P. Bedossa, and P. Marcellin. 2008. Eradication of hepatitis C virus in patients successfully treated for chronic hepatitis C. *Gastroenterology* 135(3):821-829.

McCarthy, M. 2015. Indiana declares health emergency in response to HIV outbreak. *BMJ* 350:h1708.

McCombs, J., I. Tonnu-Mihara, T. Matsuda, J. McGinnis, and S. Fox. 2015. Can hepatitis C treatment be safely delayed?: Evidence from the Department of Veterans Affairs healthcare system. *Value in Health* 18(3):A245.

Moyer, V. A. 2013. Screening for hepatitis C virus infection in adults: U.S. Preventive Services Task Force recommendation statement. *Annals of Internal Medicine* 159(5):349-357.

NASEM (National Academies of Sciences, Engineering, and Medicine). 2016. *Eliminating the public health problem of hepatitis B and C in the United States: Phase one report.* Washington, DC: The National Academies Press.

Nelson, P. K., B. M. Mathers, B. Cowie, H. Hagan, D. Des Jarlais, D. Horyniak, and L. Degenhardt. 2011. Global epidemiology of hepatitis B and hepatitis C in people who inject drugs: Results of systematic reviews. *The Lancet* 378(9791):571-583.

Nguyen, G., R. T. Garcia, N. Nguyen, H. Trinh, E. B. Keeffe, and M. H. Nguyen. 2009. Clinical course of hepatitis B virus infection during pregnancy. *Alimentary Pharmacology & Therapeutics* 29(7):755-764.

North American Syringe Exchange Network. n.d. *North American Syringe Exchange Network.* https://nasen.org (accessed February 23, 2017).

NVHR (National Viral Hepatitis Roundtable) and CHLPI (Center for Health Law & Policy Innovation). 2016. Hepatitis C: The state of Medicaid access: Preliminary findings: National summary report. *National Viral Hepatitis Roundtable and Center for Health Law & Policy Innovation, Harvard Law School.* http://www.chlpi.org/wp-content/uploads/2013/12/HCV-Report-Card-National-Summary_FINAL.pdf (accessed December 14, 2016).

Orenstein, W. A., G. T. Mootrey, K. Pazol, and A. R. Hinman. 2007. Financing immunization of adults in the United Sates. *Clinical Pharmacology & Therapeutics* 82(6):764-768.

Oster, A. M., M. Sternberg, A. Lansky, D. Broz, C. Wejnert, and G. Paz-Bailey. 2015. Population size estimates for men who have sex with men and persons who inject drugs. *Journal of Urban Health* 92(4):733-743.

Palese, P. 2016. Profile of Charles M. Rice, Ralf F. W. Bartenschlager, and Michael J. Sofia, 2016 Lasker-DeBakey Clinical Medical Research Awardees. *Proceedings of the National Academy of Sciences of the United States of America* 113(49):13934-13937.

Pan, C. Q., Z. Duan, E. Dai, S. Zhang, G. Han, Y. Wang, H. Zhang, H. Zou, B. Zhu, W. Zhao, and H. Jiang. 2016. Tenofovir to prevent hepatitis B transmission in mothers with high viral load. *New England Journal of Medicine* 374(24):2324-2334.

Patel, M. R., B. Combs, P. Hall, J. Hough, E. Chapman, A. Perez, J. T. Brooks, P. J. Peters, and D. Broz. 2015. Reduction in injection risk behaviors after institution of an emergency syring exchange program during an HIV outbreak among persons who inject drugs, Indiana 2015. *Open Forum Infectious Diseases* 2(Suppl 1):638a.

Patil, S., R. S. Rao, and A. Agarwal. 2013. Awareness and risk perception of hepatitis B infection among auxiliary healthcare workers. *Journal of International Society of Preventive & Community Dentistry* 3(2):67-71.

Pearlman, B. L., and N. Traub. 2011. Sustained virologic response to antiviral therapy for chronic hepatitis C virus infection: A cure and so much more. *Clinical Infectious Diseases* 52(7):889-900.

Peters, P. J., P. Pontones, K. W. Hoover, M. R. Patel, R. R. Galang, J. Shields, S. J. Blosser, M. W. Spiller, B. Combs, W. M. Switzer, C. Conrad, J. Gentry, Y. Khudyakov, D. Waterhouse, S. M. Owen, E. Chapman, J. C. Roseberry, V. McCants, P. J. Weidle, D. Broz, T. Samandari, J. Mermin, J. Walthall, J. T. Brooks, and J. M. Duwve. 2016. HIV infection linked to injection drug use in oxymorphone in Indiana, 2014-2015. *New England Journal of Medicine* 375(3):229-239.

Potier, C., V. Laprevote, F. Dubois-Arber, O. Cottencin, and B. Rolland. 2014. Supervised injection services: What has been demonstrated? A systematic literature review. *Drug and Alcohol Dependence* 145:48-68.

Rein, D. B., J. S. Wittenborn, B. D. Smith, D. K. Liffmann, and J. W. Ward. 2015. The cost-effectiveness, health benefits, and financial costs of new antiviral treatments for hepatitis C virus. *Clinical Infectious Diseases* 61(2):157-168.

Rich, J. D., and E. Y. Adashi. 2015. Ideological anachronism involving needle and syringe exchange programs: Lessons from the Indiana HIV outbreak. *JAMA* 314(1):23-24.

Rini, J. 2016. State changes hep C medication guidelines, avoids lawsuit. *News Journal*, June 10. http://www.delawareonline.com/story/news/health/2016/06/07/state-changes-hep-c-medication-guidelines-avoids-lawsuit/85554396/ (accessed November 11, 2016).

Rodriguez, C., and A. Reynolds. 2016. Accessing the cure: Helping patients with hepatitis C overcome barriers to care. *American Journal of Managed Care* 22(4 Suppl):S108-S112.

Rosenblatt, R. A., C. H. Andrilla, M. Catlin, and E. H. Larson. 2015. Geographic and specialty distribution of U.S. physicians trained to treat opioid use disorder. *Annals of Family Medicine* 13(1):23-26.

Rudavsky, S. 2016. State extends Scott Co. needle exchange for year. *Indianapolis Star*, May 2. http://www.indystar.com/story/news/2016/05/02/state-extends-scott-co-needle-exchange-year/83840636/ (accessed December 9, 2016).

Rudd, R. A., N. Aleshire, J. E. Zibbell, and R. M. Gladden. 2016. Increases in drug and opioid overdose deaths—United States, 2000-2014. *Morbidity and Mortality Weekly Report* 64(50-51):1378-1382.

Rural Center for AIDS/STD Prevention. 2016. *Indiana syringe exchange programming (SEP) progress and approvals: November 21, 2016.* http://www.in.gov/bitterpill/files/Counties%20moving%20toward%20syringe%20access%20in%20Indiana%2021%20November%202016.pdf (accessed December 1, 2016).

Saag, M. S. 2014. Quantum leaps, microeconomics, and the treatment of patients with hepatitis C and HIV coinfection. *JAMA* 312(4):347-348.

SAMHSA (Substance Abuse and Mental Health Services Administration). 2015a. *Behavioral health trends in the United States: Results from the 2014 National Survey on Drug Use and Health.* Rockville, MD: SAMHSA.

SAMHSA. 2015b. *Federal guidelines for opioid treatment programs.* Rockville, MD: SAMHSA.

SAMHSA. 2015c. *Methadone.* https://www.samhsa.gov/medication-assisted-treatment/treatment/methadone (accessed March 13, 2017).

SAMHSA. 2016. *Buprenorphine.* https://www.samhsa.gov/medication-assisted-treatment/treatment/buprenorphine (accessed March 13, 2017).

SAMHSA. 2017. *Buprenorphine waiver management.* https://www.samhsa.gov/medication-assisted-treatment/buprenorphine-waiver-management (accessed February 23, 2017).

Sapatkin, D. 2016. Panel recommends giving hepatitis C drugs to more Pennsylvania Medicaid patients. *Philly.com*, May 18. http://www.philly.com/philly/health/20160518_Panel_recommends_giving_Hep_C_drug_to_more_Pa__Medicaid_patients.html (accessed October 20, 2016).

Shiratori, Y., F. Imazeki, M. Moriyama, M. Yano, Y. Arakawa, O. Yokosuka, T. Kuroki, S. Nishiguchi, M. Sata, G. Yamada, S. Fujiyama, H. Yoshida, and M. Omata. 2000. Histologic improvement of fibrosis in patients with hepatitis C who have sustained response to interferon therapy. *Annals of Internal Medicine* 132(7):517-524.

Siddharta, A., S. Pfaender, A. Malassa, J. Doerrbecker, Anggakusuma, M. Engelmann, B. Nugraha, J. Steinmann, D. Todt, F. W. Vondran, P. Mateu-Gelabert, C. Goffinet, and E. Steinmann. 2016. Inactivation of HCV and HIV by microwave: A novel approach for prevention of virus transmission among people who inject drugs. *Scientific Reports* 6:36619.

Siddiqui, S. S., R. F. Armenta, J. L. Evans, M. Yu, J. Cuevas-Mota, K. Page, P. Davidson, and R. S. Garfein. 2015. Effect of legal status of pharmacy syringe sales on syringe purchases by persons who inject drugs in San Francisco and San Diego, CA. *International Journal on Drug Policy* 26(11):1150-1157.

Sidlow, R., and P. Msaouel. 2015. Improving hepatitis C virus screening rates in primary care: A targeted intervention using the electronic health record. *Journal for Healthcare Quality* 37(5):319-323.

Simon, R. E., S. D. Pearson, C. Hur, and R. T. Chung. 2015. Tackling the hepatitis C cost problem: A test case for tomorrow's cures. *Hepatology* 62(5):1334-1336.

Singer, M., R. Irizarry, and J. J. Schensul. 1991. Needle access as an AIDS prevention strategy for IV drug users: A research perspective. *Human Organization* 50:142-153.

Smith, B. D., C. Jorgensen, J. E. Zibbell, and G. A. Beckett. 2012a. Centers for Disease Control and Prevention initiatives to prevent hepatitis C virus infection: A selective update. *Clinical Infectious Diseases* 55(Suppl 1):S49-S53.

Smith, E. A., L. Jacques-Carroll, T. Y. Walker, B. Sirotkin, and T. V. Murphy. 2012b. The national perinatal hepatitis B prevention program, 1994-2008. *Pediatrics* 129(4):609-616.

Smith-Palmer, J., K. Cerri, and W. Valentine. 2015. Achieving sustained virologic response in hepatitis C: A systematic review of the clinical, economic and quality of life benefits. *BMC Infectious Diseases* 15:19.

Southern, W. N., M. L. Drainoni, B. D. Smith, C. L. Christiansen, D. McKee, A. L. Gifford, C. M. Weinbaum, D. Thompson, E. Koppelman, S. Maher, and A. H. Litwin. 2011. Hepatitis C testing practices and prevalence in a high-risk urban ambulatory care setting. *Journal of Viral Hepatitis* 18(7):474-481.

Southern, W. N., M. L. Drainoni, B. D. Smith, E. Koppelman, M. D. McKee, C. L. Christiansen, A. L. Gifford, C. M. Weinbaum, and A. H. Litwin. 2014. Physician nonadherence with a hepatitis C screening program. *Quality Management in Health Care* 23(1):1-9.

State of Indiana. n.d. *Syringe exchange.* http://www.in.gov/bitterpill/syringe-exchange.html# (accessed December 1, 2016).

Stein, B. D., R. L. Pacula, A. J. Gordon, R. M. Burns, D. L. Leslie, M. J. Sorbero, S. Bauhoff, T. W. Mandell, and A. W. Dick. 2015. Where is buprenorphine dispensed to treat opioid use disorders? The role of private offices, opioid treatment programs, and substance abuse treatment facilities in urban and rural counties. *The Milbank Quarterly* 93(3):561-583.

Steinbrook, R., and R. F. Redberg. 2014. The high price of the new hepatitis C virus drugs. *JAMA Internal Medicine* 174(7):1172.

Stopka, T. J., E. M. Geraghty, R. Azari, E. B. Gold, and K. DeRiemer. 2014. Is crime associated with over-the-counter pharmacy syringe sales? Findings from Los Angeles, California. *International Journal of Drug Policy* 25(2):244-250.

Strathdee, S. A., E. P. Ricketts, S. Huettner, L. Cornelius, D. Bishai, J. R. Havens, P. Beilenson, C. Rapp, J. J. Lloyd, and C. A. Latkin. 2006. Facilitating entry into drug treatment among injection drug users referred from a needle exchange program: Results from a community-based behavioral intervention trial. *Drug and Alcohol Dependence* 83(3):225-232.

Sun, L. 2016. White, rural drug users lack needle exchange programs to prevent HIV infections. *Washington Post*, November 29. https://www.washingtonpost.com/news/to-your-health/wp/2016/11/29/white-rural-drug-users-lack-needle-exchange-programs-to-prevent-hiv-infections/?hpid=hp_hp-cards_hp-card-national%3Ahomepage%2Fcard&utm_term=.63623df11434 (accessed December 9, 2016).

Talas, M. S. 2009. Occupational exposure to blood and body fluids among Turkish nursing students during clinical practice training: Frequency of needlestick/sharp injuries and hepatitis B immunisation. *Journal of Clinical Nursing* 18(10):1394-1403.

ter Borg, M. J., W. F. Leemans, R. A. de Man, and H. L. Janssen. 2008. Exacerbation of chronic hepatitis B infection after delivery. *Journal of Viral Hepatitis* 15(1):37-41.

Terrault, N. A., N. H. Bzowej, K. M. Chang, J. P. Hwang, M. M. Jonas, and M. H. Murad. 2016. AASLD guidelines for treatment of chronic hepatitis B. *Hepatology* 63(1):261-283.

Tetrault, J. M., and J. L. Butner. 2015. Non-medical prescription opioid use and prescription opioid use disorder: A review. *Yale Journal of Biology and Medicine* 88(3):227-233.

Tice, J. A., H. S. Chahal, and D. A. Ollendorf. 2015. Comparative clinical effectiveness and value of novel interferon-free combination therapy for hepatitis C genotype 1: Summary of California Technology Assessment Forum report. *JAMA Internal Medicine* 175(9):1559-1560.

Trooskin, S. B., H. Reynolds, and J. R. Kostman. 2015. Access to costly new hepatitis C drugs: Medicine, money, and advocacy. *Clinical Infectious Diseases* 61(12):1825-1830.

Tsochatzis, E. A., K. S. Gurusamy, S. Ntaoula, E. Cholongitas, B. R. Davidson, and A. K. Burroughs. 2011. Elastography for the diagnosis of severity of fibrosis in chronic liver disease: A meta-analysis of diagnostic accuracy. *Journal of Hepatology* 54(4):650-659.

Tsui, J. I., E. Vittinghoff, M. G. Shlipak, D. Bertenthal, J. Inadomi, R. A. Rodriguez, and A. M. O'Hare. 2007. Association of hepatitis C seropositivity with increased risk for developing end-stage renal disease. *Archives of Internal Medicine* 167(12):1271-1276.

Turner, B. J., B. S. Taylor, J. T. Hanson, M. E. Perez, L. Hernandez, R. Villarreal, P. Veerapaneni, and K. Fiebelkorn. 2015. Implementing hospital-based baby boomer hepatitis C virus screening and linkage to care: Strategies, results, and costs. *Journal of Hospital Medicine* 10(8):510-516.

UNAIDS (Joint United Nations Programme on HIV/AIDS). 2014. People who inject drugs. In *The gap report 2014.* Geneva, Switzerland: UNAIDS.

University of Washington. n.d.-a. *HCV epidemiology in the United States.* http://www. hepatitisc.uw.edu/pdf/screening-diagnosis/epidemiology-us/core-concept/all (accessed November 11, 2016).

University of Washington. n.d.-b. *Recommendations for hepatitis C screening.* http://www. hepatitisc.uw.edu/pdf/screening-diagnosis/recommendations-screening/core-concept/all (accessed November 15, 2016).

Valdiserri, R., J. Khalsa, C. Dan, S. Holmberg, J. Zibbell, D. Holtzman, R. Lubran, and W. Compton. 2014. Confronting the emerging epidemic of HCV infection among young injection drug users. *American Journal of Public Health* 104(5):816-821.

van der Meer, A. J., B. J. Veldt, J. J. Feld, H. Wedemeyer, J. F. Dufour, F. Lammert, A. Duarte-Rojo, E. J. Heathcote, M. P. Manns, L. Kuske, S. Zeuzem, W. P. Hofmann, R. J. de Knegt, B. E. Hansen, and H. L. Janssen. 2012. Association between sustained virological response and all-cause mortality among patients with chronic hepatitis C and advanced hepatic fibrosis. *JAMA* 308(24):2584-2593.

Van Handel, M. M., C. E. Rose, E. J. Hallisey, J. L. Kolling, J. E. Zibbell, B. Lewis, M. K. Bohm, C. M. Jones, B. E. Flanagan, A. E. Siddiqi, K. Iqbal, A. L. Dent, J. H. Mermin, E. McCray, J. W. Ward, and J. T. Brooks. 2016. County-level vulnerability assessment for rapid dissemination of HIV or HCV infections among persons who inject drugs, United States. *Journal of Acquired Immune Deficiency Syndromes* 73(3):323-331.

Vlahov, D., and B. Junge. 1998. The role of needle exchange programs in HIV prevention. *Public Health Reports* 113(Suppl 1):75-80.

Vlahov, D., M. H. Coady, D. C. Ompad, and S. Galea. 2007. Strategies for improving influenza immunization rates among hard-to-reach populations. *Journal of Urban Health* 84(4):615-631.

Volkow, N. D., T. R. Frieden, P. S. Hyde, and S. S. Cha. 2014. Medication-assisted therapies—Tackling the opioid-overdose epidemic. *New England Journal of Medicine* 370(22):2063-2066.

Walayat, S., Z. Ahmed, D. Martin, S. Puli, M. Cashman, and S. Dhillon. 2015. Recent advances in vaccination of non-responders to standard dose hepatitis B virus vaccine. *World Journal of Hepatology* 7(24):2503-2509.

Ward, J. 2015 (unpublished). *Placing nation on the path toward the elimination of hepatitis C.* PowerPoint presentation to the Committee on a National Strategy on the Elimination of Hepatitis B & C in Washington DC, November 30. http://nationalacademies.org/hmd/~/media/Files/Activity%20Files/PublicHealth/HepatitisBandC/1-November2015/1-%20 John%20Ward.pdf (accessed February 28, 2017).

Wasley, A., D. Kruszon-Moran, W. Kuhnert, E. P. Simard, L. Finelli, G. McQuillan, and B. Bell. 2010. The prevalence of hepatitis B virus infection in the United States in the era of vaccination. *Journal of Infectious Diseases* 202(2):192-201.

White, D. A., E. S. Anderson, S. K. Pfeil, T. K. Trivedi, and H. J. Alter. 2016. Results of a rapid hepatitis C virus screening and diagnostic testing program in an urban emergency department. *Annals of Emergency Medicine* 67(1):119-128.

WHO (World Health Organization). 2007. *Guide to starting and managing needle and syringe programmes.* Geneva, Switzerland: WHO, UNAIDS, and United Nations Office on Drugs and Crime.

WHO. 2016a. *Global health sector strategy on viral hepatitis, 2016-2021: Towards ending viral hepatitis*. Geneva, Switzerland: WHO. http://apps.who.int/iris/bitstream/10665/246177/1/WHO-HIV-2016.06-eng.pdf (accessed July 19, 2016).

WHO. 2016b. *Hepatitis B. Fact sheet*. http://www.who.int/mediacentre/factsheets/fs204/en/ (accessed December 6, 2016).

Williams, W. W., P. J. Lu, A. O'Halloran, D. K. Kim, L. A. Grohskopf, T. Pilishvili, T. H. Skoff, N. P. Nelson, R. Harpaz, L. E. Markowitz, A. Rodriguez-Lainz, and C. B. Bridges. 2016. Surveillance of vaccination coverage among adult populations—United States, 2014. *Morbidity and Mortality Weekly Report Surveillance Summaries* 65(1):1-36.

Wiseman, E., M. A. Fraser, S. Holden, A. Glass, B. L. Kidson, L. G. Heron, M. W. Maley, A. Ayres, S. A. Locarnini, and M. T. Levy. 2009. Perinatal transmission of hepatitis B virus: An Australian experience. *Medical Journal of Australia* 190(9):489-492.

Wong, J., M. Payne, and S. Hollenberg. 2014. A double-dose hepatitis B vaccination schedule in travelers presenting for late consultation. *Journal of Travel Medicine* 21(4):260-265.

Wood, E., T. Kerr, J. Stoltz, Z. Qui, R. Zhang, J. S. G. Montaner, and M. W. Tyndall. 2005. Prevalence and correlates of hepatitis C infection among users of North America's first medically supervised safer injection facility. *Public Health* 119(12):1111-1115.

Wright, N. M., and C. N. Tompkins. 2006. A review of the evidence for the effectiveness of primary prevention interventions for hepatitis C among injecting drug users. *Harm Reduction Journal* 3:27.

Younossi, Z., and L. Henry. 2014. The impact of the new antiviral regimens on patient reported outcomes and health economics of patients with chronic hepatitis C. *Digestive and Liver Disease* 46(Suppl 5):S186-S196.

Younossi, Z., and L. Henry. 2015. Systematic review: Patient-reported outcomes in chronic hepatitis C—The impact of liver disease and new treatment regimens. *Alimentary Pharmacology & Therapeutics* 41(6):497-520.

Younossi, Z. M., H. Park, S. Saab, A. Ahmed, D. Dieterich, and S. C. Gordon. 2015. Cost-effectiveness of all-oral ledipasvir/sofosbuvir regimens in patients with chronic hepatitis C virus genotype 1 infection. *Alimentary Pharmacology & Therapeutics* 41(6):544-563.

Younossi, Z. M., B. R. Bacon, D. T. Dieterich, S. L. Flamm, K. Kowdley, S. Milligan, N. Tsai, and A. Nezam. 2016. Disparate access to treatment regimens in chronic hepatitis C patients: Data from the TRIO network. *Journal of Viral Hepatitis* 23(6):447-454.

Zaller, N., A. Jeronimo, J. Bratberg, P. Case, and J. D. Rich. 2010. Pharmacist and pharmacy staff experiences with non-prescription (NP) sale of syringes and attitudes toward providing HIV prevention services for injection drug users (IDUs) in Providence, RI. *Journal of Urban Health* 87(6):942-953.

Zibbell, J. E., K. Iqbal, R. C. Patel, A. Suryaprasad, K. J. Sanders, L. Moore-Moravian, J. Serrecchia, S. Blankenship, J. W. Ward, and D. Holtzman. 2015. Increases in hepatitis C virus infection related to injection drug use among persons aged ≤30 years—Kentucky, Tennessee, Virginia, and West Virginia, 2006-2012. *Morbidity and Mortality Weekly Report* 64(17):453-458.

5

Service Delivery

Part of the challenge of eliminating hepatitis B and C in the United States is that the people suffering from or at risk for the infections are often not engaged in care and can be difficult to reach. Many hepatitis B patients are born abroad; they may not be comfortable with the U.S. health system or with English-speaking providers (Derose et al., 2009; Hacker et al., 2015). Hepatitis C is common among people who inject drugs, for whom hepatitis treatment is often not a high priority and who feel discriminated against in medical settings (Grebely et al., 2015; Mehta et al., 2011; Treloar et al., 2010). Both conditions are associated with feelings of shame and anxiety, which can be antithetical to pursuing treatment. For these reasons, the national hepatitis elimination strategy must give as much attention to the delivery of essential services as the services themselves. This piece of the strategy, what the World Health Organization (WHO) describes as "the how," considers steps that can be taken to make viral hepatitis a priority, support efficient care, and reach patients who might otherwise slip through the cracks (WHO, 2016). Overseeing such efforts should be the responsibility of the central coordinating office described in Chapter 2. This chapter discusses steps that could help improve the reach of essential hepatitis services, thereby hastening the end of hepatitis B and C in the United States.

ENCOURAGING COMPLIANCE AMONG PROVIDERS

The previous chapter discusses essential interventions for elimination of viral hepatitis in the United States. As crucial as these interventions are, they can easily be neglected in the routine practice of medicine. National survey data suggest that fewer than half of Asian Americans are tested for hepatitis B virus (HBV), for example (Hu et al., 2013). The Advisory Committee on Immunization Practices (ACIP) recommends that all infants be vaccinated against HBV before leaving the hospital, but only 72.4 percent are immunized within 3 days of birth (95 percent confidence interval [CI] 70.9 to 73.9), with state and local coverage varying from fewer than half in Vermont to nearly 90 percent in North Dakota (Hill et al., 2015; Mast et al., 2005).

There is often a gap between the practice of medicine as recommended by experts and what actually happens. Closing this gap is of concern to the National Committee for Quality Assurance (NCQA), which in the 1990s, devised a set of indicators meant to hold health plans accountable for results (Marwick, 1997; NCQA, n.d.-b). These indicators, called HEDIS,[1] are now instrumental for monitoring performance in 90 percent of American health plans (NCQA, n.d.-a). HEDIS indicators are standardized, as is the method for collecting and verifying the HEDIS data that pertain to "the most pressing clinical areas" (NCQA, 2016a). Viral hepatitis is surely one of these areas, and the addition of a few relevant HEDIS indicators would greatly aid the national elimination effort.

> **Recommendation 5-1: The National Committee for Quality Assurance should establish measures to monitor compliance with viral hepatitis screening guidelines and hepatitis B vaccine birth dose coverage and include the new measures in the Healthcare Effectiveness Data and Information Set.**

HEDIS measures compel a certain attention from providers and health plan managers because they are used to evaluate performance (NCQA, 2012). Their role in changing clinical practice can be pronounced, especially for common conditions for which there is an effective treatment but wide variability in care (Eddy et al., 2008). HEDIS measures have improved the management of hypertension (Jaffe et al., 2013). Mathematical models indicate that compliance with HEDIS for diabetes mellitus and cardiovascular disease would have prevented almost 2 million myocardial infarctions, 800,000 strokes, and 100,000 cases of end-stage renal disease between 1995 and 2005 alone (Eddy et al., 2008).

At the same time, HEDIS indicators put a burden on the health system. Emphasizing a short list of clinical actions risks creating a hierarchy wherein some services matter more than other equally meaningful ones. There are also logistical constraints. Some health plans do not have enough

---

[1] Officially, the Healthcare Effectiveness Data and Information Set.

members eligible for a given service to allow for a valid comparison of compliance (McGlynn, 1997). In selecting HEDIS indicators, NCQA considers feasibility, or the trade-off between comprehensiveness and practicality required to track an indicator (McGlynn, 1997). The indicator's scientific soundness is also taken into account, as is its relevance, with preference "given to those areas where better performance will enhance the health of the population" (McGlynn, 1997, p. 15). With these criteria in mind, the committee suggests screening and prevention measures that would benefit from NCQA's attention.

Adherence to Screening Guidelines

HBV and hepatitis C virus (HCV) are, for the most part, clinically silent infections. Fewer than a third of chronic hepatitis B patients in the United States are aware of their condition (Lin et al., 2007); about half of those with chronic hepatitis C are (Denniston et al., 2012). Diagnosis is an obvious prerequisite to any kind of service delivery. To this end, the U.S. Preventive Services Task Force recommends HBV screening for everyone at high risk of chronic infection, including people born in HBV-endemic countries, and all pregnant women during the first trimester of pregnancy (USPSTF, 2014, 2015). Similarly, the task force recommends that people at high risk of HCV infection be screened, as should anyone born between 1945 and 1965 (USPSTF, 2013). NCQA has HEDIS measures on screening for breast, cervical, and colorectal cancers, as well as chlamydia screening in young women and lead screening in children (NCQA, 2016b). Inclusion in HEDIS makes screening more of a priority for health plan managers. In order to improve chlamydia screening in adolescent girls, Kaiser of Northern California devised a system of team meetings and clinical tools to improve their screening rates (Shafer et al., 2002). About 46 percent of a sample of 37 Pennsylvania health plans implemented reminder and tracking systems in response to the introduction of HEDIS measures for colorectal screening, eliciting a 54 percentage point increase in the screening rate (Sarfaty and Myers, 2008).

A point-of-care test could facilitate wider screening. A recent systematic review and meta-analysis concluded that reliable, affordable point-of-care tests for HCV core antigen have a sensitivity and specificity greater than 90 and 98 percent respectively (Freiman et al., 2016). Core antigen tests are likely to be cheaper than traditional nucleic acid tests and may, therefore, facilitate wider use (Freiman et al., 2016). The Food and Drug Administration has not approved any point of care HBsAg tests for use in the United States, although some of the tests that are used in other countries have been found to be highly accurate (Gish et al., 2014; Njai et al., 2015; Shivkumar et al., 2012). Simple to use, point of care assays for HBsAg are used in

HBV-endemic countries, but manufacturers have little incentive to seek market authorization for such a product in the United States (Lin et al., 2008; WHO, 2001). It is possible that the addition of a HEDIS indicator on hepatitis screening would encourage manufacturers to reconsider this position. Regardless of what assay is used, an increase in screening would translate into vastly fewer undiagnosed viral hepatitis patients.

The Hepatitis B Vaccine Birth Dose

NCQA includes various measures of child and adolescent immunization as HEDIS indicators, including full immunization against HBV during the first 2 years of life (NCQA, 2009). HEDIS and Centers for Disease Control and Prevention (CDC) evaluations indicate that over 90 percent of children meet this goal, though misclassification is not uncommon (Bundy et al., 2012). This indicator does not take into account the relative importance of the timing of the first dose, however. In 2016, ACIP recommended all infants receive the first dose of the hepatitis B vaccine within 24 hours of birth (Chitnis, 2016; Jenco, 2016). Children born to HBsAg+ women or to women who have never been tested for HBV require vaccination within 12 hours of birth, and others within 24 hours (CDC, 2016b,d; Chitnis, 2016; Mast et al., 2005). The proportion of children receiving the vaccine in the first 3 days of life has improved steadily, from 53.2 percent in 2007 (95 percent CI: 51.9 to 54.5) to 72.4 percent in 2014 (95 percent CI: 70.9 to 73.9) (CDC, 2012a; Hill et al., 2015).

Starting the hepatitis B vaccine series at birth is associated with better odds of completing the three-dose series on time (Yusuf et al., 2000). Full immunization, in turn, conveys lifelong immunity to 95 percent of those vaccinated (CDC, 2016c). Emphasizing early vaccination would show a commitment to ending the vertical transmission of HBV. The risk of chronic hepatitis B is highest among those infected in early life. Up to 90 percent of people exposed to HBV in infancy and 30 percent of those exposed in early childhood develop chronic hepatitis B (Zhao and Murphy, 2013). Birth dose immunization is the first step in preventing these infections. By emphasizing the hepatitis B birth dose, as well as the completion of the three-dose series, NCQA would direct the attention of hospital and health plan administrators to this essential intervention.

REACHING PATIENTS

The viral hepatitis patient is at the center of any elimination campaign. As time passes, meeting the goals set out in Chapter 2 will depend on diagnosing and treating progressively more challenging patients. A system to manage viral hepatitis patients must include the uninsured and underinsured, people born abroad, those with mental and behavioral health problems, as well as people in prison and in unstable housing. Integrated, comprehensive primary and specialty care will be essential to the elimination effort (HHS, 2017). Making better use of primary care is one way to support this goal.

Building Capacity in Primary Care

One of the limitations of the hepatitis C models discussed in Chapter 2 is the assumption, based on published estimates, that only 260,000 hepatitis C patients could be treated every year between now and 2030. The model draws attention to this bottleneck, and the trade-off between reducing incidence of new infections or a greater reduction in liver-related deaths. Both would be possible if more patients could be treated every year. To this end, primary care providers need to be in a position to take on hepatitis C patients.

Primary care providers often build trusting relationships with their patients over the course of years (Baron, 2010). Some evidence suggests that certain kinds of patients, those with a substance use disorder for example, have better success in primary care than in specialist clinics (Bruggmann and Grebely, 2015; Bruggmann and Litwin, 2013). Primary care is also an efficient way to provide services, one the American Academy of Family Physicians describes as "the first point of entry and continuing focal point for all needed health services" (AAFP, n.d.). Viral hepatitis services should be no exception. But traditional models of primary care do not, for the most part, leave providers with much room to take on more work. Over 80 percent of primary care physicians responding to the 2016 *Survey of America's Physicians* described their practice as overextended or at full capacity (The Physicians Foundation, 2016).

Treating viral hepatitis in primary care also poses risks that providers in small practices may be reluctant to accept. Hepatitis patients are usually healthy; only about 20 to 25 percent of chronic hepatitis C patients will develop cirrhosis after two or three decades of infection (Hepatitis C Online, 2016). Similarly, more than half of all chronic hepatitis B patients will never develop any life-threatening complications (McMahon, 2009). But in a subset of patients with either infection, progression to cirrhosis and cancer can be quick. There is no good way to distinguish one kind of patient from the other early on (Hepatitis C Online, 2016; McMahon, 2009). If fibrosis progresses quickly, or if a patient develops cirrhosis, management becomes much more complicated. Cirrhotics need frequent hospitalization—about three times per person per year—usually for hepatic encephalopathy, fluid overload, and gastrointestinal hemorrhage (Ge and Runyon, 2016; Volk et al., 2012). Although such events are rare, their management may exceed

---

BOX 5-1
Project ECHO

For years New Mexico had the country's highest rate of chronic liver disease and death from cirrhosis (Arora et al., 2007; CDC, 2016a). The mostly rural state was home to an estimated 32,000 hepatitis C patients, few of whom could see specialists in any predictable way (Arora et al., 2007). Starting in 2003, the Extension for Community Healthcare Outcomes (ECHO) program facilitated collaboration between primary care providers and the specialists trained to manage hepatitis C (AHRQ, n.d.; Project ECHO, n.d.-d). The project combines medical education and patient management. Its goal is to provide primary care doctors in rural and underserved areas the skills and support to manage complex chronic conditions, such as hepatitis C (Project ECHO, n.d.-a).

In the ECHO model, specialists at academic medical centers become training mentors to primary care providers in rural and other underserved areas (Project ECHO, n.d.-a). During weekly video conferences, primary care providers from several sites present cases for discussion with specialists at the University of New Mexico and other primary care providers in different parts of the state. The use of the internet allows a primary care provider in a rural area to include experts in hepatology, pharmacology, and substance abuse in his or her daily practice.

Project ECHO now operates in 110 medical centers, for 55 conditions in 21 countries (Project ECHO, n.d.-d). The model has been adapted for behavioral health problems, diabetes and endocrinology, and pain management (Project ECHO, n.d.-c). The Centers for Disease Control and Prevention also funded an initiative to replicate the ECHO project in Utah and Arizona (Mitruka et al., 2014; Project ECHO, n.d.-b). The University of Utah and St. Joseph's Hospital in Arizona are now regional hubs for training primary care providers in hepatitis C treatment. These hubs have emphasized hepatitis testing and successful connection to care, especially among high-risk populations and in rural areas, including Navajo

---

the resources of solo practitioners in small towns or rural areas. As a result, viral hepatitis care remains out of reach for millions of patients in rural and underserved communities (Mellinger and Volk, 2013).

The University of New Mexico's ECHO[2] program aimed to reduce this disparity and make treatment for complex diseases more accessible in rural and underserved areas (Project ECHO, n.d.-d) (see Box 5-1). The program started in 2003, when hepatitis C was treated with pegylated interferon, a drug with serious side effects that required complicated medical management (Arora et al., 2011). Even so, primary care providers in the ECHO

---

[2] Officially, Extension for Community Healthcare Outcomes.

and Hopi reservations (Mitruka et al., 2014; Project ECHO, n.d.-b; St. Joseph's Hospital and Medical Center, n.d.).

Part of ECHO's success is that it is not aimed solely at patient treatment, as some other telemedicine systems are (Arora et al., 2007). Participants learn from sharing cases, serving as mentors, and participating in presentations (Arora et al., 2014). Primary care providers develop some specialty skills and are thereby able to offer their patients more complete care. Because ECHO patients stay under the purview of their primary care doctor, there are minimal opportunities for loss to follow-up and other lapses in care (Arora et al., 2014). ECHO also gives providers in rural and underserved areas a chance to continue their education, reducing feelings of professional isolation (Arora et al., 2007).

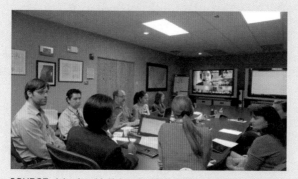

SOURCE: John Arnold, University of New Mexico Health Sciences Center.

program saw no higher rates of serious adverse events than specialists at the University of New Mexico did (Arora et al., 2011).

There are also transferable lessons from the management of other chronic conditions in primary care. Like hepatitis B and C, depression is a serious, chronic health problem, especially for older adults, many of whom have problems with adherence to treatment (Unützer et al., 2002b). Since 1999, the University of Washington's IMPACT[3] program has worked with primary care providers to improve outcomes among elderly people with depression and other complex health needs (Unützer et al., 2002b). IMPACT teams can include family doctors, nurses, pharmacists, social workers, be-

---

[3] Officially, Improving Mood–Promoting Access to Collaborative Treatment.

havioral health specialists, and various occupational and physical therapists (Hern et al., 2013; Tracy et al., 2013). The program makes good use of the internet for data management and monitoring treatment response over time (Unützer et al., 2002a,b). Patient records are kept on a secure, encrypted website in a database that is programmed to remind clinicians about follow-up or possible lapses in treatment. This feature is thought to account for the program's high rate of keeping patient assessments on schedule (Unützer et al., 2002a). The data management system encourages ongoing monitoring of both process and outcome measures, something that would be equally useful in viral hepatitis care.

> **Recommendation 5-2: The American Association for the Study of Liver Diseases and the Infectious Diseases Society of America should partner with primary care providers and their professional organizations to build capacity to treat hepatitis B and C in primary care. The program should set up referral systems for medically complex patients.**

There can be no elimination of viral hepatitis without trained providers who can manage the infections from the acute phase to cure (with HCV) or lifelong suppression (with HBV). Large-scale replication of the ECHO program's success is possible, especially with support from IDSA[4] and AASLD[5]. The program should give attention to both training and technological tools to ease collaboration. There is precedent for this level of collaboration in the management of other chronic diseases, and it is something that the Health Resources and Services Administration (HRSA) has shown support for, as with its AIDS Education and Training Centers, a feature of the Ryan White program, discussed later in this chapter. In an effort to ensure standard training across the country, IDSA and AASLD might consider developing a joint guideline, with a training curriculum, for primary care providers to use. It is generally easier for both patients and primary care providers to treat hepatitis C without a time-consuming referral process. Primary care providers have an incentive to learn new skills, especially when these are skills they can use to help patients who have problems accessing specialty care. Specialists, for their part, may find participation in a collaborative program not only an interesting educational project, but rewarding, as it allows them to reach more patients then they would in their regular practice. The rapid expansion of ECHO programs to 110 medical centers in 21 countries is evidence of the demand for such collaboration.

For the most part, the medicines used to treat viral hepatitis today have mild side effects (CDC, 2016e; VA, 2016); primary care doctors routinely

---

[4] Officially, the Infectious Diseases Society of America.
[5] Officially, the American Association for the Study of Liver Diseases.

write prescriptions for far more toxic treatments. Perhaps for this reason, specialists are often not clear how much involvement is sought or appropriate in collaboration with primary care providers (Mellinger and Volk, 2013). In the ECHO program, primary providers have predictable, weekly teleconferences with teams of specialists at an academic medical center to confer on problems such as management of cirrhosis (Arora et al., 2007). Such consults, made possible with Skype and other videoconferencing programs, help avoid ambiguity and keep lines of communication open among the involved providers.

Using phone and video conferencing (called telehealth or telemedicine) can facilitate the management of hepatitis in primary care, but telehealth laws and reimbursement practices vary widely by state (Klink et al., 2015). Of 1,557 family doctors responding to a Robert Graham Center survey, 89 percent agreed that telehealth can improve their patients' access to care, but reimbursement, liability, and training were seen as barriers to its use (Klink et al., 2015). Collaborations for viral hepatitis treatment would need to take this into account, setting up consultation networks within single states, for example. In addition to providing a system for teaching and communication, technology allows primary care and specialty providers a way to share information, similar to the internet-based clinical information system that IMPACT provides (Patel et al., 2014; Unützer et al., 2002a).

The primary goal of conferencing with specialists should be training primary care providers to manage most of the patients themselves. To this end, telehealth, as modeled in the ECHO program (that is, more a teaching tool then a patient management one) should be encouraged. As mentioned earlier, cirrhotic patients are complicated. Adherence to practice guidelines for treatment of cirrhotics is generally better among specialists (Kanwal et al., 2012; Mellinger and Volk, 2013). Provider training would need to clarify the signs and symptoms of cirrhosis and ensure that primary care providers have a way to confirm diagnosis and refer appropriately.

An information system accessible to both specialists and primary providers (similar to the one used in the IMPACT example) helps track patients over time and facilitates shared decision making (Kvamme et al., 2001). Compatible electronic systems also encourage communication between providers, who may be separated by considerable distance (Kvamme et al., 2001; Patel et al., 2014). Electronic records alone will not necessarily improve communication, however. Even in the Department of Veterans Affairs, which uses a unified patient record system, analysis of patients' records suggests unexplained breaks in communication about 10 percent of the time (Singh et al., 2011). AASLD and IDSA should ensure that their training gives clear guidelines on everyone's role in the collaboration, including expectations for responsiveness (Mellinger and Volk, 2013).

Clarifying roles will apply not just to the specialists and the primary care provider. Success in managing complex conditions in primary care depends on the cooperation of teams of health workers (Thornton et al., 2016). Educating patients on treatment adherence has long been the role of pharmacists, one that became better and more deliberately integrated into hepatitis C treatment when pegylated interferon was the standard treatment (Spooner, 2011). Nurses are also well positioned for patient counseling, and are often better at it than doctors, especially as it pertains to chronic diseases, such as hepatitis B, and behavioral change, which can be part of hepatitis C care (Bodenheimer and Bauer, 2016). Team-based care also requires support from new types of health professionals, such as care coordinators, who can have more of the routine responsibility for the logistics of clinic visits and for check-ins to help avoid hospitalization (Ge and Runyon, 2016). With more staff working to manage any patient's case, it becomes important to organize patient information and have it accessible to the care team, as in the IMPACT program.

Inclusion of Special Populations

Viral hepatitis often affects people who are hard to reach: people who were born abroad, who are underinsured, who have substance use disorders and may have other mental health problems, and who are or have been imprisoned (NASEM, 2016). Hepatitis B and C cannot be eliminated without reaching these populations, something that requires extra effort. This effort is often unrewarded. The time and resources needed to coordinate care for such patients is not accurately captured in the Medicare and Medicaid reimbursement system, which has a bias toward in-patient care and paying for clinical services (Martyn and Davis, 2014). This imbalance could undermine the viral hepatitis elimination program.

The people with the most serious need for health care, including those who are poor or have behavioral health problems, rarely have a single office to coordinate their services (Blumenthal and Abrams, 2016; Druss and Walker, 2011). Without a single entity responsible for managing care, the process can disintegrate. Case management may be the key to avoiding such problems (Johnson et al., 2016). More holistic care keeps high-risk patients engaged with the health system over time (Martyn and Davis, 2014). The right strategy to achieve such care may vary by setting and by the particular group. In any case, bringing hepatitis services to challenging populations will be an integral part of hepatitis elimination, and as such it warrants more explicit attention from the federal and state agencies involved, as well as from various local and community organizations.

The Ryan White Comprehensive AIDS Resources Emergency Act of 1990 (hereafter, the Ryan White Act) was passed in response to a similar problem with HIV services in uninsured and underinsured people (HRSA,

2016a). HRSA works with state and local health departments to administer the program, tailoring services to meet local needs (HRSA, 2015). The Ryan White Act provides a key safety net for vulnerable groups (Sood et al., 2014). It also provides states with grants to improve the organization of HIV care and support services (HRSA, 2016a). The specific services supported are chosen by state or territorial authorities in consideration of local needs, but can include case management, transportation, and language interpretation (HRSA, 2016c). A system of the same flexibility and breadth would be needed to reach the marginalized populations suffering from viral hepatitis.

> **Recommendation 5-3:** The Department of Health and Human Services should work with states to build a comprehensive system of care and support for special populations with hepatitis B and C on the scale of the Ryan White system.

The Ryan White program gives states incentives to reach vulnerable patient groups, something that would greatly benefit viral hepatitis elimination efforts. The committee recognizes that building a parallel program with the reach of the Ryan White Act for viral hepatitis might not be feasible; at best it is not within the control of any health department. It may, therefore, be most efficient to try to build outreach activities for viral hepatitis onto existing Ryan White programs, albeit using separate funding for services for HIV-negative people.

The Ryan White Act already reaches viral hepatitis patients who also have HIV, the vast majority of whom have a history of injection drug use (Grebely et al., 2013; Thomas et al., 2011). In Rhode Island, for example, an HIV clinic used Ryan White funds to improve adherence to hepatitis C treatment among people who inject drugs (Taylor, 2005). Some states use their Ryan White program to treat substance use disorder (Arkansas Department of Health, n.d.; Baltimore City Health Department, n.d.; Fischer, 2012; Honeck and Dolansky, 2011; Kansas Department of Health and Environment, n.d.; West Virginia Department of Health and Human Resources, n.d.). Between 2011 and 2014, HRSA sponsored 29 programs to treat hepatitis C in Ryan White clients (Doshi and Tinsley, 2015). In all of these instances, however, the beneficiaries have both HIV and viral hepatitis. Currently the terms of the Ryan White Act and HRSA's AIDS Drug Assistance program are clear that funding may not be used for broader prevention activities or for services for people not infected with HIV (HRSA, n.d.-a).

It would take time for the Department of Health and Human Services (HHS) to implement a Ryan White like program for hepatitis B and C. In the meantime, the CDC and HRSA would do well to build more flexibility into their grant structure to allow state and local jurisdictions to support viral hepatitis prevention and linkage to care. Especially when it comes to testing and counseling, states should be allowed to build on existing infrastructure developed for HIV.

There are also viral hepatitis patient groups who do not overlap with the Ryan White population. Federally qualified health centers (FQHCs) may be an efficient way to reach these groups. The Bureau of Primary Health Care awards FQHC designation to organizations that offer comprehensive health services to underserved populations with a sliding fee scale (HRSA, n.d.-b). The HHS report *The Community Response to Viral Hepatitis* highlighted the work of FQHCs in educating and screening high-risk groups, as well as in developing strategies to ensure patients are retained in care (HHS, 2016). The centers also have good reach into rural areas, as shown in Figure 5-1. Box 5-2 describes the hepatitis and substance use programming of an FQHC that works with homeless people in Boston.

Between 2008 and 2016 the CDC supported state viral hepatitis prevention coordinators in five cities (Chicago, Houston, Los Angeles, New York, and Philadelphia) and all states except South Dakota (CDC, 2012b).

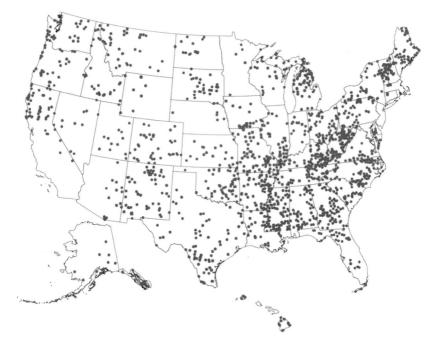

FIGURE 5-1 Federally qualified health centers in rural and suburban areas.
NOTE: Alaska and Hawaii not to scale.
SOURCES: HRSA, 2016b; Rural Health Information Hub, 2016.

BOX 5-2
Boston Health Care for the Homeless Program

Boston Health Care for the Homeless Program is a federally qualified health center that provides a variety of primary care and behavioral health services through an integrated care model to Boston's homeless population in several practice sites across the city (Boston Health Care for the Homeless Program, n.d.-b). The organization also offers special treatment and management services for hepatitis C patients (Boston Health Care for the Homeless Program, n.d.-a).

Fatal opioid overdoses increased 50 percent from 2014 to 2015 in Boston, and opioid abuse causes 80 percent of all deaths among the city's homeless (Gaeta et al., 2016; Pfeiffer, 2016). Clinic staff were called to opioid overdoses in their waiting room and in the nearby alley several times a week (Gaeta et al., 2016). In response, they opened a drop-in room for supervision of overly sedated people (Gaeta et al., 2016). The room (which is not a supervised injection site) has space for eight people to be monitored by a nurse who can provide naloxone and supplemental oxygen if needed (Gaeta et al., 2016). Clients of the room often mix a combination of opioids, such heroin and fentanyl, with various anti-anxiety and anti-convulsant medications. The resulting syndrome is more complex than a typical opioid overdose and requires several hours of close monitoring and additional medical care (Gaeta et al., 2016). People who use the supervision room are connected to the organization's services such as hepatitis C testing and care, substance use disorder treatment, harm reduction information, and peer support. The organization recorded 983 visits from 218 clients within the program's first 15 weeks, with fewer than 15 necessary transfers to the emergency room (Gaeta et al., 2016).

Boston Health Care for the Homeless Program consulted people who inject drugs, neighborhood organizations, and city and state officials before opening the drop-in room with grant funding from The Blue Cross Blue Shield of Massachusetts Foundation and other private sources (Gaeta et al., 2016). The Massachusetts Society of Addiction Medicine and the Boston Public Health Commission, which operates a syringe exchange program nearby, also support the program (Gaeta et al., 2016; Pfeiffer, 2016).

The coordinators would be an invaluable part of any effort to bring viral hepatitis services to a wider population. In Hawaii, for example, the coordinator's office developed hepatitis B education materials in the Chuukese, Ilocano, Marshallese, Samoan, and Tongan languages (CDC, 2012b). In Maine, they supported free immunization sites at sexually transmitted disease clinics, prisons, a clinic for homeless people, and five FQHCs (CDC, 2012b). However, in 2016, the CDC redirected the program that supported the viral hepatitis prevention coordinators toward improving testing and linkage at federally qualified health centers and safety-net hospitals and their affiliated clinics, and away from specific support of a hepatitis coordinator position.

Behavioral health problems often contribute to the challenge of reaching people with hepatitis, making it important to support them with a range of services, such as appointment reminders, help with insurance forms, transportation to clinics, and addiction counseling. Barriers to accessing and continuing in care fall into four main categories: logistical and child care; coordination, meaning the overall difficulty of navigating the health system; individual, referring to the patient's own mental and physical health problems that can impede functioning; and systemic, such as poverty and stigma (Broeckaert and Challacombe, 2015).

Defining the Special Populations for Viral Hepatitis Elimination

Some patients are less accessible than others. While it is not always easy to predict who will need more attention or supportive services, there are certain populations whose relative isolation and high burden of viral hepatitis make them essential targets for any hepatitis elimination campaign. Some situations worthy of concentrated outreach are described below (in no particular order).

Cultural and language barriers People born in HBV-endemic countries account for about 95 percent of new cases of chronic hepatitis B in the United States (Hu, 2008; Mitchell et al., 2011). Among the 929 Asian Americans in the NHANES[6] study, the prevalence of chronic hepatitis B is around 3 percent, 10 times higher than in the general population (Roberts et al., 2016). Among women of childbearing age, the prevalence of chronic hepatitis B was 8.9 percent among people born in Asia, compared to 0.14 percent among Asian Americans born in the United States (Smith et al., 2012). For comparison, an estimated 0.71 percent of African Americans, 0.08 percent of whites, and 0.03 percent of Hispanics have chronic hepatitis B (Smith et al., 2012). By some estimates, Asian Americans comprise more than half of the country's chronic hepatitis B cases (CDC, 2013). Nevertheless, only 35 to 60 percent of Asian Americans have been screened for HBV (CDC, 2013; Cohen et al., 2008; Hutton et al., 2007; Roberts et al., 2016; Sarpel et al., 2016).

Screening for HBV at Asian American cultural events is a strategy to identify more infected people, but one that has yielded mixed results (Hyun et al., 2016; Woo et al., 2013). Some evidence suggests that connecting the HBsAg+ patient to care is the bigger challenge (Hyun et al., 2016; Tran, 2009). Hepatitis B carries a pronounced stigma in some Asian communities

---

[6] Officially, the National Health and Nutrition Examination Survey.

(Tran, 2009; Yoo et al., 2012). In a discussion of barriers to hepatitis B treatment, Tram Tran described a Taoist preference for the natural course of things and a complementary Hmong belief in predestination and "indifference toward suffering" (Tran, 2009). She also cited the isolation of not having an English speaking family member older than 14 in a household (Tran, 2009). By this measure, almost half of Vietnamese immigrant households and more than one-third of Chinese, Hmong, Korean, and Taiwanese ones are isolated (Tran, 2009).

Health workers from the same ethnic and language groups as the target patients can help expand the reach of hepatitis B services. Such health workers have been shown to improve knowledge of hepatitis B among Chinese and Cambodian Americans, but with less effect on testing behavior (Taylor et al., 2009, 2013). Other research among Asian Americans has shown that reminders from lay health workers can motivate vaccination and linkage to care (Hyun et al., 2016; Juon et al., 2016). An ongoing randomized trial is exploring the use of patient navigators and mobile messaging to improve care for Asian Americans with chronic hepatitis B (Chak et al., 2016).

Homeless or unstable housing People who live on the street or in shelters, single room occupancy facilities, or transitional housing even occasionally are at elevated risk of death, about a three to nine times higher risk after controlling for age (Baggett et al., 2013; Hibbs et al., 1994; Zivanovic et al., 2015). At any given time, there are over half a million such people in the United States, though the biannual survey used to count them is biased in ways that invariably underestimate the true population (*The Economist*, 2016; The National Alliance to End Homelessness, 2016). Homeless people have twice the odds (as compared to housed people) of having their medical needs go untreated (Lebrun-Harris et al., 2013).

A meta-analysis of data from seven countries on the burden of infectious disease in homeless people found hepatitis C to be more common than HIV or tuberculosis (Beijer et al., 2012). In the United States, almost a third of homeless people are thought to have HCV antibody, though published estimates range from 7.5 to 52.5 percent (Edlin et al., 2015). A study in Los Angeles found that only about 30 percent of homeless, HCV-infected persons had been diagnosed and informed of their infection, though other research from the same group suggested the same proportion diagnosed as in the general population (Gelberg et al., 2012; Stein et al., 2012).

Managing hepatitis care for people in unstable housing is challenging, but recent promising examples in Boston suggest it is possible. Boston Health Care for the Homeless, the FQHC described in Box 5-2 recently developed a protocol for treating hepatitis C in its clients (Barocas et al., 2017). After 12 weeks, 97 percent had sustained virologic response (Barocas et al., 2017). The program made use of care coordinators and nurses to manage the patients' paperwork, appointments, and adherence to treatment (Beiser, 2016). Outreach workers can also be helpful in building connections with this population and encouraging the use of services (Zlotnick et al., 2013). Provider teams may also find mobile phones useful for staying in contact with transient patients (Asgary et al., 2016; McInnes et al., 2014).

Lack of stable housing can be both a cause and an effect of substance use, itself a risk factor for HBV and HCV infection (Aidala et al., 2005; Tompsett et al., 2013; Zivanovic et al., 2015). Outreach to people in unstable housing may, therefore, overlap with harm reduction and substance use treatment programs.

Ongoing substance use disorders and mental health problems The Substance Abuse and Mental Health Services Administration estimates that 43.6 million American adults have a mental illness that interferes with life activities; for about 4 percent of them the illness is considered severe, meaning it substantially limits life activities (SAMHSA, 2015). Substance use is also common, affecting 21.5 million Americans older than 12, about 8 percent of the population (SAMHSA, 2015). People diagnosed with a drug disorder often have comorbid mental health problems; compared to someone without a drug problem, they are about twice as likely to have mood (e.g, bipolar, major depressive disorder) or anxiety disorders (e.g., phobias, panic disorder) (Conway et al., 2006; NIDA, 2010).

Injection drug use is the behavioral health problem most closely associated with hepatitis B and C (CDC, 2016f). In the United States, almost three-quarters of people who inject drugs have HCV antibody; older estimates put the prevalence of HBsAg in the same group around 12 percent, roughly consistent with worldwide estimates (Grebely et al., 2015; Nelson et al., 2011). People who inject drugs can be challenging patients. They often have logistical problems making appointments, and some distrust the health system (Taylor, 2005). There is evidence that these patients do better in primary care than specialty clinics, especially if the providers treat them with compassion and respect and make an effort to build trust (Reimer and Haasen, 2009). Patient management may also require the collaboration of social workers and different kinds of providers (Bruggmann and Grebely, 2015; Bruggmann and Litwin, 2013; Hill et al., 2008).

One promising strategy for reaching this group is to treat hepatitis C in addiction clinics, involving a hepatologist or infectious disease specialist when necessary (Bruggmann and Grebely, 2015; Bruggmann and Litwin, 2013; Reimer and Haasen, 2009). Even in the days of pegylated interferon therapy, a far worse-tolerated course of treatment than direct-acting antivirals, methadone maintenance and addiction clinics had good success at treating HCV infection (Harris et al., 2010; Wilkinson et al., 2009).

Though a recent WHO review found the quality of the evidence regarding the effectiveness of most strategies to prevent viral hepatitis in people who inject drugs to be low, it encouraged syringe exchange and HBV immunization, especially with a high-dose, accelerated vaccine regimen (Walsh et al., 2014).

As discussed in Chapter 4, the opioid epidemic is drawing attention to substance use problems, including those in rural areas and small towns, and among people younger than 35, who are difficult to engage in care (Altarum Institute, 2013). Reaching these patients, and all people with substance use and mental health problems, requires sensitivity and effort; organizations working closely with the target patients may be in the best position to facilitate this.

Recently incarcerated Prisoners are often poor, and many have a history of substance use disorder. Data from the Bureau of Justice Statistics suggest a median annual income for recently incarcerated men of less than $20,000 in 2014 dollars, for recently incarcerated women of less than $14,000 (Rabuy and Kopf, 2015). During incarceration, inmates are dropped from Medicaid. A 2014 survey of medical directors found that fewer than 20 percent follow CDC recommendations for discharge planning of inmates (Solomon et al., 2014). It can take months after release to re-enroll even for the most motivated beneficiary (Solomon et al., 2014). Easing the ability of prisoners to re-enroll in Medicaid or private insurance can smooth the transition from prison life.

More than 90 percent of prisoners re-enter civilian society (Bushway, 2006; Neate, 2016; Rich et al., 2014). Release is a time of heightened risk for the inmate. In the first 2 weeks after release, the former prisoner's risk of death is almost 13 times higher than that of controls of the same age, sex, and race (Binswanger et al., 2007). Among people with a history of injection drug use (the same patients at highest risk of hepatitis B and C), death from overdose is about 12 times more likely (Binswanger et al., 2007). Viral hepatitis and accompanying substance use problems should be addressed as much as possible in the highly structured prison environment, for reasons discussed later in this chapter. Nevertheless, most prisoners, especially those with hepatitis B, will need help to ensure continued medical care.

Underinsured The Commonwealth Fund estimates that 31 million Americans are underinsured, meaning that their out-of-pocket health costs are more than 10 percent of their household income (or 5 percent of household income for people under 200 percent of the federal poverty line) (Collins et al., 2015). This includes a fifth of people with insurance from their employers, and slightly more than a fifth of Medicaid beneficiaries (Collins et al., 2015). But by far the most represented group among the underinsured is Medicare beneficiaries (people over 65 or disabled), who account for more than 40 percent of the total (Collins et al., 2015). This group has considerable burden of hepatitis B and C; the CDC estimates that people 55 and older account for over a quarter of chronic hepatitis B infections and almost 40 percent of those with hepatitis C (CDC, 2016f).

Underinsured people are more likely to forgo medical care when they need it (Collins et al., 2015; McCarthy, 2015). Forgoing hepatitis care may be particularly tempting, as HBV and HCV infections are both clinically silent until their late stages (Chen and Morgan, 2006; Post et al., 2011). The underinsured are also a less easily distinguishable group then some other high-risk patients. It is not usually obvious which patients in a practice are near poverty, on a fixed income, or have a high deductible health plan. On the other hand, outreach to underinsured patients is at least possible. By definition, all of them have some contact with the health system. With this in mind, a medical social worker or patient navigator might determine which patients in a practice were vulnerable to forgoing care and act to prevent it.

The Opportunity to Treat Incarcerated Patients

CDC estimates from the early 2000s put the prevalence of hepatitis C in jails and prisons between 12 and 35 percent, and the prevalence of chronic HBV infection between 1 and 3.7 percent (Weinbaum et al., 2003). A 2015 survey by the American Correctional Association concluded that relatively few prison systems collect the information necessary to measure prevalence, but among those that do, estimates of hepatitis C prevalence range from 8 to 10 percent on the low end and 17 percent at the high end (Maurer and Gondles, 2015). A recent, small survey in Wisconsin is representative of the lower end of this distribution, finding about 8 percent of inmates had chronic hepatitis C, and 6 percent had chronic HBV infection (Stockman et al., 2016). The northeast may have a higher disease burden. Research among Pennsylvania inmates between 2004 and 2012 found about 18 percent had HCV antibody (Larney et al., 2014). The authors did not report prevalence of chronic hepatitis C, but given spontaneous cure rates of one-fifth to one-third, a Pennsylvania prison prevalence of about 12 to 15 percent is plausible. Similarly, a 2014 study of New York City jail records found a 20 percent prevalence of HCV antibody, suggesting a similar 14 to 16 percent prevalence of chronic hepatitis C (Akiyama et al., 2016). All this is broadly consistent with *Lancet* estimates putting the prevalence of chronic hepatitis B in North American prisoners between 0.3 and 3.1 percent, and HCV antibody between 13.1 and 17.7 percent (Dolan et al., 2016).

Even at the low end of the prevalence distribution, prisoners bear a disproportionate burden of viral hepatitis. Unprotected sex and needle sharing, both risk factors for viral hepatitis, are common in correctional facilities (Macalino et al., 2004; Rubin, 2016). Therefore, prisons are sometimes seen as an amplifying reservoir for viral hepatitis (Macalino et al., 2004). The irony of this problem is that correctional facilities are, at the same time, ideal venues in which to test and vaccinate against hepatitis B and to test for and treat hepatitis C. Directly observed therapy is the norm and risk of drug diversion is low. Prisoners are disproportionately poor and male, a group often out of contact with the health system (Fox et al., 2005; Rabuy and Kopf, 2015; Weinbaum et al., 2005).

A 6-week course of ledipasvir-sofosbuvir has been shown effective at treating acute hepatitis C and well-tolerated by even the sickest patients (Deterding et al., 2016). Treating hepatitis C in its earliest stages reduces the duration of the disease and its associated morbidities, and could help limit the spread of hepatitis C in high-risk populations such as prisoners (Deterding et al., 2016). Still, only half of prison systems responding to an American Correctional Association survey reported having a clinical guideline regarding treatment of hepatitis C (Maurer and Gondles, 2015). The success of the elimination effort may well depend on reaching imprisoned patients, more than 90 percent of whom re-enter the general population (Bushway, 2006; Neate, 2016; Rich et al., 2014). Returning these inmates to their communities vaccinated against HBV and cured of hepatitis C would be an invaluable step toward elimination.

The expense of testing, vaccination, and treatment may be a limiting facor for state correctional officers (Maurer and Gondles, 2015; Weinbaum et al., 2005). Strategies to defray the costs of treatment in prisons, especially at the state and local levels, are discussed in Chapter 6.

> **Recommendation 5-4: The criminal justice system should screen, vaccinate, and treat hepatitis B and C in correctional facilities according to national clinical practice guidelines.**

Having sufficient staff to test prisoners for viral hepatitis and, depending on the result, manage prevention or treatment programs can be a problem for the correctional system. Less competitive salaries and the challenges of the work environment make it difficult to recruit health professionals to prison jobs; 90 percent of respondents to a 2016 survey of state and federal prisons and large jails reported such problems (Gondles et al., 2017). The Department of Justice review found adequate medical staffing in only about 25 percent of federal prisons (DOJ, 2016). Correctional facilities usually fill gaps by contracting with local providers (Ellis, 2009). Most state prisons also use a combination of on- and off-site providers (Chari et al., 2016). There are no comprehensive data on providers in local prisons and jails, but the use of local providers and correctional medical corporations appears to be common in jails (Shalev et al., 2011). For-profit companies may also provide about half of medical care for state and local correctional facilities (Von Zielbauer, 2005).

It is not realistic to expect any jail or prison to employ the full range of health providers their inmates may need. Off-site provider visits are necessary, but add expense and logistical complications; a guard must accompany an inmate traveling to a clinic, for example. Telehealth for specialist visits to inmates is a particularly useful strategy in correctional facilities (Schiff, 2014). Only 30 of the 45 states responding to the 2016 National Survey of Prison Health Care reported using telemedicine, however (Chari et al., 2016). Concerns about malpractice and the legality of using providers licensed in other states may be preventing some correctional health officers from using telemedicine (NCCHC, 2016). The National Commission on Correctional Health Care position supports telemedicine in correctional facilities, allowing that all providers must be properly licensed in the inmate's state, and that alternative arrangements be made for urgent and emergency care and for in-person exams when necessary (NCCHC, 2016).

The previous section discussed the efficient use of telemedicine to support primary care providers in managing hepatitis patients. The same can be done to support primary care providers who manage viral hepatitis patients in correctional facilities. The use of telemedicine is consistent with recommendations from the national commission, and a modest majority of state prisons are already moving toward phone and video health consultations (NCCHC, 1998; Schaenman et al., 2013). Viral hepatitis elimination may provide an impetus to make better use of these services for incarcerated patients.

Hepatitis B in Correctional Facilities

Prisons and jails have a constant rotation of inmates, sometimes in close quarters. The mixing of people and opportunities for disease transmission make immunization a priority for correctional health officers (Sequera et al., 2013). Hepatitis B can be a particular risk, motivating the British government's target of 80 percent of inmates being vaccinated against HBV in the first month of incarceration (Sequera et al., 2013; U.K. Department of Health, 2009). Fewer than half of British prisons reported meeting this target in a recent survey, however (U.K. Government, 2011).

Immunization in jails and prisons has proven challenging in the United States as well. A 2000 survey of 35 states and the Federal Bureau of Prisons found only Texas and Michigan routinely offered hepatitis B immunization to prisoners (Charuvastra et al., 2001). Twenty-six prison systems said they would vaccinate more widely if the vaccine were free, though nine states indicated that free hepatitis B vaccine would not be enough because of staffing and infrastructure problems (Charuvastra et al., 2001). More recent survey data suggest that about two-thirds of state prisons (covering about 84 percent of state inmates) have a hepatitis B vaccination policy; in most the policy is to vaccinate at the inmate's request or because of a risk factor for HBV acquisition (BJS, 2004). Even these policies may be observed mostly in the breach. Of the 190 prisons reporting a universal hepatitis B immunization policy, 80 percent had not vaccinated anyone in the year before the survey (BJS, 2004; Weinbaum et al., 2005).

The 2016 National Survey of Prison Care found that 32 of 45 participating states offered hepatitis B testing to incoming inmates, but 21 of those tested only if the inmate had had a clinical indication for it (Chari et al., 2016). Wider attention to testing could draw attention to the related question of immunization. If many inmates are shown to be vulnerable to infection, prison health officers might be able to make a stronger case to their state authorities for support of hepatitis B immunization.

Hepatitis C in Correctional Facilities

In 2003, the CDC recommended screening all inmates with a history of injection drug use for hepatitis C (Macalino et al., 2005; Weinbaum et al., 2003). In prisons with a relatively lower prevalence of HCV, screening only inmates who report certain risk factors may be adequate. Research in Wisconsin found that screening inmates with a history of injection drug use and those born between 1945 and 1965 would correctly identify about 92 percent of patients with a history of HCV infection (Stockman et al., 2016). In higher prevalence settings, opt-out screening may be necessary. In Rhode Island, over 65 percent of male and 44 percent of female inmates with a history of HCV infection did *not* report any prior injection drug use (Macalino et al., 2005). In California, where 43 percent of inmates reported a history of injection drug use, other notable risks for HCV infection were having a sexual relationship with a man who injects drugs and age, with older people and those imprisoned longer having elevated risk of infection (Fox et al., 2005). Pennsylvania researchers also found that screening inmates based only on risk factors for infection would have missed about three-quarters of people with HCV infection (Kuncio et al., 2015).

Concerns about adequacy of follow-up may have prevented correctional officials from pursuing wider screening in the past (Kuncio et al., 2015). Such concerns remain challenging, but the drug purchasing arrangements discussed in Chapter 6 should give prison systems access to an affordable, steady drug supply. The use of telemedicine to link inmates to specialists will also be helpful when necessary, and evidence suggests that primary care providers have no higher rate of adverse events in treating hepatitis C than specialists do (Baker et al., 2014; Ho et al., 2015, 2016).

REFERENCES

AAFP (American Academy of Family Physicians). n.d. *Primary care.* http://www.aafp.org/about/policies/all/primary-care.html (accessed October 27, 2016).

AHRQ (Agency for Healthcare Research and Quality). n.d. *Project ECHO: Bringing specialty care to rural New Mexico.* https://healthit.ahrq.gov/ahrq-funded-projects/transforming-healthcare-quality-through-health-it/project-echo-bringing (accessed November 2, 2016).

Aidala, A., J. E. Cross, R. Stall, D. Harre, and E. Sumartojo. 2005. Housing status and HIV risk behaviors: Implications for prevention and policy. *AIDS and Behavior* 9(3):251-265.

Akiyama, M. J., F. Kaba, Z. Rosner, H. Alper, R. S. Holzman, and R. MacDonald. 2016. Hepatitis C screening of the "birth cohort" (born 1945–1965) and younger inmates of New York City jails. *American Journal of Public Health* 106(7):1276-1277.

Altarum Institute. 2013. *Hepatitis C virus infection in young persons who inject drugs.* Altarum Institute. https://www.aids.gov/pdf/hcv-and-young-pwid-consultation-report.pdf (accessed December 29, 2016).

Arkansas Department of Health. n.d. *HIV/Ryan White Part B services program.* http://www.healthy.arkansas.gov/programsServices/infectiousDisease/hivStdHepatitisC/Pages/HIVServices.aspx (accessed October 25, 2016).

Arora, S., C. M. Geppert, S. Kalishman, D. Dion, F. Pullara, B. Bjeletich, G. Simpson, D. C. Alverson, L. B. Moore, D. Kuhl, and J. V. Scaletti. 2007. Academic health center management of chronic diseases through knowledge networks: Project ECHO. *Academic Medicine* 82(2):154-160.

Arora, S., K. Thornton, G. Murata, P. Deming, S. Kalishman, D. Dion, B. Parish, T. Burke, W. Pak, J. Dunkelberg, M. Kistin, J. Brown, S. Jenkusky, M. Komaromy, and C. Qualls. 2011. Outcomes of treatment for hepatitis C virus infection by primary care providers. *New England Journal of Medicine* 364(23):2199-2207.

Arora, S., K. Thornton, M. Komaromy, S. Kalishman, J. Katzman, and D. Duhigg. 2014. Demonopolizing medical knowledge. *Academic Medicine* 89(1):30-32.

Asgary, R., B. Sckell, A. Alcabes, R. Naderi, A. Schoenthaler, and G. Ogedegbe. 2016. Rates and predictors of uncontrolled hypertension among hypertensive homeless adults using New York City shelter-based clinics. *Annals of Family Medicine* 14(1):41-46.

Baggett, T., S. Hwang, J. O'Connell, B. Porneala, E. Stringfellow, and J. Orav. 2013. Mortality among homeless adults in Boston: Shifts in causes of death over a 15-year period. *JAMA Internal Medicine* 173(3):189-195.

Baker, D., M. Alavi, A. Erratt, S. Hill, A. Balcomb, R. Hallinan, S. Siriragavan, D. Richmond, J. Smart, J. Keats, N. Doong, P. Marks, J. Grebely, and G. J. Dore. 2014. Delivery of treatment for hepatitis C virus infection in the primary care setting. *European Journal of Gastroenterology & Hepatology* 26(9):1003-1009.

Baltimore City Health Department. n.d. *Ryan White program.* http://health.baltimorecity.gov/hiv-std-services/ryan-white-program (accessed October 25, 2016).

Barocas, J. A., M. Beiser, C. Leon, M. Ingemi, P. McCabe, L. Cardoso, B. P. Linas, and J. O'Connell. 2017. Real-world outcomes of HCV treatment in homeless and marginally housed adults. PowerPoint presentation at Conference on Retroviruses and Opportunistic Infections in Seattle, WA, February 13-16, 2017. Received February 23, 2017. Available by request from the National Academies of Sciences, Engineering, and Medicine Public Access Records Office. For more information, email PARO@nas.edu.

Baron, R. J. 2010. What's keeping us so busy in primary care? A snapshot from one practice. *New England Journal of Medicine* 362(17):1632-1636.

Beijer, U., A. Wolf, and S. Fazel. 2012. Prevalence of tuberculosis, hepatitis C virus, and HIV in homeless people: A systematic review and meta-analysis. *The Lancet Infectious Diseases* 12(11):859-870.

Beiser, M. 2016 (unpublished). *Enabling hepatitis C cure for individuals experiencing homelessness.* PowerPoint presentation, Boston Health Care for the Homeless Program, June 2, 2016. https://www.nhchc.org/wp-content/uploads/2016/06/enabling-hepatitis-c-cure-for-individuals-experiencing-homelessness-beiser-1.pdf (accessed February 23, 2017).

Binswanger, I. A., M. F. Stern, R. A. Deyo, P. J. Heagerty, A. Cheadle, J. G. Elmore, and T. D. Koepsell. 2007. Release from prison—A high risk of death for former inmates. *New England Journal of Medicine* 356(2):157-165.

BJS (Bureau of Justice Statistics). 2004. Hepatitis testing and treatment in state prisons. *Bureau of Justice Statistics Special Report NCJ 199173C.* http://www.bjs.gov/content/pub/pdf/httsp.pdf (accessed September 23, 2016).

Blumenthal, D., and M. K. Abrams. 2016. Tailoring complex care management for high-need, high-cost patients. *JAMA* 316(16):1657-1658.

Bodenheimer, T., and L. Bauer. 2016. Rethinking the primary care workforce—An expanded role for nurses. *New England Journal of Medicine* 375(11):1015-1017.

Boston Health Care for the Homeless Program. n.d.-a. *Hepatitis C services.* https://www.bhchp.org/specialized-services/hepc-consult-service (accessed December 7, 2016).

Boston Health Care for the Homeless Program. n.d.-b. *History.* https://www.bhchp.org/about/history (accessed December 7, 2016).

Broeckaert, L., and L. Challacombe. 2015. Does multidisciplinary care improve health outcomes among people living with HIV and/or HCV? A review of the evidence. *Prevention in Focus.* Fall. http://www.catie.ca/en/pif/fall-2015/does-multidisciplinary-care-improve-health-outcomes-among-people-living-hiv-andor-hcv- (accessed November 14, 2016).

Bruggmann, P., and J. Grebely. 2015. Prevention, treatment and care of hepatitis C virus infection among people who inject drugs. *International Journal on Drug Policy* 26(Suppl 1):S22-S26.

Bruggmann, P., and A. H. Litwin. 2013. Models of care for the management of hepatitis C virus among people who inject drugs: One size does not fit all. *Clinical Infectious Diseases* 57(Suppl 2):S56-S61.

Bundy, D. G., B. S. Solomon, J. M. Kim, and M. R. Miller. 2012. Accuracy and usefulness of the HEDIS childhood immunization measures. *Pediatrics* 129(4):648-656.

Bushway, S. D. 2006. The problem of prisoner (re)entry. Review of When prisoners come home: Parole and prisoner reentry, Joan Petersilia; But they all come back: Facing the challenges of prisoner reentry, Jeremy Travis; Prisoner reentry and crime in America, Jeremy Travis, Christy Visher. *Contemporary Sociology* 35(6):562-565.

CDC (Centers for Disease Control and Prevention). 2012a. National, state, and local area vaccination coverage among children aged 19-35 months—United States, 2011. *Morbidity and Mortality Weekly Report* 61:689-696.

CDC. 2012b. *Viral hepatitis prevention initiative: 5-years of accomplishments 2008-2012: Putting viral hepatitis on the map. PS 08-801.* CDC, National Center for HIV/AIDS, Viral Hepatitis, STD, and TB Prevention.

CDC. 2013. *Asian Americans and hepatitis B.* https://www.cdc.gov/features/aapihepatitisb (accessed January 11, 2017).

CDC. 2016a. *Chronic liver disease/cirrhosis mortality by state: 2014.* http://www.cdc.gov/nchs/pressroom/sosmap/liver_disease_mortality/liver_disease.htm (accessed November 2, 2016).

CDC. 2016b. *Hepatitis B.* http://www.cdc.gov/vaccines/pubs/pinkbook/hepb.html (accessed November 3, 2016).

CDC. 2016c. *Hepatitis B: Hepatitis B vaccine.* http://www.cdc.gov/vaccines/pubs/pinkbook/hepb.html#vaccine (accessed November 7, 2016).

CDC. 2016d. *Perinatal transmission.* http://www.cdc.gov/hepatitis/hbv/perinatalxmtn.htm (accessed November 3, 2016).

CDC. 2016e. *Possible side-effects from vaccines: Hepatitis B vaccine side-effects.* http://www.cdc.gov/vaccines/vac-gen/side-effects.htm#hepb (accessed November 7, 2016).

CDC. 2016f. *Viral hepatitis surveillance: United States, 2014.* http://www.cdc.gov/hepatitis/statistics/2014surveillance/pdfs/2014hepsurveillancerpt.pdf (accessed September 22, 2016).

Chak, E. W., S. Sarkar, and C. Bowlus. 2016. Improving healthcare systems to reduce healthcare disparities in viral hepatitis. *Digestive Diseases and Sciences* 61(10):2776-2783.

Chari, K. A., A. E. Simon, C. J. DeFrances, and L. Maruschak. 2016. National survey of prison health care: Selected findings. *National Health Statistics Reports* (96):1-23.

Charuvastra, A., J. Stein, B. Schwartzapfel, A. Spaulding, E. Horowitz, G. Macalino, and J. D. Rich. 2001. Hepatitis B vaccination practices in state and federal prisons. *Public Health Reports* 116(3):203-209.

Chen, S. L., and T. R. Morgan. 2006. The natural history of hepatitis C virus (HCV) infection. *International Journal of Medical Sciences* 3(2):47-52.

Chitnis, D. 2016. ACIP approves change to hepatitis B vaccination guidelines. *Pediatric News, MDedge.* http://www.mdedge.com/pediatricnews/article/116025/vaccines/acip-approves-change-hepatitis-b-vaccination-guidelines (accessed November 21, 2016).

Cohen, C., A. A. Evans, W. T. London, J. Block, M. Conti, and T. Block. 2008. Underestimation of chronic hepatitis B virus infection in the United States of America. *Journal of Viral Hepatitis* 15(1):12-13.

Collins, S. R., P. W. Rasmussen, S. Beutel, and M. M. Doty. 2015. The problem of underinsurance and how rising deductibles will make it worse. Findings from the Commonwealth Fund Biennial Health Insurance Survey, 2014. *Issue Brief (Commonwealth Fund)* 13:1-20.

Conway, K. P., W. Compton, F. S. Stinson, and B. F. Grant. 2006. Lifetime comorbidity of DSM-IV mood and anxiety disorders and specific drug use disorders: Results from the National Epidemiologic Survey on Alcohol and Related Conditions. *Journal of Clinical Psychiatry* 67(2):247-257.

Denniston, M. M., R. M. Klevens, G. M. McQuillan, and R. B. Jiles. 2012. Awareness of infection, knowledge of hepatitis C, and medical follow-up among individuals testing positive for hepatitis C: National Health and Nutrition Examination Survey 2001-2008. *Hepatology* 55(6):1652-1661.

Derose, K. P., B. W. Bahney, N. Lurie, and J. J. Escarce. 2009. Review: Immigrants and health care access, quality, and cost. *Medical Care Research and Review* 66(4):355-408.

Deterding, K., C. D. Spinner, E. Schott, T. M. Welzel, G. Gerken, H. Klinker, U. Spengler, J. Wiegand, J. S. Zur Wiesch, A. Pathil, M. Cornberg, A. Umgelter, C. Zollner, S. Zeuzem, A. Papkalla, K. Weber, S. Hardtke, H. von der Leyen, A. Koch, D. von Witzendorff, M. P. Manns, and H. Wedemeyer. 2016. Ledipasvir plus sofosbuvir fixed-dose combination for 6 weeks in patients with acute hepatitis C virus genotype 1 monoinfection (HepNet Acute HCV IV): An open-label, single-arm, phase 2 study. *The Lancet Infectious Diseases* 17(2):215-222.

DOJ (Department of Justice). 2016. *Review of the Federal Bureau of Prisons' medical staffing challenges.* DOJ, Office of the Inspector General, Evaluation and Inspections Division 16-02.

Dolan, K., A. L. Wirtz, B. Moazen, M. Ndeffo-mbah, A. Galvani, S. A. Kinner, R. Courtney, M. McKee, J. J. Amon, L. Maher, M. Hellard, C. Beyrer, and F. L. Altice. 2016. Global burden of HIV, viral hepatitis, and tuberculosis in prisoners and detainees. *Lancet* 388(10049):1089-1102.

Doshi, R. K., and M. Tinsley. 2015. *Hepatitis C initiative in Ryan White clinics—Findings from a special program of national significance*. https://blog.aids.gov/2015/10/hepatitis-c-initiative-in-ryan-white-clinics-findings-from-a-special-program-of-national-significance.html (accessed October 19, 2016).

Druss, B. G., and E. R. Walker. 2011. *Mental disorders and medical comorbidity. Research synthesis report no. 21*. The Synthesis Project and Robert Wood Johnson Foundation.

Eddy, D. M., L. G. Pawlson, D. Schaaf, B. Peskin, A. Shcheprov, J. Dziuba, J. Bowman, and B. Eng. 2008. The potential effects of HEDIS performance measures on the quality of care. *Health Affairs* 27(5):1429-1441.

Edlin, B. R., B. J. Eckhardt, M. A. Shu, S. D. Holmberg, and T. Swan. 2015. Toward a more accurate estimate of the prevalence of hepatitis C in the United States. *Hepatology* 62(5):1353-1363.

Ellis, A. 2009. BOP health care: What you (and your clients) need to know. *Criminal Justice* 23(4).

Fischer, L. 2012. Colorado's Ryan White screening, brief intervention, and referral to treatment collaborative project to address substance use in HIV/AIDS case management and health-care settings. *Addiction Science & Clinical Practice* 7(Suppl 1):A73.

Fox, R. K., S. L. Currie, J. Evans, T. L. Wright, L. Tobler, B. Phelps, M. P. Busch, and K. A. Page-Shafer. 2005. Hepatitis C virus infection among prisoners in the California state correctional system. *Clinical Infectious Diseases* 41(2):177-186.

Freiman, J. M., T. M. Tran, S. G. Schumacher, L. F. White, S. Ongarello, J. Cohn, P. J. Easterbrook, B. P. Linas, and C. M. Denkinger. 2016. Hepatitis C antigen testing for diagnosis of hepatitis C virus infection: A systematic review and meta-analysis. *Annals of Internal Medicine* 165(5):345-355.

Gaeta, J., B. Bock, and M. Takach. 2016. Providing a safe space and medical monitoring to prevent overdose deaths. *Health Affairs Blog*, August 31. http://healthaffairs.org/blog/2016/08/31/providing-a-safe-space-and-medical-monitoring-to-prevent-overdose-deaths (accessed December 7, 2016).

Ge, P. S., and B. A. Runyon. 2016. Treatment of patients with cirrhosis. *New England Journal of Medicine* 375(8):767-777.

Gelberg, L., M. J. Robertson, L. Arangua, B. D. Leake, G. Sumner, A. Moe, R. M. Andersen, H. Morgenstern, and A. Nyamathi. 2012. Prevalence, distribution, and correlates of hepatitis C virus infection among homeless adults in Los Angeles. *Public Health Reports* 127(4):407-421.

Gish, R. G., J. A. Gutierrez, N. Navarro-Cazarez, K. Giang, D. Adler, B. Tran, S. Locarnini, R. Hammond, and S. Bowden. 2014. A simple and inexpensive point-of-care test for hepatitis B surface antigen detection: Serological and molecular evaluation. *Journal of Viral Hepatitis* 21(12):905-908.

Gondles, E. F., K. F. Maurer, and A. Bell. 2017. A major challenge for corrections: National survey findings identify challenges in recruiting and retaining correctional health care professionals. *Corrections Today* January/February:20-27. Article courtesy of the American Correctional Association (accessed January 4, 2016).

Grebely, J., M. Oser, L. E. Taylor, and G. J. Dore. 2013. Breaking down the barriers to hepatitis C virus (HCV) treatment among individuals with HCV/HIV coinfection: Action required at the system, provider, and patient levels. *Journal of Infectious Diseases* 207(Suppl 1):S19-S25.

Grebely, J., G. Robaeys, P. Bruggmann, A. Aghemo, M. Backmund, J. Bruneau, J. Byrne, O. Dalgard, J. J. Feld, M. Hellard, M. Hickman, A. Kautz, A. Litwin, A. R. Lloyd, S. Mauss, M. Prins, T. Swan, M. Schaefer, L. E. Taylor, and G. J. Dore. 2015. Recommendations for the management of hepatitis C virus infection among people who inject drugs. *International Journal on Drug Policy* 26(10):1028-1038.

Hacker, K., M. Anies, B. L. Folb, and L. Zallman. 2015. Barriers to health care for undocumented immigrants: A literature review. *Risk Management and Health Care Policy* 8:175-183.

Harris, K. A., Jr., J. H. Arnsten, and A. H. Litwin. 2010. Successful integration of hepatitis C evaluation and treatment services with methadone maintenance. *Journal of Addiction Medicine* 4(1):20-26.

Hepatitis C Online. 2016. *Natural history of hepatitis C infection.* http://www.hepatitisc. uw.edu/pdf/evaluation-staging-monitoring/natural-history/core-concept/all (accessed November 2, 2016).

Hern, T., A. Burke Valeras, J. Banker, and G. Riebe. 2013. Collaborative partnerships within integrated behavioral health and primary care. In *Integrated behavioral health in primary care: Evaluating the evidence, identifying the essentials*, edited by M. R. Talen and A. Burke Valeras. New York: Springer. Pp. 209-227.

HHS (Department of Health and Human Services). 2016. *The community response to viral hepatitis: Contributions toward achieving the goals of the viral hepatitis action plan.* HHS, Office of the Assistant Secretary for Health, Office of HIV/AIDS and Infectious Disease Policy.

HHS. 2017. *National viral hepatitis action plan 2017-2020.* HHS, Office of the Assistant Secretary for Health, Office of HIV/AIDS and Infectious Disease Policy. https://www.hhs. gov/sites/default/files/National%20Viral%20Hepatitis%20Action%20Plan%202017-2020.pdf (accessed February 24, 2017).

Hibbs, J., L. Benner, L. Klugman, R. Spencer, I. Macchia, and A. Mellinger. 1994. Mortality in a cohort of homeless adults in Philadelphia. *New England Journal of Medicine* 331(5):304-309.

Hill, W. D., G. Butt, M. Alvarez, and M. Krajden. 2008. Capacity enhancement of hepatitis C virus treatment through integrated, community-based care. *Canadian Journal of Gastroenterology & Hepatology* 22(1):27-32.

Hill, H. A., L. D. Elam-Evans, D. Yankey, J. A. Singleton, and M. Kolasa. 2015. National, state, and selected local area vaccination coverage among children aged 19–35 months— United States, 2014. *Morbidity and Mortality Weekly Report* 64(33):889-896.

Ho, S. B., N. Bräu, R. Cheung, L. Liu, C. Sanchez, M. Sklar, T. E. Phelps, S. G. Marcus, M. M. Wasil, A. Tisi, L. Huynh, S. K. Robinson, A. L. Gifford, S. M. Asch, and E. J. Groessl. 2015. Integrated care increases treatment and improves outcomes of patients with chronic hepatitis C virus infection and psychiatric illness or substance abuse. *Clinical Gastroenterology and Hepatology* 13(11):2005-2014.

Ho, S. B., A. Dollarhide, H. Thorisdottir, J. Michelsen, C. Perry, D. Kravetz, A. Herrin, L. Carlson, S. Hadley, D. Montoya, S. Robinson, C. Sanchez, E. Enrique, and E. Groessl. 2016. A primary care-based collaborative hepatitis C clinic: Clinical structure and virologic outcomes with direct acting antiviral therapy. *Open Medicine Journal* 3(Suppl 1: M4):70-78.

Honeck, J., and T. Dolansky. 2011. The Ryan White HIV drug assistance program: A vital part of Ohio's public health infrastructure. *State Budgeting Matters* 7(8). http:// www.communitysolutions.com/assets/docs/State_Budgeting_Matters/sbmv7n8ryanwhite report100711.pdf (accessed October 25, 2016).

HRSA (Health Resources and Services Administration). 2015. *Ryan White HIV/AIDS program: Part B manual.* http://hab.hrsa.gov/sites/default/files/hab/Global/habpartbmanual 2013.pdf (accessed December 8, 2016).

HRSA. 2016a. *About the Ryan White HIV/AIDS program.* https://hab.hrsa.gov/about-ryan-white-hivaids-program/about-ryan-white-hivaids-program (accessed December 8, 2016).

HRSA. 2016b. *Federally qualified health centers (FQHC) and Federal Office of Rural Health Policy (FORHP) rural health areas.* https://datawarehouse.hrsa.gov/ExportedMaps/ORHP/HGDWMapGallery_ORHP_FQHC.pdf (accessed December 9, 2016).

HRSA. 2016c. *Part B: Grants to states & territories.* https://hab.hrsa.gov/about-ryan-white-hivaids-program/part-b-grants-states-territories (accessed December 8, 2016).

HRSA. n.d.-a. *Ryan White HIV/AIDS program services: Eligible individuals & allowable uses of funds. Policy clarification notice (PCN) #16-02.* http://hab.hrsa.gov/sites/default/files/hab/Global/service_category_pcn_16-02_final.pdf (accessed October 25, 2016).

HRSA. n.d.-b. *What are federally qualified health centers (FQHCs)?* http://www.hrsa.gov/healthit/toolbox/RuralHealthITtoolbox/Introduction/qualified.html (accessed December 8, 2016).

Hu, D. J. 2008. *Issues related to the prevention and control of hepatitis B virus (HBV) infection in the U.S.* Paper presented at Institute of Medicine Roundtable on the Prevention and Control of Viral Hepatitis Infection, Washington, DC, December 4.

Hu, D. J., J. Xing, R. A. Tohme, Y. Liao, H. Pollack, J. W. Ward, and S. D. Holmberg. 2013. Hepatitis B testing and access to care among racial and ethnic minorities in selected communities across the United States, 2009-2010. *Hepatology* 58(3):856-862.

Hutton, D. W., D. Tan, S. K. So, and M. L. Brandeau. 2007. Cost-effectiveness of screening and vaccinating Asian and Pacific Islander adults for hepatitis B. *Annals of Internal Medicine* 147(7):460-469.

Hyun, C. S., W. R. Ventura, S. S. Kim, S. Yoon, and S. Lee. 2016. A community-based hepatitis B linkage-to-care program: A case study on Asian Americans chronically infected with hepatitis B virus. *Hepatology, Medicine and Policy* 1(1).

Jaffe, M. G., G. A. Lee, J. D. Young, S. Sidney, and A. S. Go. 2013. Improved blood pressure control associated with a large-scale hypertension program. *JAMA* 310(7):699-705.

Jenco, M. 2016. ACIP updates recommendations on HPV, HepB, MenB vaccines. *American Academy of Pediatrics (AAP) News.* http://www.aappublications.org/news/2016/10/20/ACIP102016 (accessed November 21, 2016).

Johnson, N. J., M. Ip, D. D. Munoz, and F. Laraque. 2016. *Using qualitative evaluation to strengthen hepatitis B and C health promotion by patients navigators for hard-to-reach populations.* https://nphic.confex.com/cdc/nphic16/webprogram/Paper36897.html (accessed November 14, 2016).

Juon, H. S., C. Strong, F. Kim, E. Park, and S. Lee. 2016. Lay health worker intervention improved compliance and hepatitis B vaccination in Asian Americans: Randomized controlled trial. *PLoS One* 11(9):e0162683.

Kansas Department of Health and Environment. n.d. *The Kansas Ryan White Part B program.* http://www.kdheks.gov/sti_hiv/ryan_white_care.htm#MHSA (accessed October 19, 2016).

Kanwal, F., J. R. Kramer, P. Buchanan, S. M. Asch, Y. Assioun, B. R. Bacon, J. Li, and H. B. El-Serag. 2012. The quality of care provided to patients with cirrhosis and ascites in the Department of Veterans Affairs. *Gastroenterology* 143(1):70-77.

Klink, K., M. Coffman, M. Moore, A. Jetty, S. Petterson, and A. Bazemore. 2015. *Family physicians and telehealth: Findings from a national survey.* Washington, DC: Robert Graham Center.

Kuncio, D. E., E. C. Newbern, M. H. Fernandez-Vina, B. Herdman, C. C. Johnson, and K. M. Viner. 2015. Comparison of risk-based hepatitis C screening and the true seroprevalence in an urban prison system. *Journal of Urban Health* 92(2):379-386.

Kvamme, O. J., F. Olesen, and M. Samuelson. 2001. Improving the interface between primary and secondary care: A statement from the European Working Party on Quality in Family Practice (EQuiP). *Quality in Health Care* 10(1):33-39.

Larney, S., M. K. Mahowald, N. Scharff, T. P. Flanigan, C. G. Beckwith, and N. D. Zaller. 2014. Epidemiology of hepatitis C virus in Pennsylvania state prisons, 2004–2012: Limitations of 1945–1965 birth cohort screening in correctional settings. *American Journal of Public Health* 104(6):e69-e74.

Lebrun-Harris, L. A., T. P. Baggett, D. M. Jenkins, A. Sripipatana, R. Sharma, A. S. Hayashi, C. A. Daly, and Q. Ngo-Metzger. 2013. Health status and health care experiences among homeless patients in federally supported health centers: Findings from the 2009 patient survey. *Health Services Research* 48(3):992-1017.

Lin, S. Y., E. T. Chang, and S. K. So. 2007. Why we should routinely screen Asian American adults for hepatitis B: A cross-sectional study of Asians in California. *Hepatology* 46(4):1034-1040.

Lin, Y. H., Y. Wang, A. Loua, G. J. Day, Y. Qiu, E. C. Nadala, Jr., J. P. Allain, and H. H. Lee. 2008. Evaluation of a new hepatitis B virus surface antigen rapid test with improved sensitivity. *Journal of Clinical Microbiology* 46(10):3319-3324.

Macalino, G. E., D. Vlahov, S. Sanford-Colby, S. Patel, K. Sabin, C. Salas, and J. D. Rich. 2004. Prevalence and incidence of HIV, hepatitis B virus, and hepatitis C virus infections among males in Rhode Island prisons. *American Journal of Public Health* 94(7):1218-1223.

Macalino, G. E., D. Dhawan, and J. D. Rich. 2005. A missed opportunity: Hepatitis C screening of prisoners. *American Journal of Public Health* 95(10):1739-1740.

Martyn, H., and K. Davis. 2014. Care coordination for people with complex care needs in the U.S.: A policy analysis. *International Journal of Care Coordination* 17(3-4):93-98.

Marwick, C. 1997. NCQA: Quality through evaluation. *JAMA* 278(19):1555-1556.

Mast, E. E., H. S. Margolis, A. E. Fiore, E. W. Brink, S. T. Goldstein, S. A. Wang, L. A. Moyer, B. P. Bell, and M. J. Alter. 2005. A comprehensive immunization strategy to eliminate transmission of hepatitis B virus infection in the United States. Recommendations of the Advisory Committee on Immunization Practices (ACIP). Part 1: Immunization of infants, children, and adolescents. *Morbidity and Mortality Weekly Report* 54(RR-16):1-31.

Maurer, K., and E. F. Gondles. 2015. Hepatitis C in correctional settings: Challenges and opportunities. *Coalition of Correctional Health Authorities and American Correctional Association* 2(1).

McCarthy, M. 2015. A quarter of U.S. adults with health insurance are underinsured, report finds. *BMJ* 350:h2786.

McGlynn, E. A. 1997. Six challenges in measuring the quality of health care. *Health Affairs* 16(3):7-21.

McInnes, D. K., B. A. Petrakis, A. L. Gifford, S. R. Rao, T. K. Houston, S. M. Asch, and T. P. O'Toole. 2014. Retaining homeless veterans in outpatient care: A pilot study of mobile phone text message appointment reminders. *American Journal of Public Health* 104(Suppl 4):S588-S594.

McMahon, B. J. 2009. The natural history of chronic hepatitis B virus infection. *Hepatology* 49(5 Suppl):S45-S55.

Mehta, S. H., J. Astemborski, G. D. Kirk, S. A. Strathdee, K. E. Nelson, D. Vlahov, and D. L. Thomas. 2011. Changes in blood-borne infection risk among injection drug users. *Journal of Infectious Diseases* 203(5):587-594.

Mellinger, J. L., and M. L. Volk. 2013. Multidisciplinary management of patients with cirrhosis: A need for care coordination. *Clinical Gastroenterology and Hepatology* 11(3):217-223.

Mitchell, T., G. L. Armstrong, D. J. Hu, A. Wasley, and J. A. Painter. 2011. The increasing burden of imported chronic hepatitis B—United States, 1974-2008. *PLoS One* 6(12):e27717.

Mitruka, K., K. Thornton, S. Cusick, C. Orme, A. Moore, R. A. Manch, T. Box, C. Carroll, D. Holtzman, and J. W. Ward. 2014. Expanding primary care capacity to treat hepatitis C virus infection through an evidence-based care model—Arizona and Utah, 2012-2014. *Morbidity and Mortality Weekly Report* 63(18):393-398.

NASEM (National Academies of Sciences, Engineering, and Medicine). 2016. *Eliminating the public health problem of hepatitis B and C in the United States: Phase one report.* Washington, DC: The National Academies Press.

NCCHC (National Commission on Correctional Health Care). 1998. National Commission on Correctional Health Care position statement. Use of telemedicine technology in correctional facilities. *Journal of Correctional Health Care* 5(1):103-111.

NCCHC. 2016. Telemedicine technology in correctional facilities. *National Commission on Correctional Health Care.* http://www.ncchc.org/telemedicine-technology-in-correctional-facilities (accessed September 23, 2016).

NCQA (National Committee for Quality Assurance). 2009. *Childhood immunization status.* http://www.ncqa.org/portals/0/Childhood%20Immunization%20Status.pdf (accessed November 3, 2016).

NCQA. 2012. *The value of requiring health plans to report NCQA's HEDIS quality measures.* http://www.ncqa.org/portals/0/Public%20Policy/ValueinRequiringHEDIS_8.15.12.pdf (accessed November 3, 2016).

NCQA. 2016a. *HEDIS & quality measurement.* http://store.ncqa.org/index.php/performance-measurement.html (accessed November 3, 2016).

NCQA. 2016b. *Summary table of measures, product lines and changes.* http://www.ncqa.org/Portals/0/HEDISQM/HEDIS2017/HEDIS%202017%20Volume%202%20List%20of%20Measures.pdf?ver=2016-06-27-135433-350 (accessed November 7, 2016).

NCQA. n.d.-a. *HEDIS® and Quality Compass®.* http://www.ncqa.org/hedis-quality-measurement/what-is-hedis (accessed November 3, 2016).

NCQA. n.d.-b. *HEDIS® measures.* http://www.ncqa.org/hedis-quality-measurement/hedis-measures (accessed October 31, 2016).

Neate, R. 2016. Welcome to Jail Inc: How private companies make money off U.S. prisons. *Guardian*, June 16. https://www.theguardian.com/us-news/2016/jun/16/us-prisons-jail-private-healthcare-companies-profit (accessed December 28, 2016).

Nelson, P. K., B. M. Mathers, B. Cowie, H. Hagan, D. Des Jarlais, D. Horyniak, and L. Degenhardt. 2011. Global epidemiology of hepatitis B and hepatitis C in people who inject drugs: Results of systematic reviews. *Lancet* 378(9791):571-583.

NIDA (National Institute on Drug Abuse). 2010. *Research report series. Comorbidity: Addiction and other mental illnesses. NIH publication number 10-5771.* National Institutes of Health, NIDA.

Njai, H. F., Y. Shimakawa, B. Sanneh, L. Ferguson, G. Ndow, M. Mendy, A. Sow, G. Lo, C. Toure-Kane, J. Tanaka, M. Taal, U. D'Alessandro, R. Njie, M. Thursz, and M. Lemoine. 2015. Validation of rapid point-of-care (POC) tests for detection of hepatitis B surface antigen in field and laboratory settings in the Gambia, Western Africa. *Journal of Clinical Microbiology* 53(4):1156-1163.

Patel, K., M. Darling, K. Samuels, and McClellan. 2014. Transforming rural health care: High-quality, sustainable access to specialty care. *Health Affairs Blog*, December 5. http://healthaffairs.org/blog/2014/12/05/transforming-rural-health-care-high-quality-sustainable-access-to-specialty-care (accessed December 9, 2016).

Pfeiffer, S. 2016. Overwhelmed by overdoses, clinic offers a room for highs. *Boston Globe*, April 26. https://www.bostonglobe.com/business/2016/04/25/overwhelmed-overdose-epidemic-health-clinic-offers-room-for-supervised-highs/vQ61K3jao0vXNUPHK0iQhP/story.html (accessed December 7, 2016).

Post, S. E., N. K. Sodhi, C. H. Peng, K. Wan, and H. J. Pollack. 2011. A simulation shows that early treatment of chronic hepatitis B infection can cut deaths and be cost-effective. *Health Affairs* 30(2):340-348.

Project ECHO. n.d.-a. *About ECHO*. http://echo.unm.edu/about-echo/ (accessed November 2, 2016).

Project ECHO. n.d.-b. *CDC and western states consortium*. http://echo.unm.edu/initiatives/cdc-western-states-consortium (accessed October 31, 2016).

Project ECHO. n.d.-c. *Funders*. http://echo.unm.edu/about-echo/funders (accessed October 31, 2016).

Project ECHO. n.d.-d. *Our story*. http://echo.unm.edu/about-echo/our-story (accessed November 2, 2016).

Rabuy, B., and D. Kopf. 2015. Prisons of poverty: Uncovering the pre-incarceration incomes of the imprisoned. *Prison Policy Initiative*. http://www.prisonpolicy.org/reports/income.html (accessed September 23, 2016).

Reimer, J., and C. Haasen. 2009. Need-adapted HCV-treatment setting for injection drug users. *Lancet* 373(9681):2090-2091.

Rich, J. D., R. Chandler, B. A. Williams, D. Dumont, E. A. Wang, F. S. Taxman, S. A. Allen, J. G. Clarke, R. B. Greifinger, C. Wildeman, F. C. Osher, S. Rosenberg, C. Haney, M. Mauer, and B. Western. 2014. How health care reform can transform the health of criminal justice-involved individuals. *Health Affairs* 33(3):462-467.

Roberts, H., D. Kruszon-Moran, K. N. Ly, E. Hughes, K. Iqbal, R. B. Jiles, and S. D. Holmberg. 2016. Prevalence of chronic hepatitis B virus (HBV) infection in U.S. households: National Health and Nutrition Examination Survey (NHANES), 1988-2012. *Hepatology* 63(2):388-397.

Rubin, R. 2016. U.S. prisons missing opportunities to tackle HIV in inmates. *Lancet* 388(10049):1041.

Rural Health Information Hub. 2016. *Nonmetropolitan federally qualified health centers*. https://www.ruralhealthinfo.org/rural-maps/mapfiles/federally-qualified-health-centers.jpg (December 8, 2016).

SAMHSA (Substance Abuse and Mental Health Services Administration). 2015. *Behavioral health trends in the United States: Results from the 2014 National Survey on Drug Use and Health*. Rockville, MD: SAMHSA.

Sarfaty, M., and R. E. Myers. 2008. The effect of HEDIS measurement of colorectal cancer screening on insurance plans in Pennsylvania. *American Journal of Managed Care* 14(5):277-282.

Sarpel, D., E. Baichoo, and D. T. Dieterich. 2016. Chronic hepatitis B and C infection in the United States: A review of current guidelines, disease burden and cost effectiveness of screening. *Expert Review of Anti-Infective Therapy* 14(5):511-521.

Schaenman, P., E. Davies, R. Jordan, and R. Chakraborty. 2013. *Opportunities for cost savings in corrections without sacrificing service quality: Inmate health care*. Washington, DC: Urban Institute.

Schiff, M. 2014. Examining state prison health care spending: Cost drivers and policy approaches. *Health Affairs Blog*, November 4. http://healthaffairs.org/blog/2014/11/04/examining-state-prison-health-care-spending-cost-drivers-and-policy-approaches (accessed September 23, 2016).

Sequera, V. G., A. L. Garcia-Basteiro, and J. M. Bayas. 2013. The role of vaccination in prisoners' health. *Expert Review of Vaccines* 12(5):469-471.

Shafer, M. A., K. P. Tebb, R. H. Pantell, C. J. Wibbelsman, J. M. Neuhaus, A. C. Tipton, S. B. Kunin, T. H. Ko, D. M. Schweppe, and D. A. Bergman. 2002. Effect of a clinical practice improvement intervention on chlamydial screening among adolescent girls. *JAMA* 288(22):2846-2852.

Shalev, N., M. A. Chiasson, J. F. Dobkin, and G. Lee. 2011. Characterizing medical providers for jail inmates in New York state. *American Journal of Public Health* 101(4):693-698.

Shivkumar, S., R. Peeling, Y. Jafari, L. Joseph, and N. P. Pai. 2012. Rapid point-of-care first-line screening tests for hepatitis B infection: A meta-analysis of diagnostic accuracy (1980-2010). *American Journal of Gastroenterology* 107(9):1306-1313.

Singh, H., A. Esquivel, D. F. Sittig, D. Murphy, H. Kadiyala, R. Schiesser, D. Espadas, and L. A. Petersen. 2011. Follow-up actions on electronic referral communication in a multispecialty outpatient setting. *Journal of General Internal Medicine* 26(1):64-69.

Smith, E. A., L. Jacques-Carroll, T. Y. Walker, B. Sirotkin, and T. V. Murphy. 2012. The national perinatal hepatitis B prevention program, 1994-2008. *Pediatrics* 129(4):609-616.

Solomon, L., B. T. Montague, C. G. Beckwith, J. Baillargeon, M. Costa, D. Dumont, I. Kuo, A. Kurth, and J. D. Rich. 2014. Survey finds that many prisons and jails have room to improve HIV testing and coordination of postrelease treatment. *Health Affairs* 33(3):434-442.

Sood, N., T. Juday, J. Vanderpuye-Orgle, L. Rosenblatt, J. A. Romley, D. Peneva, and D. P. Goldman. 2014. HIV care providers emphasize the importance of the Ryan White program for access to and quality of care. *Health Affairs* 33(3):394-400.

Spooner, L. M. 2011. The expanding role of the pharmacist in the management of hepatitis C infection. *Journal of Managed Care Pharmacy* 17(9):709-712.

St. Joseph's Hospital and Medical Center. n.d. *Liver/hepatology.* http://www.dignityhealth.org/stjosephs/research-and-education/research/research-areas/liver-or-hepatology (accessed November 8, 2016).

Stein, J. A., R. M. Andersen, M. Robertson, and L. Gelberg. 2012. Impact of hepatitis B and C infection on health services utilization in homeless adults: A test of the Gelberg-Andersen behavioral model for vulnerable populations. *Health Psychology* 31(1):20-30.

Stockman, L. J., J. Greer, R. Holzmacher, B. Dittmann, S. A. Hoftiezer, L. E. Alsum, A. Prieve, R. P. Westergaard, S. M. Guilfoyle, and J. M. Vergeront. 2016. Performance of risk-based and birth-cohort strategies for identifying hepatitis C virus infection among people entering prison, Wisconsin, 2014. *Public Health Reports* 131(4):544-551.

Taylor, L. E. 2005. Delivering care to injection drug users coinfected with HIV and hepatitis C virus. *Clinical Infectious Diseases* 40(Suppl 5):S355-S361.

Taylor, V. M., T. G. Hislop, S. P. Tu, C. Teh, E. Acorda, M. P. Yip, E. Woodall, and Y. Yasui. 2009. Evaluation of a hepatitis B lay health worker intervention for Chinese Americans and Canadians. *Journal of Community Health* 34(3):165-172.

Taylor, V. M., N. J. Burke, C. Sos, H. H. Do, Q. Liu, and Y. Yasui. 2013. Community health worker hepatitis B education for Cambodian American men and women. *Asian Pacific Journal of Cancer Prevention* 14(8):4705-4709.

The Economist. 2016. How many homeless people are there in America? February 22. http://www.economist.com/blogs/democracyinamerica/2016/02/counting-street-sleepers (accessed October 27, 2016).

The National Alliance to End Homelessness. 2016. *The state of homelessness in America.* Washington, DC: Homelessness Research Institute.

The Physicians Foundation. 2016. *2016 survey of America's physicians: Practice patterns & perspectives.* The Physicians Foundation.

Thomas, D. L., D. Leoutsakas, T. Zabransky, and M. S. Kumar. 2011. Hepatitis C in HIV-infected individuals: Cure and control, right now. *Journal of the International AIDS Society* 14:22.

Thornton, K., P. Deming, B. Struminger, M. Sedillo, E. Castillo, M. Komaromy, S. Zalud-Cerrato, and S. Arora. 2016. Project ECHO: A revolutionary approach to expanding access to modern treatments for hepatitis C. *Current Hepatology Reports* 15(3):178-186.

Tompsett, C. J., S. E. Domoff, and P. A. Toro. 2013. Peer substance use and homelessness predicting substance abuse from adolescence through early adulthood. *American Journal of Community Psychology* 51(3-4):520-529.

Tracy, C. S., S. H. Bell, L. A. Nickell, J. Charles, and R. E. Upshur. 2013. The IMPACT clinic: Innovative model of interprofessional primary care for elderly patients with complex health care needs. *Canadian Family Physician* 59(3):e148-e155.

Tran, T. T. 2009. Understanding cultural barriers in hepatitis B virus infection. *Cleveland Clinic Journal of Medicine* 76(Suppl 3):S10-S13.

Treloar, C., J. Newland, J. Rance, and M. Hopwood. 2010. Uptake and delivery of hepatitis C treatment in opiate substitution treatment: Perceptions of clients and health professionals. *Journal of Viral Hepatitis* 17(12):839-844.

U.K. Department of Health. 2009. *Guidance notes: Prison health performance and quality indicators.* http://webarchive.nationalarchives.gov.uk/20140714084352/http://www.hpa. org.uk/webc/HPAwebFile/HPAweb_C/1232006593707 (accessed September 23, 2016).

U.K. Government. 2011. *Prison health performance and quality indicators: Annual report 2011.* https://www.gov.uk/government/uploads/system/uploads/attachment_data/file/215077/dh_133381.pdf (accessed September 23, 2016).

Unützer, J., Y. Choi, I. A. Cook, and S. Oishi. 2002a. A web-based data management system to improve care for depression in a multicenter clinical trial. *Psychiatric Services* 53(6):671-673, 678.

Unützer, J., W. Katon, C. M. Callahan, J. W. Williams, Jr., E. Hunkeler, L. Harpole, M. Hoffing, R. D. Della Penna, P. H. Noel, E. H. Lin, P. A. Arean, M. T. Hegel, L. Tang, T. R. Belin, S. Oishi, and C. Langston. 2002b. Collaborative care management of late-life depression in the primary care setting: A randomized controlled trial. *JAMA* 288(22):2836-2845.

USPSTF (U.S. Preventive Services Task Force). 2013. *Final recommendation statement: Hepatitis C: Screening.* https://www.uspreventiveservicestaskforce.org/Page/Document/RecommendationStatementFinal/hepatitis-c-screening (accessed December 8, 2016).

USPSTF. 2014. *Final update summary: Hepatitis B virus infection: Screening, 2014.* https://www.uspreventiveservicestaskforce.org/Page/Document/UpdateSummaryFinal/hepatitis-b-virus-infection-screening-2014 (accessed November 7, 2016).

USPSTF. 2015. *Final update summary: Hepatitis B in pregnant women: Screening.* https://www.uspreventiveservicestaskforce.org/Page/Document/UpdateSummaryFinal/hepatitis-b-in-pregnant-women-screening (accessed November 7, 2016).

VA (Department of Veterans Affairs). 2016. *Hepatitis C medications: A review and update for patients.* http://www.hepatitis.va.gov/products/patient/treatment-update.asp#S11X (accessed November 3, 2016).

Volk, M. L., R. S. Tocco, J. Bazick, M. O. Rakoski, and A. S. Lok. 2012. Hospital readmissions among patients with decompensated cirrhosis. *American Journal of Gastroenterology* 107(2):247-252.

Von Zielbauer, P. 2005. As health care in jails goes private, 10 days can be a death sentence. *New York Times*, February 27. http://www.nytimes.com/2005/02/27/nyregion/as-health-care-in-jails-goes-private-10-days-can-be-a-death.html?_r=0 (accessed December 27, 2016).

Walsh, N., A. Verster, M. Rodolph, and E. A. Akl. 2014. WHO guidance on the prevention of viral hepatitis B and C among people who inject drugs. *International Journal on Drug Policy* 25(3):363-371.

Weinbaum, C., R. Lyerla, and H. S. Margolis. 2003. Prevention and control of infections with hepatitis viruses in correctional settings. *Morbidity and Mortality Weekly Report* 52(RR-01):1-33.

Weinbaum, C. M., K. M. Sabin, and S. S. Santibanez. 2005. Hepatitis B, hepatitis C, and HIV in correctional populations: A review of epidemiology and prevention. *AIDS* 19(Suppl 3):S41-S46.

West Virginia Department of Health and Human Resources. n.d. *Ryan White eligibility: WV Ryan White Part B state direct services.* http://www.dhhr.wv.gov/oeps/std-hiv-hep/HIV_AIDS/caresupport/Pages/RyanWhiteEligibility.aspx (accessed October 25, 2016).

WHO (World Health Organization). 2001. *Hepatitis B surface antigen assays: Operational characteristics (phase I). Report 1.* Geneva, Switzerland: WHO.

WHO. 2016. *Global health sector strategy on viral hepatitis, 2016-2021: Towards ending viral hepatitis.* Geneva, Switzerland: WHO. http://apps.who.int/iris/bitstream/10665/246177/1/WHO-HIV-2016.06-eng.pdf (accessed July 19, 2016).

Wilkinson, M., V. Crawford, A. Tippet, F. Jolly, J. Turton, E. Sims, M. Hekker, J. Dalton, R. Marley, and G. R. Foster. 2009. Community-based treatment for chronic hepatitis C in drug users: High rates of compliance with therapy despite ongoing drug use. *Alimentary Pharmacology & Therapeutics* 29(1):29-37.

Woo, G. A., M. A. Hill, M. D. de Medina, and E. R. Schiff. 2013. Screening for hepatitis B virus and hepatitis C virus at a community fair: A single-center experience. *Gastroenterology & Hepatology* 9(5):293-299.

Yoo, G. J., T. Fang, J. Zola, and W. M. Dariotis. 2012. Destigmatizing hepatitis B in the Asian American community: Lessons learned from the San Francisco Hep B free campaign. *Journal of Cancer Education* 27(1):138-144.

Yusuf, H. R., D. Daniels, P. Smith, V. Coronado, and L. Rodewald. 2000. Association between administration of hepatitis B vaccine at birth and completion of the hepatitis B and 4:3:1:3 vaccine series. *JAMA* 284(8):978-983.

Zhao, Z., and T. V. Murphy. 2013. Which newborns missed the hepatitis B birth dose vaccination among U.S. children? *Preventive Medicine* 57(5):613-617.

Zivanovic, R., M. Milloy, K. Hayashi, H. Dong, C. Sutherland, T. Kerr, and E. Wood. 2015. Impact of unstable housing on all-cause mortality among persons who inject drugs. *BMC Public Health* 15:106.

Zlotnick, C., S. Zerger, and P. B. Wolfe. 2013. Health care for the homeless: What we have learned in the past 30 years and what's next. *American Journal of Public Health* 103(Suppl 2):S199-S205.

6

Financing Elimination

Financial backing from government has been a characteristic of successful disease elimination programs around the world. The goals set out in Chapter 2 are feasible but ambitious, set in recognition of the United States' resources and its responsibility to the global viral hepatitis elimination effort. This report describes the committee's assessment of the best strategy for meeting these targets. The previous chapters have described ways to expand preventive services and treatment, strategies for reaching new patients, and ensuring successful treatment for those already in care. Eliminating the public health problem of hepatitis B and C is still a bold goal, and reaching it will require more money for prevention and treatment. This chapter discusses strategies to increase funding for viral hepatitis elimination and ways to reduce the cost of treatment.

AN INCREASED PATIENT BURDEN

Eliminating viral hepatitis will require increasing the preventive and therapeutic services currently available. The models presented in Chapter 2 depend on improvement to the diagnosis, treatment, and care of viral hepatitis patients. There will be an expense to finding these patients, as well as to the improved harm reduction, vaccination, and prevention of mother-to-child transmission programs described in Chapter 4 and the changes in service delivery recommended in Chapter 5.

But failure to act against viral hepatitis will also come at a high cost. The burden of hepatitis C, for example, is greatest among people born between 1945 and 1965 (Smith et al., 2012; USPSTF, 2013). As these patients age, more of them will develop liver cancer and cirrhosis. Increasing cost and greater demand for treatment will put a particular strain on government payers (Pyenson et al., 2009). By a 2009 reckoning, Medicare alone stood to absorb a fivefold increase in hepatitis C expenses (from $5 to $30 billion per year) between 2009 and 2030 (Pyenson et al., 2009). The introduction of direct-acting antiviral therapies has only increased this estimate. A recent analysis estimated $136 billion in hepatitis C drug costs between 2015 and 2020 in the United States, of which government payers would fund $61 billion (Chhatwal et al., 2015).

Such estimates do not begin to account for later consequences of chronic viral hepatitis. Hepatitis C virus (HCV) infection has been a cause of about 2,000 liver transplantations a year over the last 15 years (HRSA, 2016b; Luu, 2015; Razavi, 2016). Chronic hepatitis B virus (HBV) infection, though considerably less common in the United States, accounts for another 6 percent of transplantations, over 400 annually (HRSA, 2016b; Luu, 2015). Transplantation poses complicated ethical questions to society, driven in part by the scarcity of donor organs relative to the number of transplant candidates. Action to prevent the downstream consequences of HBV and HCV infection would reduce this scarcity for the nearly 15,000 patients a year on the liver transplant list (HRSA, 2016c). Such action would clearly benefit these patients, almost 30 percent of whom die on the waiting list (Gheorghe et al., 2005; Kim et al., 2016).

A more direct estimate of the cost of inaction against viral hepatitis is shown in Chapter 2. Improving the diagnosis, treatment, and care for hepatitis B patients could result in a 50 percent cumulative reduction in HBV-related deaths by 2030. Similar measures, combined with unrestricted treatment of all hepatitis C patients, could result in a 65 percent reduction in the annual number of HCV-related deaths in 2030 compared to 2015. It is difficult to measure the cost to society of averting 90,000 deaths over the next 15 years. For the purposes of economic analysis, the Environmental Protection Agency assigns a statistical value of $7.4 million[1] to a life saved (EPA, n.d.). At this rate, the cost of neglecting hepatitis elimination is over $666 billion before 2030.

The World Health Organization (WHO) reckons that viral hepatitis elimination could cost up to $11 billion a year by 2025 (Alcorn, 2015). In theory, the United States' share of this sum should be considerably less, almost modest in the face of the human and financial costs of inaction. But the WHO estimate does not account for the high cost of health care in the United States, especially the high price of innovator pharmaceuticals. Between 2014 and the first quarter of 2016, the United States spent over $25 billion on hepatitis C direct-acting antivirals alone (Altarum Institute,

---

[1] In 2006 dollars.

2016; Roy et al., 2016). The cost of viral hepatitis elimination could easily spiral without government supervision.

While elimination of hepatitis B and C as public health problems is possible in the United States, the goal cannot be met without increased appropriations. Congress is in the best position to marshal funds to implement the strategy outline in this report. In 2016, it allocated over a billion dollars to treat hepatitis C in veterans (Leston and Finkbonner, 2016; VA, 2016b). The committee commends this decision and sees complementary spending on testing and treatment among a wider patient group as the best strategy to protect the taxpayers' investment. One way to increase spending on viral hepatitis would be a discretionary program either modeled on or adapted from the Ryan White Comprehensive AIDS Resources Emergency Act of 1990 (hereafter, the Ryan White Act).

A Discretionary Program

A discretionary program allows legislators a straightforward way to track the effects of their spending. Programs targeted to a specific disease are relatively easy to monitor over time. For viral hepatitis, the time in question is short—only 15 years. It might, therefore, be most efficient to use an existing framework to reach these patients. As discussed in Chapter 5, the Ryan White Act provides for HIV patients who cannot otherwise afford treatment, including full HCV treatment for beneficiaries who also have hepatitis C. Because there is significant overlap in risk factors for HIV and HCV, outreach and social services for people with HIV could be used for HCV patients.

About a third of HIV patients in the United States have viral hepatitis infections (CDC, 2014b). HBV and HCV are particularly dangerous to someone with HIV: the infections progress more quickly, and the risk of liver failure and liver-related death can be triple that of someone without HIV (CDC, 2014b; Grebely et al., 2013; Lo Re et al., 2014; Price and Thio, 2010; Thomas et al., 2011). With this in mind, the Health Resources and Services Administration (HRSA) recently reminded Ryan White program managers of their responsibility to screen HIV patients for HCV, and of guidelines for treating viral hepatitis with HIV coinfection (HRSA, 2015). Ryan White beneficiaries disproportionately represent groups at high risk of viral hepatitis. HRSA estimates that about 45 percent of its ~500,000 Ryan White clients are men who have sex with men; another 8.3 percent use injection drugs; roughly half fall in the 1945 to 1965 birth cohort (HRSA, 2016d). The program also reaches patients whom other assistance programs may not. As of 2013, before the Affordable Care Act was fully in effect, more than a quarter of Ryan White clients were uninsured (HRSA, 2016d).

One of the most meaningful features of the Ryan White Act is the AIDS Drug Assistance Programs it established in every state. Even states with a low disease burden received $500,000 infrastructure awards (IOM, 2004; Martin et al., 2006). Setting eligibility for assistance and enrollment in the program is a state responsibility; states purchase the drugs at discounts of 25 to 50 percent through the 340B program discussed later in this chapter. Patients enrolled in the program can seek treatment from any provider, but the state covers their medicines, an exception to the general rules of the 340B program. States have also negotiated directly with manufacturers for discounts beyond what 340B offers (*Kaiser Health News*, 2003). With help from the National Alliance of State and Territorial AIDS Directors, the states were able to reduce the cost of HIV drugs for Ryan White clients by $300 million below the 340B discount price in 2014 (ADAP Crisis Task Force, 2016). Cumulative savings between 2003 and 2014 for these patients were more than $2.3 billion (ADAP Crisis Task Force, 2016).

The drugs that cure hepatitis C infection are expensive, a problem discussed in the next section. The antivirals used to treat chronic hepatitis B are also costly. The Red Book lists a wholesale price for a year's supply of entecavir and its generic version at $16,467 and $8,252.16, respectively (Truven Health Analytics, 2017). The average annual cost for tenofovir, for which no generic version exists, is listed at $11,973 (Truven Health Analytics, 2017). For Medicare Part D beneficiaries, out-of-pocket costs for both drugs range from about $10,000 to $18,000 (Q1Medicare, 2016). Both are listed on Medicare's formulary as tier 5 specialty drugs, for which patients can expect to pay 25 to 33 percent, though some drug companies offer discounts to offset the out-of-pocket costs (Bristol-Meyers Squibb, n.d.; Gilead, n.d.; Q1Medicare, n.d.).

Since 2003, states have also been able to assist Ryan White beneficiaries with health insurance costs, such as premiums, coinsurance, co-pays, and deductibles, as long as the private insurer provides prescription drug coverage equivalent to what the state's AIDS Drug Assistance Program would offer (HRSA, 2007, n.d.-d). The goal of this adjustment is to improve efficiency and save money, and HRSA is clear that in order for a health plan to be subsidized by the state, the cost sharing strategy needs to be cheaper, at least in aggregate, than purchasing the HIV drugs directly (HRSA, 2014). More importantly, this combination of access to the 340B prices and the ability to share the cost of private insurance allows states to stretch their drug assistance funding (HRSA, 2007, 2016a).

Nevertheless, as of June 2016, the National Alliance of State and Territorial AIDS Directors found that only 20 states covered direct-acting antivirals to treat hepatitis C in their AIDS Drug Assistance Program formularies (NASTAD, 2016). Treatment of people infected only with HBV or HCV (and not HIV) is disallowed under the Ryan White Act, the last reauthorization of which expired in 2013 (Kaiser Family Foundation, 2017;

Schmid, 2016; Stand, 2015). Permission to use Ryan White funds for this purpose would have to come from a statutory change.

As Chapter 5 discussed, Ryan White is the ideal infrastructure for reaching at least those hepatitis C patients who inject drugs. State Ryan White coordinators have, for the most part, already given extensive thought to questions of outreach among these patients and strategies to improve their adherence to treatment (CDPH, n.d.; Taylor, 2005). On the other hand, direct-acting antiviral therapy takes only 2 or 3 months. The strategy of buying insurance on behalf of a patient is less necessary for someone whose treatment will last only a short time. There is no reason states could not use their savings from cost sharing with private insurance companies to treat hepatitis C, however. By the same token, hepatitis B patients, who have a chronic viral infection, might be suitable candidates for assistance with health insurance.

Any modifications to the Ryan White Act should make it clear that any services for viral hepatitis patients would be in addition to the program's goal of supporting treatment for poor and uninsured HIV patients. It is also important to remember that the Ryan White Act was passed out of concern for poor and uninsured people facing a lifetime of expensive HIV treatment. Loosening restrictions on its funding to cover expensive direct-acting agents would be entirely consistent with the spirit of the law. It would also hasten the elimination of two chronic viral infections that pose particular risk to people with HIV.

A PURCHASING STRATEGY FOR MEDICINES

Government appropriations can go a long way to meeting the increased demand for services, vaccination, and treatment that viral hepatitis elimination will pose. At the same time, the political climate can sometimes prevent congressional action on public health problems. A federal appropriation of $1.1 billion for the response to Zika, a mosquito-borne virus that causes serious birth defects, was blocked for weeks during peak mosquito season in 2016 (Herszenhorn, 2016; McCarthy, 2016). If legislators cannot allocate funding for a disease with devastating consequences for newborns, it is realistic to consider the possibility that they will not come to quick agreement on spending for a disease widely associated with illicit drug use.

The price of the direct-acting antivirals that cure HCV infection is a major obstacle to wider treatment. Introduced at a list price of about $84,000 for a course of treatment, Gilead's Sovaldi®[2] (and later Harvoni®[3] introduced at $94,500 a course) put a strain on the budgets of public and

---

[2] The U.S. proprietary name of 90 mg of the viral NS5A inhibitor ledipasvir and 400 mg of sofosbuvir, a nucleotide inhibitor of the viral RNA polymerase.

[3] The U.S. proprietary name for sofosbuvir.

private payers alike (Fegraus and Ross, 2014). By some estimates, introduction of these medicines accounted for a third of the sharp increase in prescription drug expenditures in 2014 (Martin et al., 2016). Such prices are not affordable for most payers. Faced with the unenviable task of allocating scarce treatment, payers gave first priority to the sickest patients, those with advanced fibrosis or at immediate risk of cirrhosis or end-stage liver disease (Barua et al., 2015; Brennan and Shrank, 2014; Canary et al., 2015; Graham, 2016b). Many also imposed sobriety requirements, fearing that the risk of reinfection in active injection drug users was too great to justify the expense of treating them (Barua et al., 2015; Canary et al., 2015; Ellwood, 2014; UnitedHealthcare, 2015). Such restrictions met with widespread criticism (Abram, 2015; Freyer, 2016; Harper, 2015; Ramey, 2016; Salzman, 2015). Overt drug rationing offends the American public, but it is difficult to know how else to solve the problem a recent *Washington Post* editorial described as "the de facto rationing" of "excessive drug prices" (Rizvi et al., 2016).

Repeated lawsuits, especially against Medicaid, have resulted in loosening restrictions on treatment (Graham, 2016a; NVHR and CHLPI, 2016). In November 2015, the Centers for Medicare & Medicaid Services (CMS) responded to the restrictions in Medicaid. In an open letter, CMS reminded its state contacts that they were not free to deny coverage for "medically accepted indications" of an approved drug, and that neither the state nor its managed care organizations could use a standard more restrictive than the label indication for treatment (DeBoy, 2015). In its letter, CMS acknowledged the strain direct-acting antivirals put on state budgets but pointed to increasing market competition as a force for lowering prices (DeBoy, 2015).

It is unlikely that market forces alone will lower the prices on these drugs sharply or quickly enough to meet the targets set in Chapter 2. The goals described depend on prompt, large-scale treatment of hepatitis C, and the price of these drugs is a major obstacle to unrestricted treatment, especially for institutions of limited means such as the prison system and state Medicaid offices. No direct-acting antiviral will come off patent before 2029, 1 year before the target elimination date (DrugPatentWatch, n.d.). As Chapter 2 makes clear, delaying mass treatment would result in tens of thousands of needless deaths and billions of dollars in medical costs. It is the government's role to avoid such suffering, while still respecting the innovator drug companies' rights to financial compensation for the risk they took to bring a valuable product to market (Conti et al., 2016). Bulk purchasing for volume discounts can help state Medicaid programs and other buyers manage the drug cost, though a licensing strategy loosely inspired by the Vaccines for Children program may be more effective.

Public Purchase and the Vaccines for Children Program

Vaccines were not always a universal entitlement in the United States. For decades, spotty immunization left society vulnerable to outbreaks. In 1988 a measles epidemic starting in California caused 123 deaths and more than 11,000 hospitalizations (Atkinson et al., 1992a,b; CDC, 1992; Dales et al., 1993; Orenstein, 2006). The epidemic lasted for several years; most of its 55,000 victims were preschool children living in poor, densely populated, urban neighborhoods (Hinman et al., 2004; Orenstein, 2006). The National Vaccine Advisory Committee determined that failure to immunize children aged 12 to 15 months had caused the epidemic, and recommended a federal grant program fund the purchase and delivery of vaccines for children who were not insured for them (National Vaccine Advisory Committee, 1991; Orenstein, 2006). By the mid-1990s a goal of 90 percent immunization coverage in preschool children and a measles elimination effort brought increased attention to gaps in vaccination (Orenstein, 2006).

Charging parents for immunizations put uninsured and underinsured children at risk for missing them (Orenstein, 2006). But the government was reluctant to purchase childhood vaccines outright, as many children were covered by private insurance; it seemed wasteful to spend taxpayer money to relieve insurance companies of their obligations (Orenstein, 2006). There was also concern that a single payer could force vaccine prices too low, disrupting the pharmaceutical companies' risk calculation and discouraging future innovation (Orenstein, 2006). Created in 1993, Vaccines for Children was seen as a compromise between a single payer and the status quo (Hinman et al., 2004; Orenstein, 2006). Children under 19 who are eligible for Medicaid, uninsured, or whose insurance does not cover immunization, as well as any American Indian or Alaska Native child[4] can receive free vaccination through the program (CDC, 2014c; Hinman et al., 2004).

Vaccines for Children is an entitlement, meaning it does not undergo the annual congressional appropriations process (Hinman et al., 2004). The Centers for Disease Control and Prevention's (CDC's) Advisory Council on Immunization Practices (ACIP) recommends vaccines for inclusion in the program, the CDC then negotiates prices with manufacturers and awards funding (allocated through CMS) to organizations such as state health departments that order the discounted vaccines (CDC, 2014a; Shen et al., 2009). The government contracts with a distributor to deliver vaccines to the over 44,000 private providers and public clinics registered with the program (CDC, 2014a; Shen et al., 2009). These vaccines are given free of charge, although providers can bill a standard office visit or administration fee, keeping in mind that no child can be denied a vaccine because

---

[4] As defined by the Indian Health Care Improvement Act (25 USC 1603).

his or her family cannot afford the administration fee (Shen et al., 2009). The program makes publicly purchased vaccines available in the private sector, a feature that discourages referrals from private practice to public clinics, thereby relieving strain on health departments (Lindley et al., 2009; Zimmerman et al., 2001). Eliminating referrals also makes for more efficient practice with less chance to lose patients and information in transit (Hinman et al., 2004; Lindley et al., 2009).

State Medicaid programs and health departments save money because of Vaccines for Children, as do participating private clinics. Bulk purchase guarantees lower costs, and no clinic is obliged to front money to stock vaccines. Despite early worries, the program has not harmed manufacturers. ACIP regularly recommends new (often expensive) vaccines; schools and daycare centers often require immunization, sometimes with multiple doses (Lindley et al., 2009; Rosenthal, 2014). Vaccine manufacturers support the program, which reduces volume uncertainty and ensures access for uninsured and underinsured patients, a market they could otherwise miss (Coleman et al., 2005). And Vaccines for Children does not interfere with the strong private market, profits from which allow the companies to offer lower prices to the CDC (Shen et al., 2009).

A Similar Strategy for Hepatitis C

Much as the cost of vaccination contributed to the measles outbreak of the 1980s and 1990s, so can the high price of hepatitis treatment encourage future HCV outbreaks. This committee's previous report concluded that cost is the main reason that only 7 to 14 percent of hepatitis C patients had initiated treatment with direct-acting agents by 2015 (NASEM, 2016). Access is particularly bad among patients for whom the government buys treatment. A study of 2,321 prescriptions for direct-acting antivirals written between November 1, 2014, and April 20, 2015, found 16 percent of patients received an absolute denial (Lo Re et al., 2016). The rate of denial varied by insurance type, however; 46 percent of Medicaid patients were denied treatment, compared to 5 percent of Medicare and 10 percent of private insurance patients (Lo Re et al., 2016). Similarly, a recent survey drawing on data from 41 states indicated that less than 1 percent of prison inmates known to have hepatitis C were being treated (Beckman et al., 2016).

Hepatitis C is an infectious disease. Because of the ongoing opioid epidemic, more people, many of them younger than 30, are at risk for HCV infection (CDC, 2016; Zibbell et al., 2015). As Chapter 2 made clear, without large-scale treatment, infection will continue to be a public health problem. There are, of course, differences between childhood immunization and hepatitis C treatment. Obviously, there are far more children than hepatitis C patients, although the childhood vaccines are much cheaper than direct-acting antivirals, so the overall costs may be comparable. The means by which the government should buy the product is also different. As the direct-acting agents are still on patent, licensing rights to a patent would be an excellent way to increase access to treatment without significantly increasing costs for public payers.

> **Recommendation 6-1: The federal government, on behalf of the Department of Health and Human Services, should purchase the rights to a direct-acting antiviral for use in neglected market segments, such as Medicaid, the Indian Health Service, and prisons. This could be done through the licensing or assigning of a patent in a voluntary transaction with an innovator pharmaceutical company.**

The idea of the government acquiring a patent is not new. A recent policy piece in *Health Affairs* argues that the federal government should invoke its power for "government patent use" to improve access to expensive but effective patent-protected medicines such as direct-acting antivirals (Kapczynski and Kesselheim, 2016). The authors cite 28 USC section 1498, which allows the government to use a patented product without permission in exchange for a payment of "reasonable and entire compensation" for the product (Kapczynski and Kesselheim, 2016). The Departments of Defense[5] and the Treasury[6] have invoked this provision in the manufacture of night vision goggles and fraud detection software (Kapczynski and Kesselheim, 2016).

Much the same way a single payer system for vaccines would have ended uneven immunization among children, so would government patent acquisition solve the problem of poor access to direct-acting antivirals. It could also have a chilling effect on innovation (Grabowski, 2016). Invoking section 1498 forces the patent holder to surrender market exclusivity rights at a price determined by the federal government. Patent holders have reason to doubt that they will get fair compensation when they have no ability to refuse the transaction. The innovator company could always sue the government, but the legal costs and the odds of losing the challenge may dissuade them. At the very least, legal fees could add to their expenses and detract from their overall return on investment. Fear that patent rights could be confiscated might also discourage pharmaceutical companies from investing in breakthrough research. Government takeover of a drug patent

---

[5] *Gargoyles, Inc., and Pro-Tec, Inc., v. United States*, 113 F.3d 1572 (Fed. Cir. 1997).
[6] *Advanced Software Design Corp. v. Federal Reserve Bank of St. Louis*, 583 F.3d 1371 (Fed. Cir. 2009).

would thereby increase access to direct-acting agents, but the cost to society may be too high.

There are times when the government is obliged to act in correction of market failures. With this in mind, the committee recommends a voluntary transaction between the federal government and a patent holder, wherein the companies producing direct-acting antivirals compete to license their patent to the federal government for use in neglected patients. The exact legal mechanism that would best serve this goal is debatable. The innovator companies and the government would need to determine if the situation is better suited to licensing, wherein the company issues revocable rights to a patent, or to assignment, wherein the company would permanently transfer ownership of its patent (Mendes, n.d.). One of the main differences between license and assignment is in how the rights are paid for: a licensee usually pays royalties for its rights, an assignee makes a lump sum payment (Mendes, n.d.). In practice the line between the two is not always clear, nor is it obvious how much of the "bundle of rights" guaranteed by a patent the innovator company has to transfer before an exclusive license becomes an assignment (Chapman and Fraser, 2010). In either case, the government would only have authority to use the drug in a narrow and clearly defined market.

The voluntary nature of the process guarantees the drug company reasonable compensation—the patent holder always has the option to walk away from the transaction if the price is not right. The innovator company would authorize its rights only in those market segments for which the taxpayer pays for treatment *and* access is limited, such as the uninsured, prisoners, and Medicaid beneficiaries. These are the least lucrative market segments in the United States; the buyers have serious budget constraints and access restrictions, making these markets ones the companies are not reaching otherwise. Limiting market would also control the cost to the government; it would not have to pay as much for the rights as it would if compromising the lucrative private market. Once the government acquires adequate rights, it would contract with manufacturers to produce the drugs and with distributors.

Projected Cost of the Buyout

About 700,000 people in state Medicaid programs and prisons are eligible for treatment with direct-acting agents.[7] The exact prices state Med-

---

[7] Combining the roughly 100,000 eligible prisoners (Beckman et al., 2016) and approximately 650,000 Medicaid recipients (Senate Committee on Finance, 2015), and assuming 50,000 of those were treated in 2015 and 2016, results in approximately 700,000 prisoners and state Medicaid participants eligible for treatment. Included in this estimate are the nearly

icaid programs and prisons pay for treatment are not public information, but the manufacturers' financial reports and information on Medicaid's mandatory discounts suggest costs of about $40,000 per treated patient.[8] In 2014, about 17,000 patients in prisons and Medicaid programs received treatment with direct-acting antivirals.[9] The models presented in Chapter 2 assume treatment for 260,000 patients a year (see Appendix B). Even if the United States continues treatment at the current rate, an unlikely scenario given the pressure to improve access to these drugs, there would be about 20,000 Medicaid patients and prisoners a year receiving direct-acting agents. So under the status quo, about 240,000 such patients will receive treatment in the next 12 years, generating about $10 billion in revenues for manufacturers.

Around 2028 the innovator companies' period of market exclusivity will be ending, at which time their revenue would drop precipitously. Assuming a cost of capital of about 8 percent for pharmaceutical firms,[10] the present value of this revenue stream (which takes into account that the revenues are accrued over a 12-year period) is about $6.5 billion. Currently there are five firms competing to provide direct-acting agents with varying market shares (FDA, 2016). Any of these firms should therefore be willing to license the patent for their direct-acting agent for underserved markets for less than $6.5 billion.

In practice, the expected costs would be much less than $6.5 billion as there are several firms competing in this market. Consider a firm anticipating control of one-third of the market over the next 12 years. Under the status quo, this firm expects to have a revenue stream with a present value of about $2 billion. This firm should be indifferent between the status quo and licensing its rights for $2 billion. However, if a competing firm licenses its drug to the government, then the revenue stream of the first firm would decline as it would have to compete with a cheaper generic in the same market segments. The government could, therefore, negotiate a price much lower than the present value of the revenue stream. The actual transaction amount will depend on the degree to which firms compete with each other

---

100,000 potential patients in the Indian Health Service dependent on state Medicaid programs as there are no HCV drugs on the service's formulary (CMS, n.d.; Edlin et al., 2015; Indian Health Service, 2016; Leston and Finkbonner, 2016).

[8] The estimated revenue per patient initiating therapy is $52,000 (NASEM, 2016). Applying the 23.1 percent Medicaid rebate to this revenue results in costs of about $40,000 (AASLD and IDSA, 2016).

[9] An estimated 949 prisoners (Beckman et al., 2016) and 16,200 Medicaid recipients (Senate Committee on Finance, 2015) were treated, resulting in about 17,000 patients who received treatment with direct-acting antivirals.

[10] The cost of capital is the weighted average of the cost of equity and after-tax cost of debt, weighted by the market values of equity and debt (Damodaran, 2016). Cumulative market values for the entire sector are used for the weights.

to sell to the government. Both the government and the winning firm would benefit from the outcome of the negotiation.

After the government purchases rights to the patent, it would contract manufacturer to produce the drug for supply to neglected markets, such as Medicaid, the Indian Health Service, and prisons. Prices of other direct-acting agents would be expected to fall in those markets as they would be competing with a generic. Estimates of the production costs of direct-acting agents and gross profit margins of generic suppliers suggest that the price of generic direct-acting agents will be roughly $200 per patient (Hill et al., 2014). Assuming all 700,000 hepatitis C patients in those systems receive the licensed product, the total cost of the drug itself for Medicaid programs and prisons would be only $140 million over the license cost.

This solution solves the dual problem of high costs and poor access to direct-acting antivirals in the Medicaid and prison market segments. It does so by preserving the incentives for innovation as it involves a voluntary transaction between a patent holder and the federal government at a price agreeable to both parties. Under the status quo (where the government does not have rights to patent), we expect that the federal and state governments will spend about $10 billion over the next 12 years, providing direct-acting agents to about 240,000 Medicaid beneficiaries and prisoners. These costs will be split roughly evenly between the federal and state governments, as the federal government provides matching funds to state Medicaid programs. Under the scenario where the federal government follows this recommendation and buys rights to a patent for about $2 billion, the cost to the federal government is the $2 billion for the rights and $70 million for generic drug purchases. The costs to state governments are about $70 million for generic drug purchases. Thus, overall costs are significantly lower for state governments. Costs are also lower for the federal government in the long run, but the license requires higher upfront investment. Although this investment is large, it is a small fraction of total federal spending on health. Most importantly, the patent license results in an estimated 460,000 more patients receiving treatment, essentially solving the problem of poor access to direct-acting antivirals.

Implementation Challenges

It is not clear which federal agency would be best suited to manage the licensing negotiations. HRSA is a natural choice, given its experience with the 340B program, as is the CDC, which negotiates Vaccines for Children. The Treasury may also be suitable, and the Department of Defense may have transferable expertise from other private sector negotiations. The committee does not presume to identify the best agency for the job; such a determination should be made at higher levels.

A more serious challenge lies in the potential of this recommendation to create parallel markets in one country: a market where a generic is available at lower cost and one where the same product is sold at the branded price. Innovator companies may fear that products intended for Medicaid patients would be sold illegally, undercutting their share of the private market.[11] Such concerns may be exaggerated. There have been no reports of black market diversion from developing countries where the price of direct-acting agents is orders of magnitude lower than the U.S. market (McNeil, 2015). Furthermore, there are already parallel markets in the United States. The Department of Veterans Affairs (VA), for example, pays considerably less for medicines than other federal agencies, about 42 percent of the average wholesale price, because similar products compete for listing on its closed formulary (CBO, 2005; Kesselheim et al., 2016). There has been no widespread diversion from the VA system in its almost 20 years with a closed formulary, except for a few products with street value, opioid pain killers and drugs for erectile dysfunction, for example (VA, 2015, 2016a).

Unlike Viagra® or Percocet®, there is no underground market or off-label indication for direct-acting antivirals. If a Medicaid beneficiary were to sell one, he or she would have to first find another hepatitis C patient interested in buying. Far fewer private insurance patients are denied the treatment in the first place (Lo Re et al., 2016). It is not impossible that some would want to buy on the black market, but the risks of such action are real. Selling prescription drugs is a federal crime,[12] and as long as treatment expansion proceeds as recommended in Chapter 4, the benefit is minimal. If such diversion became more than an anecdotal problem, some variant of directly observed treatment would be necessary. In Egypt, for example, where Gilead provided free sofosbuvir to 125,000 people in 2015, patients have to bring an empty pill bottle to the pharmacy to get a refill and break the seal on the new bottle in front of the pharmacist, essentially negating the product's resale value (McNeil, 2015).

Critics of this strategy may maintain that it sets a dangerous precedent. If the government can buy a patent for hepatitis C drugs, they would reason, then why should it not do the same for other medicines? This is a harder criticism to answer except to say that the U.S. government is disinclined to such action. It has not invoked its rights under section 1498 since the 1960s (Brennan et al., 2016). The U.S. government is generally extremely supportive of the pharmaceutical industry, investing heavily in the science infrastructure that supports the industry and paying considerably more for medicines than other rich countries (Conti et al., 2016).

---

[11] Arguments about product diversion are not relevant in prisons where all medicine administration is directly observed.

[12] Controlled Substances Act. 21 USC § 841(a).

Direct-acting agents may also be a special case. These products have a remarkable success rate, curing an infectious disease of public health consequence. The government has reason to improve access to these drugs, thereby reducing or eliminating the future burden of hepatitis C, something that few products can offer. There may also be a unique combination of circumstances: several innovator companies all offering patent-protected products at the same time for high prices, increasing the chances that the government can negotiate a favorable price.

Encouraging Cooperation

Negotiating a good license price depends, however, on the cooperation of the pharmaceutical industry. The companies could refuse to negotiate, though refusal would not be to their obvious financial advantage. As the previous section explained, this license would be used in an otherwise tightly restricted market, one the companies are not currently reaching. The chance to reach a relatively untapped market should be compelling. There is always a chance, however, that the firms would rather decline a new revenue stream, albeit a modest one, than license their patent rights.

Such refusal would have risks. First, it could be considered implicit collusion; the fewer companies competing to sell rights, the better the returns for the winner, after all. Such action could have serious consequences for the firms' public image. In the current political climate, high drug prices are under scrutiny (Johnson, 2017a,b; Morgenson, 2016). Were these immensely profitable companies to refuse to cooperate with the government, especially a government acting against a public health threat and in the interest of some of the poorest and least powerful people in society, this scrutiny would be likely to increase.

Furthermore, the government has the authority to exercise its rights to patent use under section 1498 at any time. The last time the government even hinted at taking such action against drug company was in 2001, when, during the anthrax scare, the manufacturer of ciprofloxacin initially refused to lower its prices to support national stockpiling (Brennan and Shrank, 2014; Kapczynski and Kesselheim, 2016). The threat alone was enough to cause the manufacturer guarantee supply at a 50 percent discount (Kapczynski and Kesselheim, 2016). The same action could be considered for a direct-acting agent, as could the pooled purchasing strategies discussed later in this chapter.

It is possible that a government's very reluctance to interfere in the pharmaceutical market emboldened Gilead to set the introductory price for sofosbuvir so high. An 18-month Senate Finance Committee investigation ended in the embarrassing publication of the company's internal pricing strategy, summarized in *The Price of Sovaldi and Its Impact on the U.S. Health Care System* (Senate Committee on Finance, 2015). The bipartisan report concluded that Gilead executives priced sofosbuvir as high as they thought the market would bear before triggering access restrictions (Senate Committee on Finance, 2015). They miscalculated that point, but did not respond to the restrictions by lowering prices (Senate Committee on Finance, 2015). Gilead offered Medicaid programs a 10 percent rebate only on the condition that they drop access restrictions, thereby increasing states' total spending on the drug (Senate Committee on Finance, 2015). "By elevating the price for the new standard of care set by Sovaldi," the report explained, "Gilead intended to raise the price floor for all future HCV treatments, including its follow-on drugs and those of its competitors" (Senate Committee on Finance, 2015, p. 118).

The government has to balance the pharmaceutical firms' right to compensation against its duty to the millions of Americans who suffer from hepatitis C, to say nothing of the taxpayers who subsidize their treatment. Voluntary licensing or assignment of patent rights could help restore equilibrium to this equation. It might also discourage future introductory drug prices similar to those for sofosbuvir. In 2015, the Senate Finance Committee openly fretted about "the budgetary effects of a future single source innovator that might not face competition as quickly [as sofosbuvir]" (Carey et al., 2015). Action now could help avoid that problem.

Pooled Purchase and Other Cost Saving Strategies

It could take time to negotiate the transaction described in Recommendation 6-1. State Medicaid and prison health officers will need a strategy to make hepatitis C treatment more affordable in the meantime. There is also room for incremental change: public and private payers can take measures immediately to improve access to medicines. Bulk purchasing brings greater bargaining power with the drug companies and is a simple strategy frequently suggested to control the cost of medicines in the United States (Kesselheim et al., 2016; Shih et al., 2016). Box 6-1 describes how such a strategy worked in Massachusetts.

Outpatient prescriptions are a major and growing financial burden, second only to long-term care as Medicaid's biggest expense (Peters, 2010). The 2003 Medicare Prescription Drug, Improvement, and Modernization Act created a drug benefit, usually referred to as Part D, which shifted some of the drug cost (those for people eligible for both Medicare and Medicaid) to Medicare (Kevles, 2014; Millar et al., 2011; Peters, 2010). Part D was created to make essential medicines more affordable for older people, but

---

BOX 6-1
HCV Drug Rebate Program in Massachusetts

Between late 2013 and early 2016, MassHealth, the Massachusetts Medicaid program, and its managed care organizations paid about $318 million for hepatitis C drugs for 4,430 of its almost 1.8 million members. In early 2016, the state attorney general threatened to sue Gilead for unfair trade practices, explaining that even after competitor drugs came on the market, the Gilead's prices remained too high, even with rebates. Her letter also pointed out the company's generosity in Egypt while, "Massachusetts taxpayers bear the full burden of Gilead's exceptionally high pricing."

In 2016, MassHealth negotiated discounts of an undisclosed amount with Gilead and Bristol-Meyers Squibb, enabling the end of restrictions on hepatitis C treatments for MassHealth and its managed care organizations. The discounts, given as rebates, will keep state spending on direct-acting antivirals around $200 million a year. *The Boston Globe* reported that, because of the discounts, another 3,400 hepatitis C patients in Massachusetts would be treated by June 2017.

The problem of treating people in the state prison system remains, however, as inmates are not eligible for Medicare or Medicaid. In 2015, state prisoners brought a class-action lawsuit against the Massachusetts Department of Corrections for restricting access to hepatitis C treatment. Their lawyers claimed that while over 1,500 inmates have hepatitis C, only three are being treated for it. State prison systems in other states are facing similar action, and all respond that treating all of the inmates with hepatitis C would quickly surpass the state's total prisoner health care budget. By some estimates treating every imprisoned person with hepatitis C in the United States would cost $33 billion, more than four times the total spending on prison health care. In Massachusetts, the attorney general is now working to extend the lower prices to the Office of Pharmacy Services which procures medicines for the state prison system.

SOURCES: Healey, 2016; Massachusetts EOHHS, 2016; Rich et al., 2014; Schoenberg, 2015; The Pew Charitable Trusts and MacArthur Foundation, 2014.

CMS is explicitly disallowed from negotiating bulk discounts for the program (Kevles, 2014).[13]

The state Medicaid programs have other ways to control drug costs. Medicaid rebates are at least 23.1 percent of the manufacturer's average wholesale price for most drugs (CMS, 2016a; Kesselheim et al., 2016). State Medicaid programs also use preferred drug lists and prior authorization to control costs (Soumerai, 2004). Drugs on the state's preferred list are fully reimbursed without review or conditions (Millar et al., 2011). Access to a

---

[13] Medicare Prescription Drug, Improvement, and Modernization Act, Public Law 108-173, 108th Cong. (2003).

medicine not on the preferred list depends on prior authorization, the process described in Chapter 4 that a prescriber or pharmacist must go through to gain approval to use a drug for which there is a cheaper alternative (Smalley et al., 1995). Prior authorization is meant to deter the careless use of an expensive medicine in cases where a cheaper one would do.

Starting in 2003, states have also used bulk buying pools to purchase Medicaid drugs (National Conference of State Legislatures, 2015) (see Box 6-2). Pooled procurement allows the states to benefit from economies of scale and can help reduce transaction costs and the administrative burden of the negotiation. Large procurements are less subject to price fluctuation over time (Andrus et al., 2009; DeRoeck et al., 2006; Huff-Rousselle, 2012). Producers also benefit from bulk purchasing arrangements, as the increased access means more people using their products.

But not all states access rebates and bulk purchasing arrangements to the same extent. Four states (Hawaii, New Jersey, New Mexico, and South Dakota) do not have Medicaid supplemental rebate programs; the rest negotiate either on their own, in pools, or some combination of single and pooled purchasing (i.e., negotiating the base rebate in a multi-state pool, and negotiating alone for an additional rebate) (CMS, 2016b; Dickson and Horn, 2016). The variation in practice among states accounts for widely different access within them (Dickson and Horn, 2016). For this reason, the Medicaid budget overview for fiscal year 2017 proposed that CMS and state Medicaid programs hire a private sector contractor to negotiate rebates for expensive medicines, a policy they estimate would save taxpayers $5.8 billion over 10 years (HHS, n.d.). The process would have to work through the private sector, as CMS is prohibited from managing such negotiations.

The 340B Program

Furthermore, not all uninsured or underinsured patients access Medicare or Medicaid. The 340B Drug Discount Program provides medicines at greatly reduced prices to safety net providers: the hospitals and clinics that serve the uninsured, Medicaid beneficiaries, and other vulnerable groups (HRSA, n.d.-c). Created in 1992, 340B aims to stretch limited federal funds for medicines. Unlike the drug rebates available to Medicaid programs, 340B discounts are generally provided up front to eligible providers, 26,907 organizations in 2014 (Fein, 2016).[14] Participating hospitals and clinics

---

[14] In some states the AIDS Drug Assistance Program may choose to receive rebates rather than front-end discounts. As of late 2016, 22 states get rebates and no discount; the others use some combination of direct purchase and rebate (Kaiser Family Foundation, 2014).

BOX 6-2
Multi-State Plans for Bulk Drug Purchase

As of January 2016, there were five different multi-state, bulk purchasing pools for medicines in the United States, as well as one separate pool specifically for hepatitis C drugs; their reach is shown in the map below (National Conference of State Legislatures, 2015).

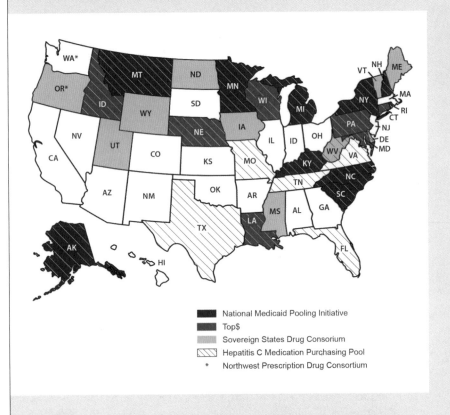

NOTE: Map does not include the states in the Minnesota Multistate Contracting Alliance for Pharmacy.
SOURCE: National Conference of State Legislatures, 2015.

Hepatitis C Medication Purchasing Pool: Missouri and 24 other state Medicaid programs formed a buying pool in early 2015 to negotiate lower costs for a hepatitis C medication, Viekira Pak®, with the manufacturer. These programs receive a 20 to 30 percent supplemental rebate when they purchase Viekira Pak® for their Medicaid beneficiaries. Missouri estimates it will save $4.2 million in 2016 after switching to Viekira Pak® from the more expensive Sovaldi® (National Conference of State Legislatures, 2015; Young, 2015).

National Medicaid Pooling Initiative: The first multi-state Medicaid purchasing pool, approved in 2004, has supplemental rebate agreements with more than 90 pharmaceutical manufacturers. As of late 2015, 10 states and the District of Columbia were participants (AK, DC, KY, MI, MN, MT, NC, NH, NY, RI, and SC) (National Conference of State Legislatures, 2015; Provider Synergies LLC, n.d.-a).

The Optimal PDL Solution (commonly abbreviated TOP$): Formed in 2005, seven state Medicaid programs participate (CT, ID, LA, MD, NE, PA, and WI) and receive supplemental rebates on a variety of medications (National Conference of State Legislatures, 2015; Provider Synergies LLC, n.d.-b).

Sovereign States Drug Consortium: A supplemental rebate program formed in 2006; rebates are based on usage data from the 10 member states (DE, IA, ME, MS, ND, OR, UT, VT, WV, and WY), with Ohio and Oklahoma scheduled to join the consortium in 2017. Unlike other multi-state pooling programs, member states own and run the consortium (National Conference of State Legislatures, 2015; SSDC, 2016).

Northwest Prescription Drug Consortium: Oregon's and Washington's non-Medicaid prescription drug programs, formed in 2007. The program offers an average discount of 42 percent of the retail price for prescriptions to Oregon and Washington residents through a large network of participating pharmacies (National Conference of State Legislatures, 2015).

Minnesota Multistate Contracting Alliance for Pharmacy: A group purchasing organization founded in 1985 and administered by the state of Minnesota. The alliance is open to states, cities, or other government health facilities, but not to Medicaid programs. There are participating organizations in almost every state (MMCAP, n.d.; National Conference of State Legislatures, 2015).

are meant to use the money they save on medicines for other services that would benefit their patients (HRSA, n.d.-a).

340B discounts are between 20 and 50 percent off average wholesale prices on prescription medicines and biologics, as well as over-the-counter drugs written as prescriptions (340B Health, n.d.; GAO, 2011). The exact 340B price for any given product is confidential, but HRSA calculates a maximum price through a formula determined by law (Apexus, n.d.).[15] Additional discounts are available to clinics participating in the prime vendor program, in which one company negotiates a bulk discount for a group of 340B facilities, but care must be taken to avoid duplicate discounts for Medicaid patients (340B Health, n.d.; HRSA, n.d.-b). Therefore, clinics serving vulnerable populations need to decide before enrolling in the program if their Medicaid patients' drugs will be purchased through 340B or through the state Medicaid program (HRSA, n.d.-b). Random audits and penalties help prevent duplicate discounts and ensure that manufacturers are honoring 340B prices. Facilities can be disqualified from 340B for mismanagement; manufacturers can be excluded from Medicaid and Medicare Part B (340B Health, n.d.).

340B is meant to stretch federal funds, so jails and prisons, usually a state responsibility, were excluded from the start. Nor are inmates Medicaid eligible, except for services provided while "a patient in a medical institution"[16] (CMS, 2016c). There is nothing to prevent correctional health officers from arranging treatment for HCV-infected inmates at 340B clinics, however. Sixteen states do this; these states tend to have some of the best priced treatments for hepatitis C drugs (Beckman et al., 2016).

340B pricing and Medicaid rebates are regulated by law (Dickson and Horn, 2016). The formulas used to calculate prices for the VA and the Department of Defense vary somewhat from those used for Medicaid, but all involve the manufacturers' reported prices to wholesalers and pharmacies (Dickson and Horn, 2016). The formulas by which these prices are calculated have been unchanged since the 1990s, despite dramatic changes in the market (Dickson and Horn, 2016). Pharmacy benefit managers and consolidated insurance companies now have influence on the market price of medicines, but the manufacturers have an incentive to hide these discounts in rebates, coupons, and other payments to insurers, not as reductions on the sticker price, because front-end discounts affect the calculation on which the government bases its pricing (Dickson and Horn, 2016). The Government Accountability Office estimates that if the formula used to calculate prices for Medicare Part B drugs (usually expensive medicines ad-

---

[15] 42 USC § 256(b).
[16] Title 1905 of the Social Security Act. 42 USC § 1396d(a)(29)(A); 42 CFR §§ 435.1009, 435.1010.

ministered by a doctor) had included rebates, coupons, and other discounts, Medicare spending on these drugs would have been $69 million lower in 2013 (Dickson and Horn, 2016; GAO, 2016).

The laws regulating the sale of medicines to the government are meant to protect the taxpayer from overpaying for an essential product. The Fair Pricing Coalition has suggested modifications to formulas through which various government agencies finance prescription drugs, most of which require legislative action (Dickson and Horn, 2016). To the extent such changes are possible, they should be supported as part of the solution to a wider problem of unaffordable prescription drugs.

REFERENCES

340B Health. n.d. *Overview of the 340B drug pricing program.* http://www.340bhealth.org/340b-resources/340b-program/overview (accessed September 26, 2016).

AASLD and IDSA (American Association for the Study of Liver Diseases and Infectious Diseases Society of America). 2016. *Overview of cost, reimbursement, and cost-effectiveness considerations for hepatitis C treatment regimens.* http://www.hcvguidelines.org/full-report/overview-cost-reimbursement-and-cost-effectiveness-considerations-hepatitis-c-treatment (accessed November 7, 2016).

Abram, S. 2015. Woman sues Anthem Blue Cross for denying hepatitis C drug Harvoni. *Los Angeles Daily News*, June 1. http://www.dailynews.com/health/20150601/woman-sues-anthem-blue-cross-for-denying-hepatitis-c-drug-harvoni (accessed October 3, 2016).

ADAP (AIDS Drug Assistance Program) Crisis Task Force. 2016. *ADAP Crisis Task Force fact sheet: March 2016.* https://www.nastad.org/sites/default/files/ADAP-Crisis-Task-Force-Fact-Sheet-March-2016.pdf (accessed October 26, 2016).

Alcorn, K. 2015. *Cost of comprehensive global viral hepatitis prevention and treatment effort might peak at $11 billion in 2025.* http://www.worldhepatitisalliance.org/en/news/sep-2015/cost-comprehensive-global-viral-hepatitis-prevention-and-treatment-effort-might-peak (accessed September 29, 2016).

Altarum Institute. 2016. *Altarum Institute Center for Sustainable Health Spending health sector trend report.* Altarum Institute. http://altarum.org/sites/default/files/uploaded-publication-files/Altarum%20RWJF%20Trend%20Report%20February%202016_2.pdf (accessed September 29, 2016).

Andrus, J. K., C. de Quadros, C. R. Matus, S. Luciani, and P. Hotez. 2009. New vaccines for developing countries: Will it be feast or famine? *American Journal of Law & Medicine* 35(2-3):311-322.

Apexus. n.d. *340B price/covered outpatient drugs.* https://www.340bpvp.com/resource-center/faqs/340b-pricing--covered-outpatient-drugs (accessed September 26, 2016).

Atkinson, W. L., S. C. Hadler, S. B. Redd, and W. A. Orenstein. 1992a. Measles surveillance—United States, 1991. *Morbidity and Mortality Weekly Report* 41(6):1-12.

Atkinson, W. L., W. A. Orenstein, and S. Krugman. 1992b. The resurgence of measles in the United States, 1989-1990. *Annual Review of Medicine* 43:4451-4463.

Barua, S., R. Greenwald, J. Grebely, G. J. Dore, T. Swan, and L. E. Taylor. 2015. Restrictions for Medicaid reimbursement of sofosbuvir for the treatment of hepatitis C virus infection in the United States. *Annals of Internal Medicine* 163(3):215-223.

Beckman, A. L., A. Bilinski, R. Boyko, G. M. Camp, A. T. Wall, J. K. Lim, E. A. Wang, R. D. Bruce, and G. S. Gonsalves. 2016. New hepatitis C drugs are very costly and unavailable to many state prisoners. *Health Affairs* 35(10):1893-1901.

Brennan, H., A. Kapczynski, C. H. Monahan, and Z. Rizvi. 2016. A prescription for excessive drug pricing: Leveraging government patent use for health. Yale Law School, Public Law Research Paper No. 577; Yale Law & Economics Research Paper No. 560. *Yale Journal of Law & Technology* 18(275). https://papers.ssrn.com/sol3/Papers. cfm?abstract_id=2832948 (accessed February 23, 2017).

Brennan, T., and W. Shrank. 2014. New expensive treatments for hepatitis C infection. *JAMA* 312(6):593-594.

Bristol-Meyers Squibb. n.d. *Co-pay assistance program and free drug program.* http://www. baraclude.bmscustomerconnect.com/Co-Pay (accessed December 14, 2016).

Canary, L. A., R. M. Klevens, and S. D. Holmberg. 2015. Limited access to new hepatitis C virus treatment under state Medicaid programs. *Annals of Internal Medicine* 163(3):226-228.

Carey, R., T. Harvey, and J. Gerber. 2015. *Wyden-Grassley Sovaldi investigation finds revenue-driven pricing strategy behind $84,000 hepatitis drug.* http://www.finance.senate. gov/ranking-members-news/wyden-grassley-sovaldi-investigation-finds-revenue-driven-pricing-strategy-behind-84-000-hepatitis-drug (accessed October 26, 2016).

CBO (Congressional Budget Office). 2005. *Prices for brand-name drugs under selected federal programs.* Congress of the United States.

CDC (Centers for Disease Control and Prevention). 1992. Public-sector vaccination efforts in response to the resurgence of measles among preschool-aged children—United States, 1989-1991. *Morbidity and Mortality Weekly Report* 41(29):522-525.

CDC. 2014a. *About VFC.* http://www.cdc.gov/vaccines/programs/vfc/about/index.html (accessed September 26, 2016).

CDC. 2014b. *HIV and viral hepatitis.* http://www.cdc.gov/hiv/pdf/library_factsheets_hiv_and_viral_hepatitis.pdf (accessed October 19, 2016).

CDC. 2014c. *VFC eligibility criteria.* http://www.cdc.gov/vaccines/programs/vfc/providers/ eligibility.html (accessed September 26, 2016).

CDC. 2016. *Viral hepatitis and young persons who inject prescription opioids and heroin.* http://www.cdc.gov/hepatitis/featuredtopics/youngpwid.htm (accessed October 26, 2016).

CDPH (California Department of Public Health). n.d. *Guidance on the use of Ryan White funds for syringe services programs.* https://www.cdph.ca.gov/programs/aids/Documents/ SALtrGuidanceRWFunds.pdf (accessed October 25, 2016).

Chapman, B. G., and K. D. Fraser. 2010. Exclusive patent license or virtual assignment. *Los Angeles Daily Journal*, July 29. https://www.ipo.org/wp-content/uploads/2013/03/ exclusivepatentlicense1.pdf (accessed February 27, 2017).

Chhatwal, J., F. Kanwal, M. S. Roberts, and M. A. Dunn. 2015. Cost-effectiveness and budget impact of hepatitis C virus treatment with sofosbuvir and ledipasvir in the United States. *Annals of Internal Medicine* 162(6):397-406.

CMS (Centers for Medicare & Medicaid Services). 2016a. *Medicaid drug rebate program.* https://www.medicaid.gov/medicaid/prescription-drugs/medicaid-drug-rebate-program/ index.html (accessed February 13, 2017).

CMS. 2016b. *Medicaid Pharmacy Supplemental Rebate Agreements (SRA).* Baltimore, MD: Center for Medicaid and CHIP Services.

CMS. 2016c. *To facilitate successful re-entry for individuals transitioning from incarceration to their communities.* https://www.medicaid.gov/federal-policy-guidance/downloads/ sho16007.pdf (accessed October 19, 2016).

CMS. n.d. *Indian health and Medicaid.* https://www.medicaid.gov/medicaid/indian-health-and-medicaid/index.html (accessed November 8, 2016).

Coleman, M. S., N. Sangrujee, F. Zhou, and S. Chu. 2005. Factors affecting U.S. manufacturers' decisions to produce vaccines. *Health Affairs* 24(3):635-642.

Conti, R. M., R. E. Gee, and J. M. Sharfstein. 2016. Pharmaceuticals and public health. *JAMA* 316(20):2083-2084.

Dales, L. G., K. W. Kizer, G. W. Rutherford, C. A. Pertowski, S. H. Waterman, and G. Woodford. 1993. Measles epidemic from failure to immunize. *The Western Journal of Medicine* 159(4):455-464.

Damodaran, A. 2016. *Cost of capital by sector (U.S.).* http://people.stern.nyu.edu/adamodar/New_Home_Page/datafile/wacc.htm (accessed October 19, 2016).

DeBoy, A. M. 2015. *Medicaid drug rebate program notice for state technical contacts.* Baltimore, MD: Center for Medicaid and CHIP Services.

DeRoeck, D., S. A. Bawazir, P. Carrasco, M. Kaddar, A. Brooks, J. Fitzsimmons, and J. Andrus. 2006. Regional group purchasing of vaccines: Review of the Pan American Health Organization EPI revolving fund and the Gulf Cooperation Council group purchasing program. *International Journal of Health Planning and Management* 21(1):23-43.

Dickson, S., and T. Horn. 2016. *Tackling drug costs: A 100 day roadmap.* New York: Fair Pricing Coalition.

DrugPatentWatch. n.d. *Sovaldi drug profile.* https://www.drugpatentwatch.com/p/tradename/SOVALDI (accessed September 30, 2016).

Edlin, B. R., B. J. Eckhardt, M. A. Shu, S. D. Holmberg, and T. Swan. 2015. Toward a more accurate estimate of the prevalence of hepatitis C in the United States. *Hepatology* 62(5):1353-1363.

Ellwood, M. 2014. *Restrictions to HCV treatment in state Medicaid programs.* http://www.chlpi.org/wp-content/uploads/2014/01/Malinda-Ellwood-Restrictions-to-HCV-Treatment-in-State-Medicaid-Programs-11.15.14.pdf (accessed September 30, 2016).

EPA (Environmental Protection Agency). n.d. *Mortality risk valuation.* https://www.epa.gov/environmental-economics/mortality-risk-valuation#means (accessed February 27, 2017).

FDA (Food and Drug Administration). 2016. *FDA drug safety communication: FDA warns about the risk of hepatitis B reactivating in some patients treated with direct-acting antivirals for hepatitis C.* https://www.fda.gov/Drugs/DrugSafety/ucm522932.htm (accessed April 19, 2017).

Fegraus, L., and M. Ross. 2014. Sovaldi, Harvoni, and why it's different this time. *Health Affairs Blog*, November 21. http://healthaffairs.org/blog/2014/11/21/sovaldi-harvoni-and-why-its-different-this-time (accessed October 5, 2016).

Fein, A. J. 2016. Challenges for managed care from 340B contract pharmacies. *Journal of Managed Care & Specialty Pharmacy* 22(3):197-203.

Freyer, F. J. 2016. Hepatitis C drug costs leave many without care. *Boston Globe*, April 9. https://www.bostonglobe.com/metro/2016/04/09/for-hepatitis-patients-cure-for-high-drug-prices/j2X4aVi7BEpU5BSL0YV0vN/story.html (accessed October 3, 2016).

GAO (Government Accountability Office). 2011. *Drug pricing: Manufacturer discounts in the 340B program offer benefits, but federal oversight needs improvement.* Washington, DC: GAO.

GAO. 2016. *Medicare Part B: Data on coupon discounts needed to evaluate methodology for setting drug payment rates.* Washington, DC: GAO.

Gheorghe, L., I. Popescu, R. Iacob, S. Iacob, and C. Gheorghe. 2005. Predictors of death on the waiting list for liver transplantation characterized by a long waiting time. *Transplant International* 18(5):572-576.

Gilead. n.d. *Welcome to the Gilead Advancing Access® co-pay program.* https://www.gilead-advancingaccess.com/copay-coupon-card (accessed December 14, 2016).

Grabowski, H. 2016. Government appropriation of breakthrough drug patent rights would deter biopharmaceutical R&D and innovation. *Health Affairs Blog*, June 20. http://healthaffairs.org/blog/2016/06/20/government-appropriation-of-breakthrough-drug-patent-rights-would-deter-biopharmaceutical-rd-and-innovation (accessed October 26, 2016).

Graham, J. 2016a. For hepatitis C patients, states' lawsuits pay off. *Kaiser Health News*, July 5. http://www.governing.com/topics/health-human-services/khn-hepatitis-drug-limits.html (accessed September 30, 2016).

Graham, J. 2016b. Medicaid, private insurers begin to lift curbs on pricey hepatitis C drugs. *Kaiser Health News*, July 5. http://khn.org/news/medicaid-private-insurers-begin-to-lift-curbs-on-pricey-hepatitis-c-drugs (accessed September 30, 2016).

Grebely, J., M. Oser, L. E. Taylor, and G. J. Dore. 2013. Breaking down the barriers to hepatitis C virus (HCV) treatment among individuals with HCV/HIV coinfection: Action required at the system, provider, and patient levels. *Journal of Infectious Diseases* 207(Suppl 1):S19-S25.

Harper, J. 2015. States deny pricey hepatitis C drugs to most Medicaid patients. *NPR* (National Public Radio), December 27. http://www.npr.org/sections/health-shots/2015/12/27/460086615/states-deny-pricey-hepatitis-c-drugs-to-most-medicaid-patients (accessed September 30, 2016).

Healey, M. 2016. *Letter from Massachusetts Attorney General Maura Healey to Gilead Chairman and CEO John C. Martin*. http://www.mass.gov/ago/docs/policy/2016/letter-to-gilead-1-22-16.pdf (accessed February 23, 2017).

Herszenhorn, D. M. 2016. Zika bill is blocked by Senate Democrats upset over provisions. *New York Times*, June 29. http://www.nytimes.com/2016/06/29/us/politics/congress-zika-funding.html?_r=0 (accessed September 30, 2016).

HHS (Department of Health and Human Services). n.d. *HHS FY 2017 budget in brief - CMS - Medicaid*. http://www.hhs.gov/about/budget/fy2017/budget-in-brief/cms/medicaid/index.html (accessed December 9, 2016).

Hill, A., S. Khoo, J. Fortunak, B. Simmons, and N. Ford. 2014. Minimum costs for producing hepatitis C direct-acting antivirals for use in large-scale treatment access programs in developing countries. *Clinical Infectious Diseases* 58(7):928-936.

Hinman, A. R., W. A. Orenstein, and L. Rodewald. 2004. Financing immunizations in the United States. *Clinical Infectious Diseases* 38(10):1440-1446.

HRSA (Health Resources and Services Administration). 2007. *Policy notice-07-05: The use of the Ryan White HIV/AIDS program Part B AIDS Drug Assistance Program (ADAP) funds to purchase health insurance*. https://hab.hrsa.gov/sites/default/files/hab/Global/partbadapfundspn0705.pdf (accessed October 19, 2016).

HRSA. 2014. *Clarifications regarding use of Ryan White HIV/AIDS program funds for premium and cost-sharing assistance for private health insurance. Policy Clarification Notice (PCN) #13-05*. http://hab.hrsa.gov/sites/default/files/hab/Global/pcn1305premium costsharing.pdf (accessed October 25, 2016).

HRSA. 2015. *Letter to Ryan White HIV/AIDS program Part B AIDS Drug Assistance Programs*. http://hab.hrsa.gov/sites/default/files/hab/Global/hcvmeds022015.pdf (accessed October 25, 2016).

HRSA. 2016a. *AIDS Drug Assistance Program (ADAP) manual, 2016*. http://hab.hrsa.gov/sites/default/files/hab/Global/adapmanual.pdf (accessed October 28, 2016).

HRSA. 2016b. *Organ Procurement and Transplantation Network. Data*. https://optn.transplant.hrsa.gov/data (accessed September 29, 2016).

HRSA. 2016c. *Organ Procurement and Transplantation Network. National data*. https://optn.transplant.hrsa.gov/data/view-data-reports/national-data/# (accessed September 29, 2016).

HRSA. 2016d. *The United States—Ryan White HIV/AIDS program client characteristics.* http://hab.hrsa.gov/stateprofiles/Client-Characteristics.aspx (accessed October 19, 2016).

HRSA. n.d.-a. *340B drug pricing program.* http://www.hrsa.gov/opa (accessed September 26, 2016).

HRSA. n.d.-b. *340B drug pricing program: Duplicate discount prohibition.* http://www.hrsa.gov/opa/programrequirements/medicaidexclusion (accessed September 26, 2016).

HRSA. n.d.-c. *340B drug pricing program: Eligibility and registration.* http://www.hrsa.gov/opa/eligibilityandregistration (accessed September 26, 2016).

HRSA. n.d.-d. *Closing the gap: Financing insurance services with ADAP.* ftp://ftp.hrsa.gov/hab/report_06_03.pdf (accessed October 25, 2016).

Huff-Rousselle, M. 2012. The logical underpinnings and benefits of pooled pharmaceutical procurement: a pragmatic role for our public institutions? *Social Science & Medicine* 75(9):1572-1580.

Indian Health Service. 2016. *Formulary.* https://www.ihs.gov/nptc/formulary (accessed February 10, 2017).

IOM (Institute of Medicine). 2004. *Measuring what matters: Allocation, planning, and quality assessment for the Ryan White CARE Act.* Washington, DC: The National Academies Press.

Johnson, C. Y. 2017a. Lawmakers slam new $89,000 price tag on rare disease treatment: "Unconscionable." *Washington Post,* February 13. https://www.washingtonpost.com/news/wonk/wp/2017/02/13/outrage-over-a-drug-price-controversy-is-building-in-congress-again/?utm_term=.fd25c396520e (accessed February 23, 2017).

Johnson, C. Y. 2017b. Trump on drug prices: Pharma companies are "getting away with murder." *Washington Post,* January 11. https://www.washingtonpost.com/news/wonk/wp/2017/01/11/trump-on-drug-prices-pharma-companies-are-getting-away-with-murder/?utm_term=.41c64b4d177f (accessed February 23, 2017).

Kaiser Family Foundation. 2014. *AIDS Drug Assistance Programs (ADAPs).* http://kff.org/hivaids/fact-sheet/aids-drug-assistance-programs (accessed December 29, 2016).

Kaiser Family Foundation. 2017. *The Ryan White HIV/AIDS Program: The basics.* http://kff.org/hivaids/fact-sheet/the-ryan-white-hivaids-program-the-basics (accessed February 8, 2017).

Kaiser Health News. 2003. States, territories negotiate $65M in annual price concessions for HIV/AIDS drugs from eight pharmaceutical companies. August 6. http://khn.org/morning-breakout/dr00019217 (accessed October 25, 2016).

Kapczynski, A., and A. S. Kesselheim. 2016. "Government patent use": A legal approach to reducing drug spending. *Health Affairs* 35(5):791-797.

Kesselheim, A. S., J. Avorn, and A. Sarpatwari. 2016. The high cost of prescription drugs in the United States: Origins and prospects for reform. *JAMA* 316(8):858-871.

Kevles, D. 2014. Medicare, Medicaid, and pharmaceuticals: The price of innovation. *Health Affairs Blog,* November 20. http://healthaffairs.org/blog/2014/11/20/medicare-medicaid-and-pharmaceuticals-the-price-of-innovation (accessed October 26, 2016).

Kim, W. R., J. R. Lake, J. M. Smith, M. A. Skeans, D. P. Schladt, E. B. Edwards, A. M. Harper, J. L. Wainright, J. J. Snyder, A. K. Israni, and B. L. Kasiske. 2016. OPTN/SRTR annual data report: Liver. *American Journal of Transplantation* 16(S2):69-98.

Leston, J., and J. Finkbonner. 2016. The need to expand access to hepatitis C virus drugs in the Indian Health Service. *JAMA* 316(8):817-818.

Lindley, M. C., A. K. Shen, W. A. Orenstein, L. E. Rodewald, and G. S. Birkhead. 2009. Financing the delivery of vaccines to children and adolescents: Challenges to the current system. *Pediatrics* 124(Suppl 5):S548-S557.

Lo Re, V. III, M. J. Kallan, J. P. Tate, A. R. Localio, J. K. Lim, M. B. Goetz, M. B. Klein, D. Rimland, M. C. Rodriguez-Barradas, A. A. Butt, C. L. Gibert, S. T. Brown, L. Park, R. Dubrow, K. R. Reddy, J. R. Kostman, B. L. Strom, and A. C. Justice. 2014. Hepatic decompensation in antiretroviral-treated patients co-infected with HIV and hepatitis C virus compared with hepatitis C virus-monoinfected patients: A cohort study. *Annals of Internal Medicine* 160(6):369-379.

Lo Re, V. III, C. Gowda, P. N. Urick, J. T. Halladay, A. Binkley, D. M. Carbonari, K. Battista, C. Peleckis, J. Gilmore, J. A. Roy, J. A. Doshi, P. P. Reese, K. R. Reddy, and J. R. Kostman. 2016. Disparities in absolute denial of modern hepaitits C therapy by type of insurance. *Clinical Gastroenterology and Hepatology* 14(7):1035-1043.

Luu, L. 2015. *Liver transplants.* http://emedicine.medscape.com/article/776313-overview (accessed September 29, 2016).

Martin, A. B., M. Hartman, J. Benson, and A. Catlin. 2016. National health spending in 2014: Faster growth driven by coverage expansion and presciption drug spending. *Health Affairs* 35(1):150-160.

Martin, E. G., H. A. Pollack, and A. D. Paltiel. 2006. Fact, fiction, and fairness: Resource allocation under the *Ryan White CARE Act. Health Affairs* 25(4):1103-1112.

Massachusetts EOHHS (Executive Office of Health and Human Services). 2016. *MassHealth implements new drug rebate program, extends access to hep C treatment.* http://www.mass.gov/eohhs/gov/newsroom/press-releases/eohhs/masshealth-implements-new-drug-rebate-program.html (accessed November 9, 2016).

McCarthy, M. 2016. U.S. Congress fails to agree Zika virus funding before summer break. *BMJ* 354:i3991.

McNeil, D. G., Jr. 2015. Curing hepatitis C, in an experiment the size of Egypt. *New York Times*, December 25. http://www.nytimes.com/2015/12/16/health/hepatitis-c-treatment-egypt.html?_r=0 (accessed October 26, 2016).

Mendes, P. n.d. *To license a patent – or, to assign it: Factors influencing the choice.* http://www.wipo.int/export/sites/www/sme/en/documents/pdf/license_assign_patent.pdf (accessed February 27, 2017).

Millar, T. P., S. Wong, D. H. Odierna, and L. A. Bero. 2011. Applying the essential medicines concept to U.S. preferred drug lists. *American Journal of Public Health* 101(8):1444-1448.

MMCAP (Minnesota Multistate Contracting Alliance for Pharmacy). n.d. *What is MMCAP and membership.* http://www.mmd.admin.state.mn.us/MMCAP/background/MMCAP_Mission_Model_Vision.aspx (accessed October 14, 2016).

Morgenson, G. 2016. To stop price spikes on prescription drugs, a widening radar. *New York Times*, December 23. https://www.nytimes.com/2016/12/23/business/drug-price-medicare-mallinckrodt-acthar.html?_r=0 (accessed February 23, 2016).

NASEM (National Academies of Sciences, Engineering, and Medicine). 2016. *Eliminating the public health problem of hepatitis B and C in the United States: Phase one report.* Washington, DC: The National Academies Press.

NASTAD (National Alliance of State and Territorial AIDS Directors). 2016. *Consultation summary: Strategies to increase hepatitis C treatment within ADAPs.* Washington, DC: NASTAD.

National Conference of State Legislatures. 2015. *Pharmaceutical bulk purchasing: Multi-state and inter-agency plans.* http://www.ncsl.org/research/health/bulk-purchasing-of-prescription-drugs.aspx (accessed August 26, 2016).

National Vaccine Advisory Committee. 1991. The measles epidemic: The problems, barriers, and recommendations. *JAMA* 266(11):1547-1552.

NVHR and CHLPI (National Viral Hepatitis Roundtable and Center for Health & Policy Innovation). 2016. Hepatitis C: The state of Medicaid access: Preliminary findings: National summary report. *National Viral Hepatitis Roundtable and Center for Health Law & Policy Innovation, Harvard Law School.* http://www.chlpi.org/wp-content/uploads/2013/12/HCV-Report-Card-National-Summary_FINAL.pdf (accessed December 14, 2016).

Orenstein, W. A. 2006. The role of measles elimination in development of a national immunization program. *The Pediatric Infectious Disease Journal* 25(12):1093-1101.

Peters, C. P. 2010. *Medicaid payment for generic drugs: Achieving savings and access. Issue brief no. 839.* Washington, DC: National Health Policy Forum.

Price, J. C., and C. L. Thio. 2010. Liver disease in the HIV-infected individual. *Clinical Gastroenterology and Hepatology* 8(12):1002-1012.

Provider Synergies LLC. n.d.-a. *NMPI—National Medicaid Pooling Initiative.* http://www.providersynergies.com/services/medicaid/default.asp?content=NMPI (accessed October 14, 2016).

Provider Synergies LLC. n.d.-b. *TOP$—The optimal PDL solution.* http://www.providersynergies.com/services/medicaid/default.asp?content=TOPS (accessed October 14, 2016).

Pyenson, B., K. Fitch, and K. Iwasaki. 2009. *Consequences of hepatitis C virus (HCV): Costs of a baby boomer epidemic of liver disease.* New York: Milliman Inc.

Q1Medicare. 2016. *2017 drug finder: Search for your prescription drug across all Medicare Part D or Medicare Advantage Plans.* https://q1medicare.com/PartD-SearchPDPMedicarePartDDrugFinder.php (accessed December 14, 2016).

Q1Medicare. n.d. *What are 'tiers or categories' on a Medicare drug plan's drug list (formulary)?* https://q1medicare.com/PartD-WhatAreDrugListTiersOrCategories.php (accessed December 14, 2016).

Ramey, C. 2016. Insurers probed on hepatitis C drug coverage. *Wall Street Journal*, March 2. http://www.wsj.com/articles/insurers-probed-on-hepatitis-c-drug-coverage-1456965087 (accessed October 3, 2016).

Razavi, H. 2016. *Modeling the elimination of hepatitis C in the United States.* Paper commissioned by the Committee on a National Strategy for the Elimination of Hepatitis B and C (see Appendix B).

Rich, J. D., S. A. Allen, and B. A. Williams. 2014. Responding to hepatitis C through the criminal justice system. *New England Journal of Medicine* 370(20):1871-1874.

Rizvi, Z., A. Kapczynski, and A. Kesselheim. 2016. A simple way for the government to curb inflated drug prices. *Washington Post*, May 12. https://www.washingtonpost.com/opinions/a-simple-way-for-the-government-to-curb-inflated-drug-prices/2016/05/12/ed89c9b4-16fc-11e6-aa55-670cabef46e0_story.html?utm_term=.581745400a4e (accessed September 30, 2016).

Rosenthal, E. 2014. The price of prevention: Vaccine costs are soaring. *New York Times*, July 2. http://www.nytimes.com/2014/07/03/health/Vaccine-Costs-Soaring-Paying-Till-It-Hurts.html?_r=1 (accessed September 28, 2016).

Roy, V., D. Chokshi, S. Kissler, and P. Singh. 2016. Making hepatitis C a rare disease in the United States. *Health Affairs Blog*, June 15. http://healthaffairs.org/blog/2016/06/15/making-hepatitis-c-a-rare-disease-in-the-united-states (accessed September 29, 2016).

Salzman, S. 2015. How insurance providers deny hepatitis C patients lifesaving drugs. *Al Jazeera America*, October 16. http://america.aljazeera.com/articles/2015/10/16/insurance-providers-deny-hepatitis-drugs.html (accessed October 3, 2016).

Schmid, C. 2016. *Integrating hepatitis services into HIV prevention and care programs.* http://theaidsinstitute.org/sites/default/files/attachments/Carl%20USCA%202016Hepatitis%20Presentation.pdf (accessed October 25, 2016).

Schoenberg, S. 2015. Inmates' suit claims Massachusetts denies prisoners hepatitis C drugs. *MassLive*, June 15. http://www.masslive.com/politics/index.ssf/2015/06/inmates_sue_massachusetts_for.html (accessed February 23, 2017).

Senate Committee on Finance. 2015. *The price of Sovaldi and its impact on the U.S. health care system*. (97-329 PDF/S. Prt. 114-20). Washington, DC: Government Publishing Office.

Shen, A. K., L. E. Rodewald, and G. S. Birkhead. 2009. Perspective of vaccine manufacturers on financing pediatric and adolescent vaccines in the United States. *Pediatrics* 124(Suppl 5):S540-S547.

Shih, C., J. Schwartz, and A. Coukell. 2016. *How would government negotiation of Medicare Part D drug prices work? Health Affairs Blog*, February 1. http://healthaffairs.org/blog/2016/02/01/how-would-government-negotiation-of-medicare-part-d-drug-prices-work (accessed October 26, 2016).

Smalley, W. E., M. R. Griffin, R. L. Fought, L. Sullivan, and W. A. Ray. 1995. Effect of a prior-authorization requirement on the use of nonsteroidal anti-inflammatory drugs by Medicaid patients. *New England Journal of Medicine* 332(24):1612-1617.

Smith, B. D., R. L. Morgan, G. A. Beckett, Y. Falck-Ytter, D. Holtzman, and J. W. Ward. 2012. Hepatitis C virus testing of persons born during 1945–1965: Recommendations from the Centers for Disease Control and Prevention. *Annals of Internal Medicine* 157(11):817-822.

Soumerai, S. B. 2004. Benefits and risks of increasing restrictions on access to costly drugs in Medicaid. *Health Affairs* 23(1):135-146.

SSDC (Sovereign States Drug Consortium). 2016. *CMS approved Medicaid supplemental drug rebate pool—Fact sheet*. https://www.rxssdc.org (accessed October 14, 2016).

Stand, L. 2015. *Integrating hepatitis services into HIV programs: Setting the federal policy stage*. http://www.theaidsinstitute.org/sites/default/files/attachments/Hepatitis%20Presentation%20-%20Lisa%20Stand.pdf (accessed October 25, 2016).

Taylor, L. E. 2005. Delivering care to injection drug user coinfected with HIV and hepatitis C virus. *Clinical Infectious Diseases* 40(Suppl 5):S355-S361.

The Pew Charitable Trusts and MacArthur Foundation. 2014. *State prison health care spending: An examination*. The Pew Charitable Trusts and the John D. and Catherine T. MacArthur Foundation. http://www.pewtrusts.org/~/media/assets/2014/07/stateprison-healthcarespendingreport.pdf (accessed February 23, 2017).

Thomas, D. L., D. Leoutsakas, T. Zabransky, and M. S. Kumar. 2011. Hepatitis C in HIV-infected individuals: Cure and control, right now. *Journal of the International AIDS Society* 14(1):22.

Truven Health Analytics. 2017. *Red Book*. http://micromedex.com/products/product-suites/clinical-knowledge/redbook (accessed January 12, 2017).

UnitedHealthcare. 2015. *Harvoni prior authorization/medical necessity*. https://www.unitedhealthcareonline.com/ccmcontent/ProviderII/UHC/en-US/Assets/ProviderStaticFiles/ProviderStaticFilesPdf/Tools%20and%20Resources/Pharmacy%20Resources/Med_Nec_Harvoni.pdf (accessed October 3, 2016).

USPSTF (U.S. Preventive Services Task Force). 2013. *Final recommendation statement. Hepatitis C: Screening*. https://www.uspreventiveservicestaskforce.org/Page/Document/RecommendationStatementFinal/hepatitis-c-screening#consider (accessed September 30, 2016).

VA (Department of Veterans Affairs). 2015. *Semiannual report to Congress. Issue 73. October 1, 2014-March 31, 2015*. Washington, DC: Office of Inspector General. http://www.va.gov/oig/pubs/sars/vaoig-sar-2015-1.pdf (accessed October 26, 2016).

VA. 2016a. *Department of Veterans Affairs: Office of Inspector General: August 2016 highlights.* http://www.va.gov/oig/pubs/highlights/VAOIG-highlights-201608.pdf (accessed October 26, 2016).

VA. 2016b. *VA expands hepatitis C drug treatment.* http://www.va.gov/opa/pressrel/pressrelease.cfm?id=2762 (accessed November 17, 2016).

Young, V. 2015. Missouri to drop expensive hepatitis C drug Sovaldi, use alternative. *St. Louis Post-Dispatch*, January 27. http://www.stltoday.com/news/local/govt-and-politics/virginia-young/missouri-to-drop-expensive-hepatitis-c-drug-sovaldi-use-alternative/article_0f2a8964-d4bc-5362-8d41-b10e65d13408.html (accessed October 26, 2016).

Zibbell, J. E., K. Iqbal, R. C. Patel, A. Suryaprasad, K. J. Sanders, L. Moore-Moravian, J. Serrecchia, S. Blankenship, J. W. Ward, and D. Holtzman. 2015. Increases in hepatitis C virus infection related to injection drug use among persons aged ≤30 years—Kentucky, Tennessee, Virginia, and West Virginia, 2006–2012. *Morbidity and Mortality Weekly Report* 64(17):453-458.

Zimmerman, R. K., M. P. Nowalk, T. A. Mieczkowski, H. M. Mainzer, I. K. Jewell, and M. Raymund. 2001. The Vaccines for Children program: Policies, satisfaction, and vaccine delivery. *American Journal of Preventive Medicine* 21(4):243-249.

7

Research

This committee's first report was clear that eliminating viral hepatitis as a public health problem is a bold goal, and not one that can be realized without significant improvements in prevention, screening, and treatment (NASEM, 2016a). There are still gaps in our understanding of the viruses that can hold back progress on meeting the targets set in Chapter 2. For this reason, the World Health Organization (WHO) identified research as one of the essential pieces of any country's national viral hepatitis elimination program. For the United States, a comparative advantage in science and technology compels special attention to such questions. Advancing understanding of the hepatitis B and C viruses and their treatment and prevention in a range of settings is a crucial contribution to the elimination effort in this country and the world.

The National Institutes of Health (NIH) has been criticized for failing to align its funding priorities with measures of disease burden in the United States or the world (Gillum et al., 2011). Viral hepatitis research is no exception. Chronic hepatitis B virus (HBV) and hepatitis C virus (HCV) infection affects 3 to 5 times more Americans than HIV, for example;[1] worldwide, it is about 10 times more.[2] But NIH funding for viral hepatitis between 2012 and 2017 has been between $195 and $273 million a year,

---

[1] The Centers for Disease Control and Prevention (CDC) estimates 1.2 million cases of HIV in the United States, 2.7 to 3.9 million chronic hepatitis C, and 850,000 to 2.2 million chronic hepatitis B (CDC, 2016a,b).
[2] The WHO estimates 36.7 million cases of HIV, 240 million chronic hepatitis B, and 130 to 150 million chronic hepatitis C (WHO, 2016a,b,c).

compared to nearly $3 billion a year (roughly 12 times more) for HIV (NIH, 2016b).[3] Despite being the seventh leading cause of death in the world, viral hepatitis research accounts for less than 1 percent of NIH's $31 billion research budget (IHME, 2015; NIH, 2016b,c; Stanaway et al., 2016).

Viral hepatitis elimination would do well to copy the success of the fight against HIV, starting with its success in research. Many of the breakthroughs that stopped transmission of HIV, from the development of AIDS therapies to the use of treatment to prevent sexual transmission, came from NIH-funded studies (Cohen et al., 2011b; NCI, n.d.; NIH, 2011). In the early 1980s, most HIV research was within the purview of the National Institute of Allergy and Infectious Diseases and the National Cancer Institute, but as the virus emerged as an international epidemic, NIH leaders realized that no one institute's mission was sufficient to encompass the necessary research agenda (NIH, n.d.). The Office of AIDS Research was established in response to this problem. The office works across the NIH to ensure that a range of biomedical and behavioral research questions get sufficient attention, coordinating the budget and setting priorities for HIV research (NIH, n.d.).

This report has already argued that eliminating viral hepatitis as a public health threat is a complicated proposition and one that will require attention from various federal, state, and local government offices, as well as coordination with various private sector organizations. Coordinating these organizations will be challenging, and may do well to try to replicate the success of the HIV research program.

The creation of the Office of AIDS Research in 1993 was accompanied by a full review of NIH's investment in HIV and AIDS research (Cohen, 1996). It could be helpful to conduct a similar review of viral hepatitis activities, considering them against the care continuum introduced in Chapter 4. The diagram shown in Chapter 4 represents an ideal continuum with very few drop-offs. In the real world, patients are frequently lost to follow-up and fail to respond to treatment. Attrition at any step is a barrier to elimination, so each drop along the continuum should be considered for possible research opportunities.

The NIH Division of Program Coordination, Planning, and Strategic Initiatives manages research on topics that naturally straddle more than one institute, including behavioral science, women's health, and AIDS (NIH, 2016a). The office also handles the Trans-NIH Committee on Viral Hepatitis, a group formed to implement the goals articulated in the Department of Health and Human Services viral hepatitis action plan (HHS,

---

[3] As indicated by a search for the terms "hepatitis" and "HIV" in 2016 on the NIH's Research Portfolio Online Reporting Tools.

2015; NIH, 2013). The committee involves members from nine centers and institutes and the Office of AIDS Research (NIH, 2013; Viral Hepatitis Implementation Group, 2011). It is possible that the committee, or some other coordinating entity, might be able to lead an expanded viral hepatitis research program across agencies that fund viral hepatitis research. Special priorities for NIH and other research funding organizations are discussed in the next section.

RESEARCH ACROSS THE CARE CONTINUUM

A diagram of the hepatitis C care continuum shows multiple opportunities for improvement (see Figure 7-1). A recent study in New York City found that only 20 percent of people tested for HCV antibody have a confirmatory HCV RNA test, and among those who received a confirmatory HCV RNA test, the median wait time for testing was 13 days (IQR, 2 to 52 days) (Norton et al., 2016). Figure 7-2 suggests similar gaps in hepatitis B care.

There are new opportunities to better understand where and why people drop off the care continuum. The Department of Veterans Affairs (VA) program to treat all HCV-infected patients in its health system is one such opportunity. The VA has a good clinical records system that is the same across the country (Kane and Chesanow, 2014). VA beneficiaries have relatively reliable access to care, something that one would expect to be maintained after HCV treatment is over. The cohort is also large; over 174,000 veterans have chronic HCV infection (VA, 2014). Therefore, this population is an ideal one in which to study the long-term risk of liver disease in people cured of hepatitis C. It would also be possible to investigate results from different models of care or subpopulations of infected veterans.

Meeting people at every step of the care continuum will get more challenging over time; the patients who are easiest to manage will have already been found. The challenges of the later stages of elimination could be headed off now by developing new tools and clarifying the most efficient strategies for reaching different patient groups. To this end, the committee has identified a set of pressing research questions key to the elimination effort. These topics are divided broadly into mechanistic questions dealing with the basic science of the viruses and ways to diagnose and cure them, and operations and implementation research questions concerned with identifying the best strategies to prevent and treat viral hepatitis. The research questions identified below are not necessarily new, in many cases the body of knowledge described builds off other recent studies. This is, rather, the committee's best summary of important questions in the field. Attention to these topics would serve the large goal of elimination of hepatitis B and C.

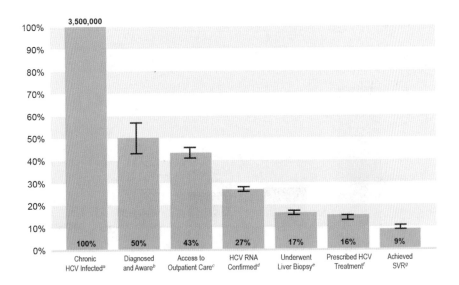

FIGURE 7-1 The treatment cascade for chronic hepatitis C virus infection in the United States.

NOTES: Only non-VA studies are included in the above HCV treatment cascade. HCV = hepatitis C virus; RNA = ribonucleic acid; SVR = sustained virologic response; VA = Department of Veterans Affairs.

[a] Chronic HCV infected; n = 3,500,000.

[b] Calculated as estimated number chronic HCV-infected (3,500,000) × estimated percentage diagnosed and aware of their infection (49.8%); n = 1,743,000.

[c] Calculated as estimated number diagnosed and aware (1,743,000) × estimated percentage with access to outpatient care (86.9%); n = 1,514,667.

[d] Calculated as estimated number with access to outpatient care (1,514,667) × estimated percentage HCV RNA confirmed (62.9%); n = 952,726.

[e] Calculated as estimated number with access to outpatient care (1,514,667) × estimated percentage who underwent liver biopsy (38.4%); n = 581,632.

[f] Calculated as estimated number with access to outpatient care (1,514,667) × estimated percentage prescribed HCV treatment (36.7%); n = 555,883.

[g] Calculated as estimated number prescribed HCV treatment (555,883) × estimated percentage who achieved SVR (58.8%); n = 326,859.

SOURCE: Yehia et al., 2014.

Mechanistic Research

There can be no elimination of HBV and HCV infections without enhanced understanding of the fundamental biology of these viruses and novel therapeutic targets (Palese, 2016). To this end, there should more research on viral life cycle, including the entry of the virus into host cells,

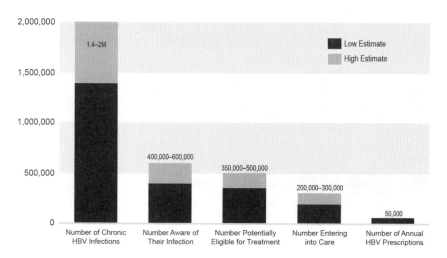

FIGURE 7-2 Gradient of the number of chronic hepatitis B infections to the number of individuals receiving treatment in the United States with ranges based on low and high estimates of hepatitis B prevalence.
NOTE: HBV = hepatitis B virus.
SOURCE: Cohen et al., 2011a.

host protein interactions, viral replication, persistence, release, and virion maturation. Virology research has always been intertwined with discovery of host biology, particularly immunology, providing dividends that extend well beyond the particular virus studied (Tortorella et al., 2000). Between 1901 and 2014, 14 Nobel Prizes in medicine were awarded for virology research; Table 7-1 gives examples of breakthroughs with broader applications that have come from studying viral hepatitis (Nobelprize.org, n.d.).

Molecular Epidemiology and Phylodynamic Methods

As elimination efforts proceed and viral hepatitis prevalence decreases, case finding will become more difficult and the study of ongoing transmission networks more important. Modern molecular epidemiology, including the use of phylodynamics to describe transmission dynamics and reconstruct transmission histories, would complement classical epidemiological research (Pybus and Rambaut, 2009). Sequencing of HBV and HCV genomes would advance this goal, as would investing in epidemiological and clinical data to link the genomic analysis (Pillay et al., 2015). Understanding the risk of transmission requires linking sequences in the viral genome to clinical and epidemiological data (Pillay et al., 2015). To be successful,

TABLE 7-1 Virology Breakthroughs from Viral Hepatitis Research

Virus	Discovery	Reference
HBV	First vaccine to prevent human cancer (the hepatitis B vaccine)	Chang et al., 2009; NAS, 2000
HBV	First radioimmunoassay (RIA)	Ling and Overby, 1972
HBV	First model to elucidate the causative role of inflammation in carcinogenesis	Nakamoto et al., 1998
HCV	Discovery of human polymorphism (initially IL28B, ultimately interferon λ4) governing outcome of acute HCV infection and response to interferon	O'Brien et al., 2014
HCV	Discovery of MAVS, a key adaptor protein in RIG-I signaling	Meylan et al., 2005
HCV	First microRNA dependent virus, first microRNA targeted drug	Lindow and Kauppinen, 2012
HCV	First cure of an infectious disease using an immune checkpoint inhibitor (anti-D-1)	Gardiner et al., 2013

NOTE: HBV = hepatitis B virus; HCV = hepatitis C virus; MAVS = mitochondrial antiviral-signaling protein.

elimination efforts will have to adapt to address remaining transmission, which is likely to vary by location, population, and behavior—variables that can be informed by phylodynamics.

Rapid Diagnostic Testing for HBV DNA and HCV RNA

Rapid or point-of-care tests can help avoid attrition on the viral hepatitis care continuum from the start. With rapid tests, people receive counseling and test results all in one interaction, limiting opportunity for loss to follow-up. In some settings, rapid point-of-care tests also enhance the ability to screen family members and other contacts of infected cases.

Hepatitis C antibody testing alone is not sufficient to diagnose hepatitis C. As discussed earlier in this report, rapid tests for HCV RNA in addition to existing antibody tests would improve patient management, especially in places catering to patients at elevated risk for hepatitis C such as syringe exchange centers (Smith et al., 2011).

In addition to individual testing for screening and disease management, there is a need for population-level assessment of progress toward elimination goals. Understanding incidence is crucial to this goal, but the cohort studies needed to document incidence are expensive and logistically complicated. Recently, serological testing research has demonstrated the accuracy of cross-sectional incidence testing for HIV, and similar work with HCV is promising (Brookmeyer et al., 2013; Patel et al., 2016). Further work with HBV and HCV could result in tests that detect recent infection in a single blood sample, which would greatly enhance efforts to identify new infections.

Immune Response to HBV

More complete understanding of the human immune response to HBV would have broad benefits. Immune responses can protect against transmission of HBV and play a key role in successful antiviral therapy (Bertoletti and Ferrari, 2012). Immune response also contributes to fibrosis progression (Bertoletti and Ferrari, 2012; Bertoletti et al., 2010). Deeper understanding of anti-HBV immune responses could open new avenues for additional vaccine development, informing antigen and adjuvant selection. Of particular interest would be research to simplify the hepatitis B vaccine schedule and reduce vaccine failure, and ways to shorten or enhance success of antiviral therapy, and further reduce mother-to-child transmission of HBV.

Hepatitis B in Pregnancy

Recent evidence suggests that it is possible to prevent chronic hepatitis B in newborns born to highly viremic, HBeAg+ women with prophylactic antiviral therapy in addition to standard newborn prophylaxis with hepatitis B immune globulin and vaccine (Pan et al., 2016). There is considerable uncertainty as to what the HBV DNA threshold should be to start antiviral therapy in pregnant women who would not otherwise require treatment. Suggested cut points range from 200,000 to 10 million IU/ml (ASHM, 2014; Terrault et al., 2016). It is also unclear when in pregnancy the therapy should be started or stopped, or even if the goal of such therapy should be preventing newborn viremia or preventing chronic infection in the newborn. All of these questions warrant wider attention.

Vaccine Against HCV

The well-tolerated direct-acting antiviral treatments for chronic HCV infection make it possible to even consider eliminating viral hepatitis in the United States, but curative tools alone seem limited in service to a goal as ambitious as elimination. Control of other infectious diseases such as tuberculosis and syphilis is still extremely challenging, and cures for these infections have been available for decades. Vaccines are almost invariably essential for eliminating infectious diseases, and an HCV vaccine has been elusive (Palese, 2016).

It is not surprising that HCV vaccine development has been challenging. HCV is extensively diverse genetically, the virus cannot be cultured (with a few genetically restricted exceptions), and there is no immunocompetent small animal model that supports HCV replication (Bukh, 2016).

In spite of early setbacks, there is growing evidence that it may be possible to make an effective vaccine for HCV, especially if the goal is to enhance spontaneous clearance rather than prevent infection (Man John Law et al., 2013). It is well known that about 25 percent of people acutely infected with HCV clear the infection spontaneously (Grebely et al., 2012; Micallef et al., 2006). People who have cleared HCV infection once are far more likely to do so again, with progressively lower levels and duration of viremia (Grebely et al., 2006; Osburn et al., 2010). People who clear infection spontaneously develop cell-mediated and neutralizing antibody responses (Dowd et al., 2009; Keoshkerian et al., 2016; Pestka et al., 2007). Chimpanzee studies have shown that depletion of CD4+ and CD8+ T cells resulted in HCV persistence (Grakoui et al., 2003; Shoukry et al., 2003). Both findings indicate immune response is an essential element in clearance (Dowd et al., 2009; Grakoui et al., 2003; Keoshkerian et al., 2016; Pestka et al., 2007; Shoukry et al., 2003). Studies are now emerging in humans, but additional vaccine candidates and correlates of protection are likely to be necessary to prevent HCV infection (Swadling et al., 2014).

Studies of humoral and cellular immunity have advanced understanding of HCV and suggest that a vaccine to prevent chronic infection is feasible (Bukh, 2016; Liang, 2013). Though the HCV envelope is highly variable, broadly neutralizing antibody responses have been identified during early infection (Osburn et al., 2014), and some epitopes of broadly neutralizing antibodies are evolutionarily constrained (Rodrigo et al., 2017). Though the crystal structure of the HCV envelope proteins remains elusive, structural studies of core domains are advancing (McCaffrey et al., 2017). Such studies can inform the design of rational humoral vaccine. Recent molecular dynamic studies have also illuminated a mechanistic basis for prior failures to elicit broadly neutralizing antibody responses, opening new avenues for rational design (Kong et al., 2016). As with antibody response, broadly directed T cell responses appear early in natural infection, but are rapidly lost in chronic infection (Schulze Zur Wiesch et al., 2012). A candidate prophylactic vaccine currently in clinical trials elicited strong T cell responses in phase I and II testing, but lacks an envelope protein component (NIAID, 2017; Swadling et al., 2014).

Taken together, the current status of HCV vaccine development is intermediate but promising; given the importance of vaccine prophylaxis in other elimination campaigns, this area of research should receive additional attention.

Curative Therapy for HBV

The lack of a cure for HBV infection is an obstacle to elimination. Fundamental study of the virus would identify therapeutic targets that might facilitate development of curative rather than suppressive therapy. Such research should aim to clarify the mechanisms of viral persistence, host and viral determinants of the stability of cccDNA, and the role of integrated portions of the HBV genome in the host genome.

The treatment of HBV infection might be improved by novel antiviral combinations and sequential therapy. Clinical trials of such treatments are necessary to determine the best treatment strategy, as well as the best format for answering questions regarding the discontinuation of therapy, treatment of low-level viremia in persons with cirrhosis, and treatment in patients at particular risk of complications, such as HIV patients. Clinical trials would also help determine the best frequency and way to monitor treatment outcomes. Clinical outcomes such as cirrhosis and liver cancer are the gold standard in trials, but it takes a large study size and years of follow-up to track such outcomes. Some key clinical outcomes have been shown to correlate strongly with intermediate outcomes, such as HBV DNA suppression, normalization of liver enzymes, HBeAg to anti-HBe conversion, and regression of cirrhosis (Lok et al., 2016). Therapeutic trials may make faster progress by giving attention to some of these intermediate outcomes, though some authorities have indicated a need for studies on long-term health outcomes, which would require a large prospective cohort study (USPSTF, 2014).

HBV Reactivation During Immunosuppressant Therapy

The mechanisms contributing to reactivation of HBV are poorly understood. Both reactivation of HBV during therapy for autoimmune disease or cancer and reactivation of HBV during or after treatment of HCV infection may occur (Balagopal and Thio, 2015; Collins et al., 2015; Paul et al., 2016; Perez-Alvarez et al., 2011). It will be difficult to eliminate chronic hepatitis B in the face of potential reactivation of HBV infection. Widespread treatment for hepatitis C could trigger complications in people with both infections. Greater understanding of what predicts reactivation at the host, and viral levels, as well as ways to prevent and treat HBV reactivation is necessary.

Detection and Management of Fibrosis, Cirrhosis, Hepatocellular Carcinoma

The complications of chronic HBV and HCV infection arise mainly from progressive liver fibrosis. Even after cure or sustained suppression of the virus, liver fibrosis and cirrhosis continue to be associated with end-stage liver disease and hepatocellular carcinoma (Lok et al., 2016; Tholey and Ahn, 2015). Basic research on the pathogenesis of fibrosis has led to some candidate anti-fibrotic therapies (Lee et al., 2015). Such treatment has the potential to benefit everyone with liver disease, not only viral hepatitis patients, but no treatment for reversal of liver fibrosis has been approved.

As Chapter 1 made clear, everyone with chronic viral hepatitis is at increased risk of hepatocellular carcinoma, which is the second most common cause of cancer death worldwide (Ferlay et al., 2015; Makarova-Rusher et al., 2016; Welzel et al., 2013). The incidence of liver cancer in the United States increased 38 percent between 2003 and 2012; liver cancer deaths increased 56 percent in the same time (Ryerson et al., 2016).

The environmental, host, and viral determinants that predict the transition from chronic viral hepatitis to liver cancer are not completely understood (El-Serag, 2012; Westbrook and Dusheiko, 2014). Guidelines for detection of hepatocellular carcinoma in persons at risk, including those with HBV or HCV infection, are well-established despite limited data, but adherence to the guidelines is poor, even among specialists (Bruix and Sherman, 2011; Hearn et al., 2015; Sharma et al., 2011; Wu et al., 2014). Part of the challenge lies in the available screening tools.

Current screening methods call for liver imaging every 6 months. However, liver ultrasound without bubble contrast has limited sensitivity, particularly in obese patients (Chou et al., 2015; Giannini et al., 2013; Hennedige and Venkatesh, 2013). There are logistical challenges with the more accurate abdominal computed tomography (CT), magnetic resonance imaging (MRI), and ultrasound with contrast imaging (Chou et al., 2015). (CT scan exposes the patient to radiation; both MRI and CT scans are expensive, require special equipment, and, when being used to diagnose hepatocellular carcinoma, both scans require contrast.) In any case, repeated imaging appointments are a burden to patients and providers. In the 2010 update to the AASLD[4] guidelines, alpha-fetoprotein testing was abandoned due to poor sensitivity and specificity, and no serum biomarker has replaced it (Bruix and Sherman, 2011).

The effectiveness of current screening methods for hepatocellular carcinoma, in terms of reducing mortality, is disputed (El-Serag and Davila, 2011; Marrero and El-Serag, 2011). A recent meta-analysis in cirrhotic

---

[4] Officially, the American Association for the Study of Liver Diseases.

patients showed hepatocellular carcinoma surveillance is associated with significant improvements in early tumor detection, curative treatment rates and overall survival (Singal et al., 2014). Additional study of pathogenesis, correlates, and biomarkers of hepatocellular carcinoma could significantly improve the accuracy and availability of screening tests and the ability to diagnose liver cancer at a treatable stage. Longitudinal study of these correlates should help identify people at minimal risk of liver cancer for whom frequent screening may not be necessary.

Hepatocellular carcinoma remains a risk among hepatitis B patients whose HBV DNA is suppressed and in hepatitis C patients with cirrhosis who have not been cured (de Oliveria Andrade et al., 2009; El-Serag, 2012; Fernandez-Rodriguez and Gutierrez-Garcia, 2014). It is not clear if such patients need to be monitored for cancer for the rest of their lives. A prospective cohort study to determine their residual risk over time would be valuable.

New treatments for liver cancer are also needed. Without early detection, most hepatocellular carcinoma patients have poor outcomes. Surgical treatment is associated with 5-year survival rates of up to 70 percent, but only 10 to 20 percent of patients are diagnosed with resectable tumors (Dhir et al., 2012; NCI, 2016; Shah et al., 2011; Sonnenday et al., 2007; Tiong and Maddern, 2011). In patients with unresectable disease, systemic or targeted chemotherapy or embolization with or without radiofrequency ablation yield a median survival of about 1 to 2 years (Tiong and Maddern, 2011). Genetically targeted cancer therapy and immunotherapy should offer more effective avenues for treating hepatocellular carcinoma (Bernicker, 2016; Roychowdhury and Chinnaiyan, 2016; Yang, 2015).

The cure of hepatitis C poses a valuable opportunity to study the long-term risk of complications after the agent causing damage to the liver is removed. Follow-up studies of people cured of chronic hepatitis C, with and without HIV, have revealed reduced, but non-zero, rates of hepatic decompensation, hepatocellular carcinoma, and death (Labarga et al., 2015; Moon et al., 2015; Morgan et al., 2010, 2013; Papastergiou et al., 2013). Cohort studies on cured patients could give insight into the management of liver fibrosis and identify genetic and environmental risks that may guide education, monitoring, and treatment after successful antiviral therapy.

Implementation Research

A better understanding of how and under what circumstances interventions work in the real world is the purview of implementation research (Peters et al., 2013). Much of the challenge of viral hepatitis elimination will lie in ensuring that preventative services and care reach the widest possible audience. This section identifies some implementation science questions that would serve the viral hepatitis elimination effort, both by adding to the tools available to prevent infection and by clarifying the best manner in which to implement programs that work.

Health in Jails and Prisons

As discussed in Chapter 5, prisons bear a disproportionate burden of viral hepatitis (Dolan et al., 2016; Maurer and Gondles, 2015; Weinbaum et al., 2003). They also have a serious burden of other infectious diseases, as well as mental and behavioral health problems (Freudenberg, 2001). In order for society to reap the full benefit of treating chronic hepatitis C in correctional facilities, better effort must be made to treat substance use disorder among prisoners, as this is the root cause of most viral hepatitis (CDC, 2016c; Grebely et al., 2015; Nelson et al., 2011). Failing to treat substance use risks exposing the cured inmate to reinfection, undermining the investment in his or her treatment. Drug relapse is more common during the transition from prison to civilian life (Vestal, 2016).

Estimates of the prevalence of drug dependence in jails and prisons range from 10 to 60 percent, partly because of varying definitions of drug dependence in this setting (Fazel et al., 2006). The National Institute on Drug Abuse encourages treatment of substance use disorder in prison, with provisions for outpatient treatment made after the inmate's release, but this is not common practice (NIH, 2014) (see Figure 7-3). Fewer than 0.1 percent of inmates in the United States receive opioid agonist therapy, the modern treatment standard for opioid addiction (Larney et al., 2011; WHO, 2009). Reasons for this inconsistency range from the philosophical (the belief that substance use is a weakness rather than a medical disorder or that the appropriate role of the criminal justice system is to punish offenders, not medicate them) to the practical (a lack of funds or concern that the medicines could not be securely stored in the prison infirmary) (NIDA, 2011; Nunn et al., 2009; Pecoraro and Woody, 2011).

Inconsistency in treatment of drug use in prisons has consequences for society, which routine treatment of hepatitis C in prisons will underscore. Treating substance use disorder in prisons would minimize the threat of reinfection after cure. It is not clear what the best strategies to manage such treatment may be. An evidence base on the value of treating substance use (including opioid dependence), considering outcomes such as blood-borne disease, and also violence and recidivism, would be of value to policy makers, as would information about the comparative effectiveness of modern opioid agonist methods compared to the current standard of care in most states.

Research in incarcerated people poses special challenges. The imprisoned participant is, by definition, being held against his or her will, so ques-

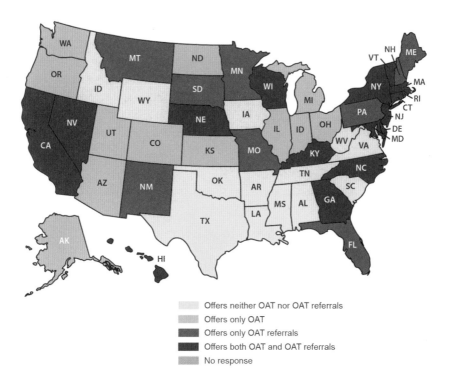

FIGURE 7-3 Opioid agonist therapy and referrals to community programs upon release from state prisons.
NOTE: OAT = opioid agonist therapy.
SOURCE: Nunn et al., 2009.

tions of coercion and informed consent become paramount (Chandler et al., 2009; Gostin, 2007). Prison research must be designed to ensure benefit to the participant, either individually or to prisoners as a group (IOM, 2007). Research on how best to implement substance use treatment programs in prisons meets both criteria. Prisoners would benefit from having research done on their behalf, as would society benefit from better understanding the safest and most efficient strategies to return inmates to their communities in the best health possible.

The transition from prison to civilian life, particularly the health risks of this transition, would also benefit from research attention. As Chapter 5 discussed, fewer than 20 percent of prison medical directors follow CDC recommendations for discharge planning with inmates (Solomon et al., 2014). Operations research would also be useful to determine the best ways to ensure a smooth transition from correctional health to Medicaid or another insurance program.

Strategies to Reach Key Populations

Chapter 5 discussed various populations that viral hepatitis services must reach in order for elimination to work. This includes people with substance use problems, mental illness, in unstable housing or living on the streets, and people facing cultural, language, or financial barriers to accessing care, including undocumented immigrants. These groups can be described as sensitive or hard to reach, terms used in the literature for populations that meet three criteria: the exact size of the group is not known, preventing articulation of a clear sampling frame; recognition as a member of the group risks prosecution or stigma; and members in the groups may be distrustful or uncooperative with outsiders (Benoit et al., 2005; Heckathorn, 1997). It is not clear how to best overcome these barriers and ensure that viral hepatitis prevention and care services reach the people who need them most.

Complex adaptive systems research, a field that aims to understand how different parts of a systems work together and influence each other, is a promising way to clarify what strategies work best to reach these populations (Paina and Peters, 2012). The complex adaptive systems strategy has been successful in studying health programs, especially at determining why some strategies work and others do not, as well as modeling the likely outcomes of different strategies (Jordon et al., 2010; Paina and Peters, 2012). On a practical note, connecting with community organizations that have existing, trusting relationships with the groups in question often eases the research logistics (Benoit et al., 2005).

Strategies to Alleviate Stigma

As this committee's first report discussed, stigma is a barrier to elimination of viral hepatitis (NASEM, 2016a). Stigma is also a difficult problem to tackle, partly because it can occur at many levels ranging from the laws and policies in place in a society, to negative attitudes toward certain groups or behaviors, to a person's internalized sense of shame or guilt (NASEM, 2016b). The best strategy to reduce stigma depends on the type of stigma targeted.

Part of the challenge relating to viral hepatitis is that it is difficult to disentangle the stigma of the infection from that of substance use often associated with liver disease in general, viral hepatitis in particular. Qualitative research could clarify the relative contributions of each among different communities and HBV- and HCV-infected people. This information would be a first step to understanding the problem.

Evidence regarding what strategies work best to fight stigma is murkier. There is an emerging consensus in mental health that media campaigns are not effective (Livingston et al., 2014; NASEM, 2016b). It is not clear if the same would be true for infectious disease, or what might work better. Research into this topic is sorely needed, and should consider, as the recent National Academies report concluded, "captur[ing] both direct and indirect effects, [. . .] intended and unintended consequences" (NASEM, 2016b, p. 10).

Harm Reduction in Emerging Settings and Populations

The 2010 Institute of Medicine report on viral hepatitis recommended the expansion of access to sterile injecting equipment for people who inject drugs (IOM, 2010). In the years since that report was published, injection drug use has exploded in rural and suburban areas (Des Jarlais et al., 2015). Less is known about the best strategies for harm reduction outside of cities, as Chapter 5 discussed. The relative merits of mobile syringe services, unstaffed exchange methods (i.e., vending machines), and over-the-counter sale of injecting equipment should all be examined (Duplessy and Reynaud, 2014; Strathdee and Beyrer, 2015). A recent meta-analysis found plausible evidence that combining harm reduction and substance use treatment was effective at preventing transmission of HCV, but the authors acknowledged that very few studies used HCV seroconversion as an outcome measure (Hagan et al., 2011). Future researchers should be encouraged to measure HCV seroconversion among people who inject drugs.

Another feature of the epidemic of injection drug use described in Chapter 5 that warrants particular research attention is injection drug use in people younger than 30. Young adults and adolescents who inject drugs are thought to be fueling spikes in HCV infection in the United States, but less is known about how to reach this group with harm reduction and other health services (Page et al., 2013; Stockings et al., 2016). Research on networks of drug users may be an efficient strategy to understand this population (Bryant, 2014).

Understanding Networks of Drug Users

As this report has made clear, people who inject drugs are a difficult but important population to engage in a viral hepatitis elimination program. Chapter 4 described how opioid drug use is reaching more and different populations than it did a generation ago (Des Jarlais et al., 2015; Havens et al., 2013). Our understanding, albeit limited, of social relationships among people who inject drugs and how these relationships influence disease transmission may not be relevant to rural or suburban settings.

Social network research aims to understand the influence of a person's social group on his or her behavior and risk (De et al., 2007; Weeks et al., 2009). The quality and types of relationships members have with other drug users and with the wider community are all thought to affect such behavior (De et al., 2007; Young et al., 2013). Research among drug users has shown that people in large, dense networks are more likely to share injecting equipment (De et al., 2007). It is not clear if or how social dynamics would differ in rural areas. On one hand, there is little in-migration to rural areas, so social ties tend to be long-lasting and strong. At the same time, distance and reliance on cars could contribute to isolation, especially among people already feeling isolated by substance use. A better understanding of how these dynamics unfold could help behavioral scientists tailor interventions to stop transmission of viral hepatitis and bring infected people who inject drugs into care.

Prevention of the Transition to Injecting Drugs

It is not clear what factors influence people who may have an addiction to drugs that are smoked or ingested to switch to injection. The user's social milieu is thought to play a role: relatives, friends, and sexual partners may encourage the switch, as does living in a neighborhood where injection drug use is common (Neaigus et al., 2006; Sherman et al., 2002). The user's physiological addiction can also drive him or her to more potent injectable drugs, as does the drug's cost, and the user's relative wealth (Mars et al., 2014; Neaigus et al., 2006; Sherman et al., 2002). Homelessness is also a risk factor (Neaigus et al., 2006).

A better understanding of why people start injecting drugs would inform efforts to prevent it. Self-administered questionnaires for people who inject drugs have been used in the past to measure risk of HIV (University of Pennsylvania, n.d.; Ward et al., 1990). A more recent tool, the Behavioral Risk Assessment for Infectious Diseases, looks specifically at drug use other than injection (Dunn et al., 2016). Research using these tools, alone or in combination, may help identify common threads driving the switch to the higher risk injection behavior.

REFERENCES

ASHM (Australasian Society for HIV, Viral Hepatitis and Sexual Health Medicine). 2014. *10.0 managing hepatitis B virus infection in pregnancy and children.* http://hepatitisb. org.au/10-0-managing-hepatitis-b-virus-infection-in-pregnancy-and-children (accessed November 21, 2016).

Balagopal, A., and C. L. Thio. 2015. Editorial commentary: Another call to cure hepatitis B. *Clinical Infectious Diseases* 61(8):1307-1309.

Benoit, C., M. Jansson, A. Millar, and R. Phillips. 2005. Community-academic research on hard-to-reach populations: Benefits and challenges. *Qualitative Health Research* 15(2):263-282.

Bernicker, E. 2016. Next-generation sequencing and immunotherapy biomarkers: A medical oncology perspective. *Archives of Pathology & Laboratory Medicine* 140(3):245-248.

Bertoletti, A., and C. Ferrari. 2012. Innate and adaptive immune responses in chronic hepatitis B virus infections: Towards restoration of immune control of viral infection. *Gut* 61(12):1754-1764.

Bertoletti, A., M. K. Maini, and C. Ferrari. 2010. The host-pathogen interaction during HBV infection: Immunological controversies. *Antiviral Therapy* 15(3):15-24.

Brookmeyer, R., O. Laeyendecker, D. Donnell, and S. H. Eshleman. 2013. Cross-sectional HIV incidence estimation in HIV prevention research. *Journal of Acquired Immune Deficiency Syndromes* 63(Suppl 2):S233-S239.

Bruix, J., and M. Sherman. 2011. Management of hepatocellular carcinoma: An update. *Hepatology* 53(3):1020-1022.

Bryant, J. 2014. Using respondent-driven sampling with 'hard to reach' marginalised young people: Problems with slow recruitment and small network size. *International Journal of Social Research Methodology* 17(6):599-611.

Bukh, J. 2016. The history of hepatitis C virus (HCV): Basic research reveals unique features in phylogeny, evolution and the viral life cycle with new perspectives for epidemic control. *Journal of Hepatology* 65(1 Suppl):S2-S21.

CDC (Centers for Disease Control and Prevention). 2016a. *Living with HIV.* https://www.cdc.gov/hiv/basics/livingwithhiv/index.html (accessed December 15, 2016).

CDC. 2016b. *Viral hepatitis–Statistics & surveillance.* https://www.cdc.gov/hepatitis/statistics/index.htm (accessed December 15, 2016).

CDC. 2016c. *Viral hepatitis surveillance: United States, 2014.* http://www.cdc.gov/hepatitis/statistics/2014surveillance/pdfs/2014hepsurveillancerpt.pdf (accessed Setpember 22, 2016).

Chandler, R. K., B. W. Fletcher, and N. D. Volkow. 2009. Treating drug abuse and addiction in the criminal justice system: Improving public health and safety. *JAMA* 301(2):183-190.

Chang, M. H., S. L. You, C. J. Chen, C. J. Liu, C. M. Lee, S. M. Lin, H. C. Chu, T. C. Wu, S. S. Yang, H. S. Kuo, and D. S. Chen. 2009. Decreased incidence of hepatocellular carcinoma in hepatitis B vaccinees: A 20-year follow-up study. *Journal of the National Cancer Institute* 101(19):1348-1355.

Chou, R., C. Cuevas, R. Fu, B. Devine, N. Wasson, A. Ginsburg, B. Zakher, M. Pappas, E. Graham, and S. D. Sullivan. 2015. Imaging techniques for the diagnosis of hepatocellular carcinoma: A systematic review and meta-analysis. *Annals of Internal Medicine* 162(10):697-711.

Cohen, C., S. D. Holmberg, B. J. McMahon, J. M. Block, C. L. Brosgart, R. G. Gish, W. T. London, and T. M. Block. 2011a. Is chronic hepatitis B being undertreated in the United States? *Journal of Viral Hepatitis* 18(6):377-383.

Cohen, J. 1996. AIDS politics: OAR gets by with a little help from new guard friends. *Science* 272(5270):1878.

Cohen, M. S., Y. Q. Chen, M. McCauley, T. Gamble, M. C. Hosseinipour, N. Kumarasamy, J. G. Hakim, J. Kumwenda, B. Grinsztejn, J. H. S. Pilotto, S. V. Godbole, S. Mehendale, S. Chariyalertsak, B. R. Santos, K. H. Mayer, I. F. Hoffman, S. H. Eshleman, E. Piwowar-Manning, L. Wang, J. Makhema, L. A. Mills, G. de Bruyn, I. Sanne, J. Eron, J. Gallant, D. Havlir, S. Swindells, H. Ribaudo, V. Elharrar, D. Burns, T. E. Taha, K. Nielsen-Saines, D. Celentano, M. Essex, and T. R. Fleming. 2011b. Prevention of HIV-1 infection with early antiretroviral therapy. *New England Journal of Medicine* 365(6):493-505.

Collins, J. M., K. L. Raphael, C. Terry, E. J. Cartwright, A. Pillai, F. A. Anania, and M. M. Farley. 2015. Hepatitis B virus reactivation during successful treatment of hepatitis C virus with sofosbuvir and simeprevir. *Clinical Infectious Diseases* 61(8):1304-1306.

De, P., J. Cox, J. F. Boivin, R. W. Platt, and A. M. Jolly. 2007. The importance of social networks in their association to drug equipment sharing among injection drug users: A review. *Addiction* 102(11):1730-1739.

de Oliveria Andrade, L. J., A. D'Oliveira, R. C. Melo, E. C. De Souza, C. A. Costa Silva, and R. Parana. 2009. Association between hepatitis C and hepatocellular carcinoma. *Journal of Global Infectious Diseases* 1(1):33-37.

Des Jarlais, D. C., A. Nugent, A. Solberg, J. Feelemyer, J. Mermin, and D. Holtzman. 2015. Syringe service programs for persons who inject drugs in urban, suburban, and rural areas—United States, 2013. *Morbidity and Mortality Weekly Report* 64(48):1337-1341.

Dhir, M., E. R. Lyden, L. M. Smith, and C. Are. 2012. Comparison of outcomes of transplantation and resection in patients with early hepatocellular carcinoma: A meta-analysis. *HPB (Oxford)* 14(9):635-645.

Dolan, K., A. L. Wirtz, B. Moazen, M. Ndeffo-mbah, A. Galvani, S. A. Kinner, R. Courtney, M. McKee, J. J. Amon, L. Maher, M. Hellard, C. Beyrer, and F. L. Altice. 2016. Global burden of HIV, viral hepatitis, and tuberculosis in prisoners and detainees. *Lancet* 388(10049):1089-1102.

Dowd, K. A., D. M. Netski, X. H. Wang, A. L. Cox, and S. C. Ray. 2009. Selection pressure from neutralizing antibodies drives sequence evolution during acute infection with hepatitis C virus. *Gastroenterology* 136(7):2377-2386.

Dunn, K. E., F. S. Barrett, E. S. Herrmann, J. G. Plebani, S. C. Sigmon, and M. W. Johnson. 2016. Behavioral risk assessment for infectious diseases (BRAID): Self-report instrument to assess injection and noninjection risk behaviors in substance users. *Drug and Alcohol Dependence* 168:69-75.

Duplessy, C., and E. G. Reynaud. 2014. Long-term survey of a syringe-dispensing machine needle exchange program: Answering public concerns. *Harm Reduction Journal* 11:16.

El-Serag, H. B. 2012. Epidemiology of viral hepatitis and hepatocellular carcinoma. *Gastroenterology* 142(6):1264-1273.

El-Serag, H. B., and J. A. Davila. 2011. Surveillance for hepatocellular carcinoma: In whom and how? *Therapeutic Advances in Gastroenterology* 4(1):5-10.

Fazel, S., P. Bains, and H. Doll. 2006. Substance abuse and dependence in prisoners: A systematic review. *Addiction* 101(2):181-191.

Ferlay, J., I. Soerjomataram, R. Dikshit, S. Eser, C. Mathers, M. Rebelo, D. M. Parkin, D. Forman, and F. Bray. 2015. Cancer incidence and mortality worldwide: Sources, methods and major patterns in GLOBOCAN 2012. *International Journal of Cancer* 136(5):e359-e386.

Fernandez-Rodriguez, C. M., and M. L. Gutierrez-Garcia. 2014. Prevention of hepatocellular carcinoma in patients with chronic hepatitis B. *World Journal of Gastrointestinal Pharmacology and Therapeutics* 5(3):175-182.

Freudenberg, N. 2001. Jails, prisons, and the health of urban populations: A review of the impact of the correctional system on community health. *Journal of Urban Health* 78(2):214-235.

Gardiner, D., J. Lalezari, E. Lawitz, M. DiMicco, R. Ghalib, K. R. Reddy, K. M. Chang, M. Sulkowski, S. O. Marro, J. Anderson, B. He, V. Kansra, F. McPhee, M. Wind-Rotolo, D. Grasela, M. Selby, A. J. Korman, and I. Lowy. 2013. A randomized, double-blind, placebo-controlled assessment of BMS-936558, a fully human monoclonal antibody to programmed death-1 (PD-1), in patients with chronic hepatitis C virus infection. *PLoS One* 8(5):e63818.

Giannini, E. G., A. Cucchetti, V. Erroi, F. Garuti, F. Odaldi, and F. Trevisani. 2013. Surveillance for early diagnosis of hepatocellular carcinoma: How best to do it? *World Journal of Gastroenterology* 19(47):8808-8821.

Gillum, L. A., C. Gouveia, E. R. Dorsey, M. Pletcher, C. D. Mathers, C. E. McCulloch, and S. C. Johnston. 2011. NIH disease funding levels and burden of disease. *PLoS One* 6(2):e16837.

Gostin, L. O. 2007. Biomedical research involving prisoners: Ethical values and legal regulation. *JAMA* 297(7):737-740.

Grakoui, A., N. H. Shoukry, D. J. Woollard, J. H. Han, H. L. Hanson, J. Ghrayeb, K. K. Murthy, C. M. Rice, and C. M. Walker. 2003. HCV persistence and immune evasion in the absence of memory T cell help. *Science* 302(5645):659-662.

Grebely, J., B. Conway, J. D. Raffa, C. Lai, M. Krajden, and M. W. Tyndall. 2006. Hepatitis C virus reinfection in injection drug users. *Hepatology* 44(5):1139-1145.

Grebely, J., M. Prins, M. Hellard, A. L. Cox, W. O. Osburn, G. Lauer, K. Page, A. R. Lloyd, and G. J. Dore. 2012. Hepatitis C virus clearance, reinfection, and persistence, with insights from studies of injecting drug users: Towards a vaccine. *The Lancet Infectious Diseases* 12(5):408-414.

Grebely, J., G. Robaeys, P. Bruggmann, A. Aghemo, M. Backmund, J. Bruneau, J. Byrne, O. Dalgard, J. J. Feld, M. Hellard, M. Hickman, A. Kautz, A. Litwin, A. R. Lloyd, S. Mauss, M. Prins, T. Swan, M. Schaefer, L. E. Taylor, and G. J. Dore. 2015. Recommendations for the management of hepatitis C virus infection among people who inject drugs. *International Journal on Drug Policy* 26(10):1028-1038.

Hagan, H., E. R. Pouget, and D. C. Des Jarlais. 2011. A systematic review and meta-analysis of interventions to prevent hepatitis C virus infection in people who inject drugs. *Journal of Infectious Diseases* 204(1):74-83.

Havens, J. R., M. R. Lofwall, S. D. Frost, C. B. Oser, C. G. Leukefeld, and R. A. Crosby. 2013. Individual and network factors associated with prevalent hepatitis C infection among rural Appalachian injection drug users. *American Journal of Public Health* 103(1):e44-e52.

Hearn, B., R. Chasan, K. Bichoupan, M. Suprun, E. Bagiella, D. T. Dieterich, P. Perumalswami, A. D. Branch, and S. Huprikar. 2015. Low adherence of HIV providers to practice guidelines for hepatocellular carcinoma screening in HIV/hepatitis B coinfection. *Clinical Infectious Diseases* 61(11):1742-1748.

Heckathorn, D. D. 1997. Respondent-driven sampling: A new approach to the study of hidden populations. *Social Problems* 44(2):174-199.

Hennedige, T., and S. K. Venkatesh. 2013. Imaging of hepatocellular carcinoma: Diagnosis, staging and treatment monitoring. *Cancer Imaging* 12:530-547.

HHS (Department of Health and Human Services). 2015. *Action plan for the prevention, care, and treatment of viral hepatitis: 2014-2016.* HHS, Office of the Assistant Secretary for Health, Office of HIV/AIDS and Infectious Disease Policy. https://www.aids.gov/pdf/viral-hepatitis-action-plan.pdf (accessed October 26, 2016).

IHME (Institute for Health Metrics and Evaluation). 2015. *GBD compare.* http://vizhub.healthdata.org/gbd-mortality (accessed February 23, 2016).

IOM (Institute of Medicine). 2007. *Ethical considerations for research involving prisoners.* Washington, DC: The National Academies Press.

IOM. 2010. *Hepatitis and liver cancer: A national strategy for prevention and control of hepatitis B and C.* Washington, DC: The National Academies Press.

Jordon, M., H. J. Lanham, R. A. Anderson, and R. R. McDaniel, Jr. 2010. Implications of complex adaptive systems theory for interpreting research about health care organizations. *Journal of Evaluation in Clinical Practice* 16(1):228-231.

Kane, L., and N. Chesanow. 2014. *Medscape EHR report 2014: Top rated EHRs by practice situation.* http://www.medscape.com/features/slideshow/public/ehr2014#11 (accessed December 15, 2016).

Keoshkerian, E., M. Hunter, B. Cameron, N. Nguyen, P. Sugden, R. Bull, A. Zekry, L. Maher, N. Seddiki, J. Zaunders, A. Kelleher, and A. R. Lloyd. 2016. Hepatitis C-specific effector and regulatory CD4 T-cell responses are associated with the outcomes of primary infection. *Journal of Viral Hepatitis* 23(12):985-993.

Kong, L., D. E. Lee, R. U. Kadam, T. Liu, E. Giang, T. Nieusma, F. Garces, N. Tzarum, V. L. Woods, Jr., A. B. Ward, S. Li, I. A. Wilson, and M. Law. 2016. Structural flexibility at a major conserved antibody target on hepatitis C virus E2 antigen. *Proceedings of the National Academy of Sciences of the United States of America* 113(45):12768-12773.

Labarga, P., J. V. Fernandez-Montero, C. de Mendoza, P. Barreiro, J. Pinilla, and V. Soriano. 2015. Liver fibrosis progression despite HCV cure with antiviral therapy in HIV-HCV-coinfected patients. *Antiviral Therapy* 20(3):329-334.

Larney, S., B. Toson, L. Burns, and K. Dolan. 2011. *Opioid substitution treatment in prison and post-release: Effects on criminal recidivism and mortality.* Canberra, Australian Capital Territory: National Drug and Alcohol Research Centre, University of New South Wales.

Lee, Y. A., M. C. Wallace, and S. L. Friedman. 2015. Pathobiology of liver fibrosis: A translational success story. *Gut* 64(5):830-841.

Liang, T. J. 2013. Current progress in development of hepatitis C virus vaccines. *Nature Medicine* 19(7):869-878.

Lindow, M., and S. Kauppinen. 2012. Discovering the first microRNA-targeted drug. *Journal of Cell Biology* 199(3):407-412.

Ling, C. M., and L. R. Overby. 1972. Prevalence of hepatitis B virus antigen as revealed by direct radioimmune assay with 125 I-antibody. *Journal of Immunology* 109(4):834-841.

Livingston, J. D., M. Cianfrone, K. Korf-Uzan, and C. Coniglio. 2014. Another time point, a different story: One year effects of a social media intervention on the attitudes of young people towards mental health issues. *Social Psychiatry and Psychiatric Epidemiology* 49(6):985-990.

Lok, A. S. F., B. J. McMahon, R. S. Brown, J. B. Wong, A. T. Ahmed, W. Farah, J. Almasri, F. Alahdab, K. Benkhadra, M. A. Mouchli, S. Singh, E. A. Mohamed, A. M. Abu Dabrh, L. J. Prokop, Z. Wang, M. H. Murad, and K. Mohammed. 2016. Antiviral therapy for chronic hepatitis B viral infection in adults: A systematic review and meta-analysis. *Hepatology* 63(1):284-306.

Makarova-Rusher, O. V., S. F. Altekruse, T. S. McNeel, S. Ulahannan, A. G. Duffy, B. I. Graubard, T. F. Greten, and K. A. McGlynn. 2016. Population attributable fractions of risk factors for hepatocellular carcinoma in the United States. *Cancer* 122(11):1757-1765.

Man John Law, L., A. Landi, W. C. Magee, D. Lorne Tyrrell, and M. Houghton. 2013. Progress towards a hepatitis C virus vaccine. *Emerging Microbes & Infections* 2:e79.

Marrero, J. A., and H. B. El-Serag. 2011. Alpha-fetoprotein should be included in the hepatocellular carcinoma surveillance guidelines of the American Association for the Study of Liver Diseases. *Hepatology* 53(3):1060-1061; author reply 1061-1062.

Mars, S. G., P. Bourgois, G. Karandinos, F. Montero, and D. Ciccarone. 2014. "Every 'never' I ever said came true": Transitions from opioid pills to heroin injecting. *International Journal of Drug Policy* 25(2):257-266.

Maurer, K., and E. F. Gondles. 2015. Hepatitis C in correctional settings: Challenges and opportunities. *Coalition of Correctional Health Authorities and American Correctional Association* 2(1).

McCaffrey, K., I. Boo, C. M. Owczarek, M. P. Hardy, M. A. Perugini, L. Fabri, P. Scotney, P. Poumbourios, and H. E. Drummer. 2017. An optimized hepatitis C virus E2 glycoprotein core adopts a functional homodimer that efficiently blocks virus entry. *Journal of Virology* 91(5).

Meylan, E., J. Curran, K. Hofmann, D. Moradpour, M. Binder, R. Bartenschlager, and J. Tschopp. 2005. Cardif is an adaptor protein in the RIG-I antiviral pathway and is targeted by hepatitis C virus. *Nature* 437(7062):1167-1172.

Micallef, J. M., J. M. Kaldor, and G. J. Dore. 2006. Spontaneous viral clearance following acute hepatitis C infection: A systematic review of longitudinal studies. *Journal of Viral Hepatitis* 13(1):34-41.

Moon, C., K. S. Jung, D. Y. Kim, O. Baatarkhuu, J. Y. Park, B. K. Kim, S. U. Kim, S. H. Ahn, and K. H. Han. 2015. Lower incidence of hepatocellular carcinoma and cirrhosis in hepatitis C patients with sustained virological response by pegylated interferon and ribavirin. *Digestive Diseases and Sciences* 60(2):573-581.

Morgan, R. L., B. Baack, B. D. Smith, A. Yartel, M. Pitasi, and Y. Falck-Ytter. 2013. Eradication of hepatitis C virus infection and the development of hepatocellular carcinoma: A meta-analysis of observational studies. *Annals of Internal Medicine* 158(5 Pt 1):329-337.

Morgan, T. R., M. G. Ghany, H. Y. Kim, K. K. Snow, M. L. Shiffman, J. L. De Santo, W. M. Lee, A. M. Di Bisceglie, H. L. Bonkovsky, J. L. Dienstag, C. Morishima, K. L. Lindsay, and A. S. Lok. 2010. Outcome of sustained virological responders with histologically advanced chronic hepatitis C. *Hepatology* 52(3):833-844.

Nakamoto, Y., L. G. Guidotti, C. V. Kuhlen, P. Fowler, and F. V. Chisari. 1998. Immune pathogenesis of hepatocellular carcinoma. *Journal of Experimental Medicine* 188(2):341-350.

NAS (National Academy of Sciences). 2000. *Beyond discovery: The hepatitis B story.* http://www.nasonline.org/publications/beyond-discovery/hepatitis-b-story.pdf (accessed January 3, 2017).

NASEM (National Academies of Sciences, Engineering, and Medicine). 2016a. *Eliminating the public health problem of hepatitis B and C in the United States: Phase one report.* Washington, DC: The National Academies Press.

NASEM. 2016b. *Ending discrimination against people with mental and substance use disorders: The evidence for stigma change.* Washington, DC: The National Academies Press.

NCI (National Cancer Institute). 2016. *Adult primary liver cancer treatment (PDQ®)–Health professional version.* https://www.cancer.gov/types/liver/hp/adult-liver-treatment-pdq (accessed October 28, 2016).

NCI. n.d. *HIV and AIDS Malignancy Branch.* https://ccr.cancer.gov/HIV-and-AIDS-Malignancy-Branch (accessed December 15, 2016).

Neaigus, A., V. A. Gyarmathy, M. Miller, V. M. Frajzyngier, S. R. Friedman, and D. C. Des Jarlais. 2006. Transitions to injecting drug use among noninjecting heroin users: Social network influence and individual susceptibility. *Journal of Acquired Immune Deficiency Syndromes* 41(4):493-503.

Nelson, P. K., B. M. Mathers, B. Cowie, H. Hagan, D. Des Jarlais, D. Horyniak, and L. Degenhardt. 2011. Global epidemiology of hepatitis B and hepatitis C in people who inject drugs: Results of systematic reviews. *Lancet* 378(9791):571-583.

NIAID (National Institute of Allergy and Infectious Diseases). 2017. Staged phase I/II hepatitis C prophylactic vaccine. In: ClinicalTrials.gov. Bethesda, MD: National Library of Medicine. Available from: https://clinicaltrials.gov/ct2/show/NCT01436357 (accessed February 23, 2017).

NIDA (National Institute on Drug Abuse). 2011. *More opioid replacement therapy in correctional facilities might yield public safety and health benefits.* https://www.drugabuse.gov/news-events/nida-notes/2011/07/prison-use-medications-opioid-addiction-remains-low (accessed December 15, 2016).

NIH (National Institutes of Health). 2011. *HIV study named 2011 breakthrough of the year by* Science. https://www.nih.gov/news-events/news-releases/hiv-study-named-2011-breakthrough-year-science (accessed December 15, 2016).

NIH. 2013. *Committees, working groups, and tasks forces.* https://dpcpsi.nih.gov/collaborations/committees.aspx?TID=2&FY=2013 (accessed February 23, 2017).

NIH. 2014. *Drug addiction treatment in the criminal justice system: Drug use, crime, and incarceration.* https://www.drugabuse.gov/related-topics/criminal-justice/drug-addiction-treatment-in-criminal-justice-system (accessed December 15, 2016).

NIH. 2016a. *About DPCPSI.* https://dpcpsi.nih.gov/about (accessed February 23, 2017).

NIH. 2016b. *Estimates of funding for various research, condition, and disease categories (RCDC).* https://report.nih.gov/categorical_spending.aspx (accessed December 15, 2016).

NIH. 2016c. *NIH budget history: Total NIH budget authority: FY 2016 enacted.* https://report.nih.gov/NIHDatabook/Charts/Default.aspx?showm=Y&chartId=5&catId=1 (accessed March 6, 2017).

NIH. n.d. *OAR history.* https://www.oar.nih.gov/about_oar/history.asp (accessed December 15, 2016).

Nobelprize.org. n.d. *The Nobel Prize in physiology or medicine fields.* https://www.nobelprize.org/nobel_prizes/medicine/fields.html (accessed January 3, 2017).

Norton, B. L., W. N. Southern, M. Steinman, J. Deluca, Z. Rosner, A. H. Litwin, B. L. Norton, M. Steinman, J. Deluca, Z. Rosner, A. H. Litwin, W. N. Southern, and B. D. Smith. 2016. No differences in achieving hepatitis C virus care milestones between patients identified by birth cohort or risk-based screening. *Clinical Gastroenterology and Hepatology* 14(9):1356-1360.

Nunn, A., N. Zaller, S. Dickman, C. Trimbur, A. Nijhawan, and J. D. Rich. 2009. Methadone and buprenorphine prescribing and referral practices in U.S. prison systems: Results from a nationwide survey. *Drug and Alcohol Dependence* 105(1-2):83-88.

O'Brien, T. R., L. Prokunina-Olsson, and R. P. Donnelly. 2014. IFN- 4: The paradoxical new member of the interferon lambda family. *Journal of Interferon & Cytokine Research* 34(11):829-838.

Osburn, W. O., B. E. Fisher, K. A. Dowd, G. Urban, L. Liu, S. C. Ray, D. L. Thomas, and A. L. Cox. 2010. Spontaneous control of primary hepatitis C virus infection and immunity against persistent reinfection. *Gastroenterology* 138(1):315-324.

Osburn, W. O., A. E. Snider, B. L. Wells, R. Latanich, J. R. Bailey, D. L. Thomas, A. L. Cox, and S. C. Ray. 2014. Clearance of hepatitis C infection is associated with the early appearance of broad neutralizing antibody responses. *Hepatology* 59(6):2140-2151.

Page, K., M. D. Morris, J. A. Hahn, L. Maher, and M. Prins. 2013. Injection drug use and hepatitis C virus infection in young adult injectors: Using evidence to inform comprehensive prevention. *Clinical Infectious Diseases* 57(Suppl 2):S32-S38.

Paina, L., and D. H. Peters. 2012. Understanding pathways for scaling up health services through the lens of complex adaptive systems. *Health Policy and Planning* 27(5):365-373.

Palese, P. 2016. Profile of Charles M. Rice, Ralf F. W. Bartenschlager, and Michael J. Sofia, 2016 Lasker-DeBakey Clinical Medical Research Awardees. *Proceedings of the National Academy of Sciences of the United States of America* 113(49):13934-13937.

Pan, C. Q., Z. Duan, E. Dai, S. Zhang, G. Han, Y. Wang, H. Zhang, H. Zou, B. Zhu, W. Zhao, and H. Jiang. 2016. Tenofovir to prevent hepatitis B transmission in mothers with high viral load. *New England Journal of Medicine* 374(24):2324-2334.

Papastergiou, V., M. Stampori, P. Lisgos, C. Pselas, K. Prodromidou, and S. Karatapanis. 2013. Durability of a sustained virological response, late clinical sequelae, and long-term changes in aspartate aminotransferase to the platelet ratio index after successful treatment with peginterferon/ribavirin for chronic hepatitis C: A prospective study. *European Journal of Gastroenterology & Hepatology* 25(7):798-805.

Patel, E. U., A. L. Cox, S. H. Mehta, D. Boon, C. E. Mullis, J. Astemborski, W. O. Osburn, J. Quinn, A. D. Redd, G. D. Kirk, D. L. Thomas, T. C. Quinn, and O. Laeyendecker. 2016. Use of hepatitis C virus (HCV) immunoglobulin G antibody avidity as a biomarker to estimate the population-level incidence of HCV infection. *Journal of Infectious Diseases* 214(3):344-352.

Paul, S., A. Saxena, N. Terrin, K. Viveiros, E. M. Balk, and J. B. Wong. 2016. Hepatitis B virus reactivation and prophylaxis during solid tumor chemotherapy: A systematic review and meta-analysis. *Annals of Internal Medicine* 164(1):30-40.

Pecoraro, A., and G. E. Woody. 2011. Medication-assisted treatment for opioid dependence: Making a difference in prisons. *F1000 Medicine Reports* 3:1.

Perez-Alvarez, R., C. Diaz-Lagares, F. Garcia-Hernandez, L. Lopez-Roses, P. Brito-Zeron, M. Perez-de-Lis, S. Retamozo, A. Bove, X. Bosch, J. M. Sanchez-Tapias, X. Forns, and M. Ramos-Casals. 2011. Hepatitis B virus (HBV) reactivation in patients receiving tumor necrosis factor (TNF)-targeted therapy: Analysis of 257 cases. *Medicine* 90(6):359-371.

Pestka, J. M., M. B. Zeisel, E. Blaser, P. Schurmann, B. Bartosch, F. L. Cosset, A. H. Patel, H. Meisel, J. Baumert, S. Viazov, K. Rispeter, H. E. Blum, M. Roggendorf, and T. F. Baumert. 2007. Rapid induction of virus-neutralizing antibodies and viral clearance in a single-source outbreak of hepatitis C. *Proceedings of the National Academy of Sciences of the United States of America* 104(14):6025-6030.

Peters, D. H., O. Alonge, T. Adam, I. A. Agyepong, and N. Tran. 2013. Implementation research: What it is and how to do it. *BMJ* 347:f6753.

Pillay, D., J. Herbeck, M. S. Cohen, T. de Oliveira, C. Fraser, O. Ratmann, A. L. Brown, and P. Kellam. 2015. PANGEA-HIV: Phylogenetics for generalised epidemics in Africa. *The Lancet Infectious Diseases* 15(3):259-261.

Pybus, O. G., and A. Rambaut. 2009. Evolutionary analysis of the dynamics of viral infectious disease. *Nature Reviews Genetics* 10(8):540-550.

Rodrigo, C., M. R. Walker, P. Leung, A. A. Eltahla, J. Grebely, G. J. Dore, T. Applegate, K. Page, S. Dwivedi, J. Bruneau, M. D. Morris, A. L. Cox, W. Osburn, A. Y. Kim, J. Schinkel, N. H. Shoukry, G. M. Lauer, L. Maher, M. Hellard, M. Prins, F. Luciani, A. R. Lloyd, and R. A. Bull. 2017. Limited naturally occurring escape in broadly neutralizing antibody epitopes in hepatitis C glycoprotein E2 and constrained sequence usage in acute infection. *Infection, Genetics and Evolution* 49:88-96.

Roychowdhury, S., and A. M. Chinnaiyan. 2016. Translating cancer genomes and transcriptomes for precision oncology. *CA: A Cancer Journal for Clinicians* 66(1):75-88.

Ryerson, A. B., C. R. Eheman, S. F. Altekruse, J. W. Ward, A. Jemal, R. L. Sherman, S. J. Henley, D. Holtzman, A. Lake, A. Noone, R. N. Anderson, J. Ma, K. N. Ly, K. A. Cronin, L. Penberthy, and B. A. Kohler. 2016. Annual report to the nation on the status of cancer, 1975-2012, featuring the increasing incidence of liver cancer. *Cancer* 122(9):1312-1337.

Schulze Zur Wiesch, J., D. Ciuffreda, L. Lewis-Ximenez, V. Kasprowicz, B. E. Nolan, H. Streeck, J. Aneja, L. L. Reyor, T. M. Allen, A. W. Lohse, B. McGovern, R. T. Chung, W. W. Kwok, A. Y. Kim, and G. M. Lauer. 2012. Broadly directed virus-specific CD4+ T cell responses are primed during acute hepatitis C infection, but rapidly disappear from human blood with viral persistence. *The Journal of Experimental Medicine* 209(1):61-75.

Shah, S. A., J. K. Smith, Y. Li, S. C. Ng, J. E. Carroll, and J. F. Tseng. 2011. Underutilization of therapy for hepatocellular carcinoma in the medicare population. *Cancer* 117(5):1019-1026.

Sharma, P., S. D. Saini, L. B. Kuhn, J. H. Rubenstein, D. S. Pardi, J. A. Marrero, and P. S. Schoenfeld. 2011. Knowledge of hepatocellular carcinoma screening guidelines and clinical practices among gastroenterologists. *Digestive Diseases and Sciences* 56(2):569-577.

Sherman, S. G., L. Smith, G. Laney, and S. A. Strathdee. 2002. Social influences on the transition to injection drug use among young heroin sniffers: A qualitative analysis. *International Journal of Drug Policy* 13(2):113-120.

Shoukry, N. H., A. Grakoui, M. Houghton, D. Y. Chien, J. Ghrayeb, K. A. Reimann, and C. M. Walker. 2003. Memory CD8+ T cells are required for protection from persistent hepatitis C virus infection. *Journal of Experimental Medicine* 197(12):1645-1655.

Singal, A. G., A. Pillai, and J. Tiro. 2014. Early detection, curative treatment, and survival rates for hepatocellular carcinoma surveillance in patients with cirrhosis: A meta-analysis. *PLoS Medicine* 11(4):e1001624.

Smith, B. D., J. Drobeniuc, A. Jewett, B. M. Branson, R. S. Garfein, E. Teshale, S. Kamili, and C. M. Weinbaum. 2011. Evaluation of three rapid screening assays for detection of antibodies to hepatitis C virus. *Journal of Infectious Diseases* 204(6):825-831.

Solomon, L., B. T. Montague, C. G. Beckwith, J. Baillargeon, M. Costa, D. Dumont, I. Kuo, A. Kurth, and J. D. Rich. 2014. Survey finds that many prisons and jails have room to improve HIV testing and coordination of postrelease treatment. *Health Affairs* 33(3):434-442.

Sonnenday, C. J., J. B. Dimick, R. D. Schulick, and M. A. Choti. 2007. Racial and geographic disparities in the utilization of surgical therapy for hepatocellular carcinoma. *Journal of Gastrointestinal Surgery* 11(12):1636-1646; discussion 1646.

Stanaway, J. D., A. D. Flaxman, M. Naghavi, C. Fitzmaurice, T. Vos, I. Abubakar, L. J. Abu-Raddad, R. Assadi, N. Bhala, B. Cowie, M. H. Forouzanfour, J. Groeger, K. M. Hanafiah, K. H. Jacobsen, S. L. James, J. MacLachlan, R. Malekzadeh, N. K. Martin, A. A. Mokdad, A. H. Mokdad, C. J. L. Murray, D. Plass, S. Rana, D. B. Rein, J. H. Richardus, J. Sanabria, M. Saylan, S. Shahraz, S. So, V. V. Vlassov, E. Weiderpass, S. T. Wiersma, M. Younis, C. Yu, M. El Sayed Zaki, and G. S. Cooke. 2016. The global burden of viral hepatitis from 1990 to 2013: Findings from the Global Burden of Disease Study 2013. *Lancet* 388(10049):1081-1088.

Stockings, E., W. D. Hall, M. Lynskey, K. I. Morley, N. Reavley, J. Strang, G. Patton, and L. Degenhardt. 2016. Prevention, early intervention, harm reduction, and treatment of substance use in young people. *The Lancet Psychiatry* 3(3):280-296.

Strathdee, S. A., and C. Beyrer. 2015. Threading the needle—How to stop the HIV outbreak in rural Indiana. *New England Journal of Medicine* 373(5):397-399.

Swadling, L., S. Capone, R. D. Antrobus, A. Brown, R. Richardson, E. W. Newell, J. Halliday, C. Kelly, D. Bowen, J. Fergusson, A. Kurioka, V. Ammendola, M. Del Sorbo, F. Grazioli, M. L. Esposito, L. Siani, C. Traboni, A. Hill, S. Colloca, M. Davis, A. Nicosia, R. Cortese, A. Folgori, P. Klenerman, and E. Barnes. 2014. A human vaccine strategy based on chimpanzee adenoviral and MVA vectors that primes, boosts, and sustains functional HCV-specific T cell memory. *Science Translational Medicine* 6(261):261ra153.

Terrault, N. A., N. H. Bzowej, K. M. Chang, J. P. Hwang, M. M. Jonas, and M. H. Murad. 2016. AASLD guidelines for treatment of chronic hepatitis B. *Hepatology* 63(1):261-283.

Tholey, D. M., and J. Ahn. 2015. Impact of hepatitis C virus infection on hepatocellular carcinoma. *Gastroenterology Clinics of North America* 44(4):761-773.

Tiong, L., and G. J. Maddern. 2011. Systematic review and meta-analysis of survival and disease recurrence after radiofrequency ablation for hepatocellular carcinoma. *British Journal of Surgery* 98(9):1210-1224.

Tortorella, D., B. E. Gewurz, M. H. Furman, D. J. Schust, and H. L. Ploegh. 2000. Viral subversion of the immune system. *Annual Review of Immunology* 18:861-926.

University of Pennsylvania. n.d. *Risk assessment battery (RAB): Overview.* University of Pennsylvania Perelman School of Medicine, Department of Psychiatry, HIV/AIDS Prevention Research Division. http://www.med.upenn.edu/hiv/rab_overview.html (accessed December 14, 2016).

USPSTF (U.S. Preventive Services Task Force). 2014. *Final recommendation statement: Hepatitis B virus infection: Screening, 2014.* https://www.uspreventiveservicestask force.org/Page/Document/RecommendationStatementFinal/hepatitis-b-virus-infection-screening-2014 (accessed October 31, 2016).

VA (Department of Veterans Affairs). 2014. *State of care for veterans with hepatitis C 2014.* Veterans Health Administration.

Vestal, C. 2016. Helping drug-addicted inmates break the cycle. *Pew Charitable Trusts,* January 13. http://www.pewtrusts.org/en/research-and-analysis/blogs/stateline/2016/01/13/helping-drug-addicted-inmates-break-the-cycle (accessed December 15, 2016).

Viral Hepatitis Implementation Group. 2011. *Status report on the implementation of the viral hepatitis action plan.* https://www.aids.gov/pdf/status-report-on-implementation-of-vhap.pdf (accessed February 24, 2017).

Ward, J., S. Darke, and W. Hall. 1990. *The HIV Risk-taking Behavior Scale (HRBS) manual. Technical report no. 10.* National Drug and Alcohol Research Centre. https://ndarc.med.unsw.edu.au/sites/default/files/ndarc/resources/TR.010.PDF (accessed December 14, 2016).

Weeks, M. R., M. Convey, J. Dickson-Gomez, J. Li, K. Radda, M. Martinez, and E. Robles. 2009. Changing drug users' risk environments: Peer health advocates as multi-level community change agents. *American Journal of Community Psychology* 43(3-4):330-344.

Weinbaum, C., R. Lyerla, and H. S. Margolis. 2003. Prevention and control of infections with hepatitis viruses in correctional settings. *Morbidity and Mortality Weekly Report* 52(RR-01):1-33.

Welzel, T. M., B. I. Graubard, S. Quraishi, S. Zeuzem, J. A. Davila, H. B. El-Serag, and K. A. McGlynn. 2013. Population-attributable fractions of risk factors for hepatocellular carcinoma in the United States. *American Journal of Gastroenterology* 108(8):1314-1321.

Westbrook, R. H., and G. Dusheiko. 2014. Natural history of hepatitis C. *Journal of Hepatology* 61(1 Suppl):S58-S68.

WHO (World Health Organization). 2009. *Guidelines for the psychosocially assisted pharmacological treatment of opioid dependence.* Geneva, Switzerland: WHO.

WHO. 2016a. *Hepatitis B: Fact sheet.* http://www.who.int/mediacentre/factsheets/fs204/en (accessed December 6, 2016).

WHO. 2016b. *Hepatitis C: Fact sheet.* http://www.who.int/mediacentre/factsheets/fs164/en (accessed December 15, 2016).

WHO. 2016c. *HIV/AIDS: Factsheet.* http://www.who.int/mediacentre/factsheets/fs360/en (accessed December 15, 2016).

Wu, Y., K. B. Johnson, G. Roccaro, J. Lopez, H. Zheng, A. Muiru, N. Ufere, R. Rajbhandari, O. Kattan, and R. T. Chung. 2014. Poor adherence to AASLD guidelines for chronic hepatitis B management and treatment in a large academic medical center. *American Journal of Gastroenterology* 109(6):867-875.

Yang, Y. 2015. Cancer immunotherapy: Harnessing the immune system to battle cancer. *Journal of Clinical Investigation* 125(9):3335-3337.

Yehia, B. R., A. J. Schranz, C. A. Umscheid, and V. Lo Re III. 2014. The treatment cascade for chronic hepatitis C virus infection in the United States: A systematic review and meta-analysis. *PLoS One* 9(7):e101554.

Young, A. M., A. B. Jonas, and J. R. Havens. 2013. Social networks and HCV viraemia in anti-HCV-positive rural drug users. *Epidemiology & Infection* 141(2):402-411.

Appendix A

Population Health Impact and Cost-Effectiveness of Chronic Hepatitis B Diagnosis, Care, and Treatment in the United States

Mehlika Toy
Asian Liver Center
Department of Surgery
Stanford University School of Medicine

ABSTRACT

To study the population health impact and cost-effectiveness of increasing chronic hepatitis B (CHB) diagnosis, care, and antiviral treatment on risks of hepatocellular carcinoma, cirrhosis, and hepatitis B virus (HBV)-related deaths, a Markov model was constructed with disease progression estimates, liver transplantation, and background mortality rates. Age-specific HBsAg prevalence was estimated by race, ethnicity, and nativity, and a 2015 study cohort was constructed from age-group prevalence of HBsAg, HBeAg, chronic active hepatitis, and cirrhosis. Among the estimated 1.29 million people (confidence interval [CI]: 855,000 to 2.02 million) or 0.4 percent of the population living with CHB in the United States in 2015, an estimated 25.8 percent or 333,978 would be eligible for antiviral treatment because they either have chronic active hepatitis or cirrhosis. The scenarios analyzed included Base 2015 current practice with diagnosis, care, and treatment rates at 34.6, 33.3, and 45 percent; Department of Health and Human Services (HHS) 2020 target increasing diagnosis to 66 percent; HHS 2020 target with increased care and treatment at 80 percent; hypothetical 80/80/80 scenario; World Health Organization (WHO) 2030 target at 90/90/80; and idealistic 100/100/100 scenario. If the current diagnosis, care, and treatment cascade remains unchanged, as many as 6 percent of the cohort would develop hepatocellular carcinoma, 10.3 percent cirrhosis, and 9.4 percent would die from HBV-related death by 2030. Compared to current practice, the HHS 2020 diagnosis target would only reduce death by 4.5 percent if care and treatment are not increased.

The hypothetical 80/80/80 scenario and WHO 2030 target will prevent new cases of hepatocellular carcinoma and cirrhosis, and HBV-related deaths in 15 years by 26, 34, and 36 percent and 35, 45, and 50 percent, respectively. Increasing CHB diagnosis, care, and antiviral treatment is cost-effective. The incremental cost-effectiveness ratio (ICER) of the hypothetical and WHO 2030 target are $17,748 to $43,745 and $26,242 to $60,147, respectively, compared to current practice.

INTRODUCTION

Viral hepatitis is increasingly recognized as a leading cause of death and disability worldwide. In 2013 viral hepatitis took the lives of about 1.45 million people and was the seventh leading cause of death in the world (Stanaway et al., 2016). Chronic infection with HBV and hepatitis C virus (HCV) accounts for 95 percent of the deaths and causes 80 percent of hepatocellular carcinoma, the most common type of liver cancer worldwide. Among the estimated 400 million people living with chronic viral hepatitis, 250 million have CHB, which carries a 15 to 25 percent risk of premature death from liver cirrhosis and liver cancer without care and antiviral treatment. In 2016, in response to the 2030 Agenda for Sustainable Development to combat viral hepatitis, the WHO issued the first ever global health sector strategy on viral hepatitis (WHO, 2016). Apart from setting important prevention and vaccination targets, the strategy's global targets for CHB aimed to have a 30 percent diagnosis rate, 5 million people on treatment, and a 10 percent reduction in liver-related deaths by 2020, with the ultimate goal of a 90 percent diagnosis rate, 80 percent treatment rate of eligible persons for treatment, and 65 percent reduction in liver-related deaths by 2030.

In the United States, there are an estimated 850,000 to 2.2 million people living with CHB according to the Centers for Disease Control and Prevention (CDC) (CDC, 2015). After the successful adoption of the hepatitis B vaccine into the routine infant immunization schedule, CHB infection acquired from domestic infection is uncommon. By CDC estimates, as many as 53,800 CHB cases were imported to the United States yearly between 2004 and 2008 through immigration and about 95 percent of new cases of CHB infection in the United States are imported (Mitchell et al., 2011). Persons born in high endemic regions such as Asia and Africa and countries with a prevalence of CHB infection of 2 percent or greater are at the highest risk for chronic infection (Din et al., 2011; Kowdley et al., 2012). Asian Americans alone account for over half of the CHB cases (Roberts et al., 2016). At present, there are no CHB curative therapies. However, diagnosis, monitoring, and viral suppression with recommended antiviral therapy when indicated can reduce the risk of cirrhosis, hepatocellular carcinoma, and liver-related death (Lok et al., 2016; Terrault et al., 2016). Hutton et al. found it is cost effective to screen adult Asian Americans for CHB, treat those who are chronically infected and ring vaccinate their unprotected household contacts or sex partners (Hutton et al., 2007). Since 2014, USPSTF[1] recommended routine hepatitis B screening beyond pregnant women to include persons born in countries with CHB prevalence of 2 percent or greater (USPSTF, 2016). Routine hepatitis B screening in the primary care setting in accordance to USPSTF recommendation also became officially covered by the Centers for Medicare & Medicaid Services in 2016 (CMS, n.d.). In the United States, only an estimated one-third of those living with CHB are diagnosed (Lin et al., 2007), and among them, a third are receiving care (Hu et al., 2013) and 45 percent of those who are eligible for treatment based on treatment guidelines are receiving treatment (Kim et al., 2014). One of the four overarching goals of the HHS *Action Plan for the Prevention, Care, and Treatment of Viral Hepatitis* is to double the proportion of persons aware of their CHB infection from 33 to 66 percent by 2020 (HHS, 2015).

The National Academies of Sciences, Engineering, and Medicine convened a consensus committee to analyze the question of hepatitis B and C elimination in the United States. The committee concluded in its phase one report (NASEM, 2016) published in 2016 that hepatitis B and C could both be eliminated as public health problems, but that would take considerable will and resources; disease control might be more manageable in the short term. The aim of this study is to model the potential population health impact of increasing CHB diagnosis, care, and treatment in reducing the risks of hepatocellular carcinoma, cirrhosis, and HBV-related deaths in the United States and the cost-effectiveness of the various target scenarios compared with current practice.

MATERIALS AND METHODS

Overview

We developed a Markov model to simulate long-term outcomes, such as cirrhosis, hepatocellular carcinoma, and CHB-related death, under each scenario. Patients begin the simulation in one of the starting states (see Figure A-1): inactive CHB, active CHB HBeAg+, active CHB HBeAg–, and cirrhosis. The proportion of patients in each state depends on the rates for each scenario tested and whether there is a larger proportion of patients who remain undiagnosed and will follow the natural history of disease.

---

[1] Officially, the U.S. Preventive Services Task Force.

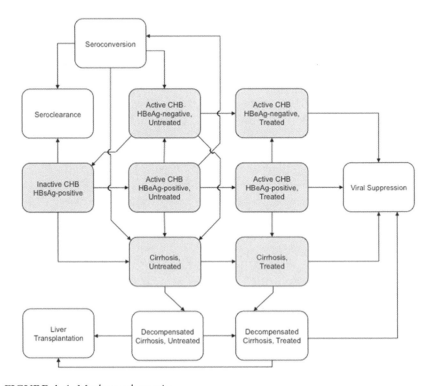

FIGURE A-1 Markov schematic.
NOTES: Starting health states in the Markov model are Inactive HBsAg+, Active chronic hepatitis B HBeAg+ and HBeAg−, and Cirrhosis. The model assumes that individuals in the decompensated health state are being treated with antivirals depending on the scenario they are in. All health states are subject to background mortality and death due to hepatocellular carcinoma. CHB = chronic hepatitis B; HBeAg = hepatitis B e antigen; HBsAg = hepatitis B surface antigen.

Following the recent AASLD[2] guidelines (Terrault et al., 2016), disease activity is defined by an elevation of ALT >2 ULN or evidence of significant histological disease plus elevated HBV DNA above 2,000 IU/mL for HBeAg− and above 20,000 IU/mL for HBeAg+. In the model once people with inactive CHB develop active hepatitis, depending on the level of care and treatment they receive, they would be less likely to develop liver-related complications such as hepatocellular carcinoma and cirrhosis.

---

[2] Officially, the American Association for the Study of Liver Diseases.

Study Cohort

The population in the United States in 2015 by age, race, ethnicity, and nativity was obtained from the Census Bureau (Census Bureau, n.d.). The 2015 CHB study cohort was estimated based on race, ethnicity and nativity, and age-specific HBsAg prevalence studies for the various racial and ethnic groups in the United States (Din et al., 2011; Hyun et al., 2016; Jung et al., 2016; Lin et al., 2007; Roberts et al., 2016; Shuler et al., 2009; Tanaka et al., 2011; Ugwu et al., 2008). CHB disease activity was categorized by HBeAg+ rate of 26.3 percent and chronic active hepatitis in 14 percent who are HBeAg+ and in 26 percent who are HBeAg–, based on data from the Hepatitis B Research Network study (Ghany et al., 2015) that collected data on clinical characteristics of adult CHB infections who were enrolled in a multisite North America cohort study. The proportion of the CHB cohort with cirrhosis was based on studies by Iloeje et al. (2006) and Kim et al. (2014). Estimated new cases of CHB due to migration of Asian and Pacific Islander and black people into the United States from year 2015 to 2060 was calculated from the U.S. census migration projection estimates (Census Bureau, n.d.) by nativity and race/ethnicity.

Model

The Markov model was developed using TreeAge Pro 2014 (TreeAge Software, Williamstown, Massachusetts). The model was adapted from our previous study on the population health impact and cost-effectiveness of CHB treatment in Shanghai, China (Toy et al., 2014). Transitions in the Markov model were calculated in 1-year cycles and were governed by disease progression estimates (see Table A-1) and treatment-related estimates (see Table A-2). The natural history disease progression estimates were derived from recent cohort studies and meta-analysis mainly from North America (Campsen et al., 2013; Chen et al., 2010; Chu and Liaw, 2007, 2009; Fattovich et al., 2008; Kanwal et al., 2006; Lin et al., 2005; Raffetti et al., 2016; Thiele et al., 2014). Treatment effectiveness estimates were expressed as reductions in progression risks and are shown in Table A-2 (Heathcote et al., 2011; Lok et al., 2016; Papatheodoridis et al., 2015; Tenney et al., 2009; Wong et al., 2013). The nucleoside analogue entecavir and nucleotide analogue tenofovir are both highly potent antivirals and have high barriers to viral resistance (Lok et al., 2016; Marcellin et al., 2013). We assumed that the effectiveness for both these drugs were similar and are equally effective in prevention progression from chronic active hepatitis to cirrhosis in both HBeAg+ or HBeAg– patients and they are used as first line treatment in the United States. The model also assumed that the few patients who developed drug resistance to entecavir will be switched to

TABLE A-1 Annual Transition Estimates for Natural History of Chronic Hepatitis B by Initial State

Transition	Age Group	Estimate (%)	Range	References
From inactive, HBsAg+				
To seroclearance	<30 years	0.8	(0.38-1.15)	Chu and Liaw, 2007
	30-39 years	1.1	(0.53-1.60)	
	40-49 years	1.7	(0.82-2.47)	
	50+ years	1.8	(0.91-2.74)	
To active CHB, HBeAg+	<30 years	0.9	(0.4-1.3)	Chu and Liaw, 2007, 2009
	30-39 years	1.4	(0.7-2.1)	
	40-49 years	2.8	(1.4-4.1)	
	50+ years	2	(1.0-3.0)	
To cirrhosis	<30 years	0.038	(0.019-0.057)	Chu and Liaw, 2009
	30-39 years	0.049	(0.024-0.073)	
	40-49 years	0.068	(0.034-0.102)	
	50+ years	0.15	(0.052-0.202)	
To HCC	All ages	0.17	(0.02-0.62)	Raffetti et al., 2016
From active CHB, HBeAg+				
To seroconversion	All ages	7	(2.0-23)	Kanwal et al., 2006
To active CHB, HBeAg–	All ages	1.9	(1.0-3.8)	Fattovich et al., 2008
To cirrhosis	All ages	2.4	(2.1-2.6)	Lin et al., 2005
To HCC	All ages	0.48	(0.22-0.91)	Raffetti et al., 2016
To HBV-related death	All ages	0.11	(0.09-0.14)	Thiele et al., 2014
From active CHB, HBeAg–				
To inactive CHB, HBsAg+	All ages	1.6	(0.0-11)	Kanwal et al., 2006
To cirrhosis	All ages	2.4	(1.3-3.4)	Lin et al., 2005
To HCC	All ages	0.48	(0.22-0.91)	Raffetti et al., 2016
To HBV-related death	All ages	0.11	(0.09-0.14)	Thiele et al., 2014
From seroconversion				Chen et al., 2010
To active CHB, HBeAg–	<30 years	2.9	(1.4-4.3)	
	31-40 years	3.8	(1.9-5.7)	
	40+ years	8.6	(4.3-12.9)	

TABLE A-1 Continued

Transition	Age Group	Estimate (%)	Range	References
To cirrhosis	<30 years	0.2	(0.1-0.3)	
	31-40 years	1	(0.5-1.5)	
	40+ years	4.2	(2.1-6.3)	
To HCC	<30 years	0.1	(0.05-0.15)	
	31-40 years	0.2	(0.1-0.3)	
	40+ years	0.6	(0.3-0.9)	
To seroclearance	<30 years	0.8	(0.4-1.2)	
	31-40 years	0.7	(0.3-1.0)	
	40+ years	0.3	(0.1-0.4)	
From seroclearance				
To HCC	All ages	1.55	(0.092-2.61)	Liu et al., 2012
From cirrhosis				
To decompensated cirrhosis	All ages	3.9	(3.2-4.6)	Lin et al., 2005
To HCC	All ages	3.16	(2.58-3.74)	Thiele et al., 2014
To HBV-related death	All ages	4.89	(3.16-6.63)	Thiele et al., 2014
From decompensated cirrhosis				
To liver transplantation	All ages	1.2	(1.0-3.0)	HRSA, n.d.
To HCC	All ages	7.1	(3.5-10.0)	Lin et al., 2005
To HBV-related death	All ages	15	(9.9-20.0)	Lin et al., 2005
From HCC				
To liver transplantation	All ages	7	(5.0-9.0)	HRSA, n.d.
To HBV-related death	All ages	35.1	(18.0-45.0)	Hutton et al., 2007
From liver transplantation				Campsen et al., 2013
To HBV-related death year 1	All ages	5.7	(4.5-6.8)	
To HBV-related death year 3	All ages	12.9	(10.3-15.5)	
To HBV-related death year 5	All ages	14.7	(11.8-17.6)	

NOTE: CHB = chronic hepatitis B; HBeAg = hepatitis B e antigen; HBsAg = hepatitis B surface antigen; HBV = hepatitis B virus; HCC = hepatocellular carcinoma; HCV = hepatitis C virus.

TABLE A-2 Annual Transition Estimates for Treatment Strategies with First Line Antiviral Therapy

Transition	Annual probability, % (range)	Reference
From active CHB, long-term treatment		
To active CHB, drug resistant	0.012 (0.0-0.01)	Heathcote et al., 2011; Lok et al., 2016; Tenney et al., 2009
To HCC	0.2 (0.1-0.5)	Papatheodoridis et al., 2015; Wong et al., 2013
From cirrhosis, long-term treatment		
To cirrhosis, drug resistant	0.012 (0.0-0.01)	Heathcote et al., 2011; Lok et al., 2016; Tenney et al., 2009
To decompensated cirrhosis	1.8 (0.9-3.8)	Wong et al., 2013
To HCC	1.6 (0.8-3.2)	Papatheodoridis et al., 2015; Wong et al., 2013
To HBV-related death	2.4 (1.6-3.3)	Papatheodoridis et al., 2015; Wong et al., 2013
From decompensated cirrhosis, long-term treatment		
To HCC	3.5 (1.7-5.0)	Papatheodoridis et al., 2015; Wong et al., 2013
To HBV-related death	7.5 (4.9-10.0)	Papatheodoridis et al., 2015; Wong et al., 2013

NOTE: CHB = chronic hepatitis B; HBV = hepatitis B virus; HCC = hepatocellular carcinoma.

tenofovir and continue treatment. The primary goal of antiviral treatment is to suppress replication of HBV, thereby preventing progression to cirrhosis and reducing the risk of hepatocellular carcinoma. Based on recent findings, we assumed that it was possible to develop hepatocellular carcinoma while on treatment, but with a 50 percent reduction in the rate decrease from natural history (Arends et al., 2015; Marcellin et al., 2013). Causes of death that were not related to CHB were included in the model, based on age-specific mortality rates from the National Vital Statistics Report, United States Life Tables (Arias, 2015). Annual probabilities of receiving a liver transplant for decompensated cirrhosis and hepatocellular carcinoma if CHB-infected (1.2 and 7 percent, respectively) were calculated based on data from the Organ Procurement and Transplantation Network (OPTN) (HRSA, n.d.). If progression rates were reported, these were transformed into annual probabilities using a standard formula ($P=1-e^{-r\times t}$), where P is the probability, e is the base of the natural logarithm, r is the event rate, and t is the time interval.

Cost and Utility Estimates

The annual wholesale prices for entecavir 0.5mg were $8,400 for the generic drug (range $4,740 to $12,796) and $16,464 for the brand drug, and tenofovir 300mg (only brand available) was $11,964 (Truven Health Analytics, 2016). We obtained medical management costs for CHB, cirrhosis, decompensated cirrhosis, and hepatocellular carcinoma from Liu et al. (Liu et al., 2012), liver transplantation cost from OPTN, and annual monitoring cost from Hutton et al. (Hutton et al., 2007) (see Table A-3). All costs were adjusted for inflation using the U.S. consumer price index to reflect 2015 U.S. dollars (Bureau of Labor Statistics, n.d.). An assumption in the model pertaining to costs was that patients achieving seroconversion from the CHB active state continued to incur annual costs for CHB management. The utilities were obtained from a health state utility and quality of life study on CHB (Woo et al., 2012) (see Table A-3). Outcomes included 15 year and lifetime disease and HBV-related death risk, discounted costs, quality-adjusted life years (QALYs) gained, and incremental cost-effectiveness ratios (ICERs) for each scenario. Results are presented as weighted averages over age. All costs and QALYs were discounted at a rate of 3 percent per year.

Scenarios

The following diagnosis, care, and treatment scenarios were examined (see Table A-4):

- Base 2015 Current Practice: According to the literature we assumed that 34.6 percent of CHB is diagnosed in the United States (Lin et al., 2007), 33.3 percent receive care (Hu et al., 2013), and 45 percent receive treatment if eligible according to treatment guidelines (Kim et al., 2014), where 85 percent adhere to treatment (Chotiyaputta et al., 2011). We assume here that 35.1 percent of patients adhere to monitoring recommendations, which has the observed level of adherence to monitoring at least once every 12 months (Juday et al., 2011).
- HHS 2020 Screening Target: One of the national goals (HHS, 2015) for reducing the burden of viral hepatitis by 2020 was to increase the proportion of persons who are aware of their hepatitis B infection from 33 to 66 percent. In this scenario we examined the

TABLE A-3 Cost and Utility Estimates

Variable	Base Case	Range
Cost (U.S. dollars) $		
Entecavir (0.5mg) (generic)	$8,400	$4,740-$12,796
Entecavir (0.5mg)	$16,464	$16,464-$19,752
Tenofovir (300mg)	$11,964	$11,964-$14,364
Annual monitoring	$710	$347-$1,390
Chronic hepatitis B	$1,483	$154-$5,956
Cirrhosis	$4,414	$154-$5,408
Decompensated cirrhosis	$11,690	$3,735-$28,256
Hepatocellular carcinoma	$46,538	$22,443-$67,321
Liver transplantation 1st year	$159,220	$127,376-$191,064
Liver transplantation 2nd year	$22,820	$18,256-$27,384
Health state utilities		
Active CHB	0.85	(0.80-0.92)
Cirrhosis	0.87	(0.78-0.88)
Inactive CHB	0.95	(0.90-0.99)
Decompensated cirrhosis	0.82	(0.49-0.82)
Hepatocellular carcinoma	0.84	(0.77-0.85)
Liver transplantation	0.86	(0.72-0.84)
Seroclearance	0.99	(0.90-1.00)
Viral suppression	1	(0.95-1.00)

NOTES: All costs are adjusted for inflation using the U.S. consumer price index to reflect 2015 U.S. dollars. CHB = chronic hepatitis B.
SOURCES: Hutton et al., 2007; Liu et al., 2012; Truven Health Analytics, 2016. Red Book drug prices accessed January 13, 2017.

impact of only increasing diagnosis to 66 percent, but care, treatment, adherence to monitoring, and treatment remain unchanged.

- HHS 2020 Target with Improved Care and Treatment: In this hypothetical scenario we increased the rates for care and treatment by 80 percent along with the 66 percent of diagnosis target. Adherence to monitoring and treatment was kept at 35.1 and 85 percent, respectively.
- Hypothetical scenario: In this scenario, we assume that the diagnosis, care, treatment, and adherence to monitoring increased to 80 percent and adherence to treatment to 95 percent.
- WHO 2030 Target: The WHO has made viral hepatitis a priority

TABLE A-4 Scenario Analysis Rates

Scenario	Diagnosed	Received HBV Care	Treatment Rate Among Treatment Eligible Patients	Adherence to Monitoring	Adherence to Treatment
Natural History	—	—	—	—	—
Current Practice	34.6%[a]	33.3%[b]	45%[c]	35.1%[d]	85%[e]
HHS 2020 Target	66%	33.3%	45%	35.1%	85%
HHS 2020 Target + Improved Rx	66%	80%	80%	35.1%	85%
Hypothetical Scenario	80%	80%	80%	80%	95%
WHO 2030 Target	90%	90%	80%	100%	100%
Idealistic (Utopian)	100%	100%	100%	100%	100%

NOTE: HBV = hepatitis B virus; HHS = Department of Health and Human Services; WHO = World Health Organization.
[a] Lin et al., 2007.
[b] Hu et al., 2013.
[c] Kim et al., 2014.
[d] Juday et al., 2011.
[e] Chotiyaputta et al., 2011.

and has set targets to eliminate viral hepatitis as a public health threat by year 2030 (WHO, 2016). We adopted these targets into this scenario where diagnosis and care is increased to 90 percent and treatment to 80 percent and assumed 100 percent adherence to monitoring and treatment.

- Idealistic scenario: In this scenario we examined the impact if that all (100 percent) CHB cases are diagnosed, cared for and treated, and adhere to monitoring and treatment.

Sensitivity Analysis

Sensitivity analyses were performed using the low and high ranges of the transition estimates (see Tables A-1, A-2, and A-3). The best case scenario was assessed by applying the low ranges to the estimate of disease progression and costs and applying the low estimates to the utilities. The worst case scenario was assessed by applying the high ranges to the estimates of disease progression and costs and applying the low estimates to the utilities. We also performed a probabilistic sensitivity analysis to examine the effect of uncertainty around the cost-effectiveness outcomes of the various scenarios.

RESULTS

In 2015, an estimated 1.29 million (CI: 855,000 to 2.02 million) or 0.40 percent (CI: 0.27 to 0.63 percent) of the population in the United States lived with CHB, with the highest prevalence among ages 30 to 59 years (see Table A-5). Among them, 25.8 percent or 333,978 would be eligible for antiviral treatment because they either have chronic active hepatitis (295,556 [47,638 HBeAg+ and 247,918 HBeAg–]) or cirrhosis (38,422). HBsAg prevalence estimates by race and nativity are shown in Table A-6. An estimated 72.6 percent were foreign born Asian and Pacific Islander and black. Based on census projected migration data of black and Asian and Pacific Islander to the United States in the next 15 years, the number of CHB cases is estimated to increase by 23,370 (CI: 17,800 to 31,660) annually due to migration alone. By year 2030, the number of people living with CHB in the United States is projected to increase to an estimated 1.64 million. Table A-7 shows the baseline population distributions for the entry of the Markov model.

If the current diagnosis, care, and treatment practices remain unchanged, as many as 6 percent of the 2015 CHB cohort will have developed hepatocellular carcinoma, 10.31 percent will have developed cirrhosis, and 9.40 percent will have died from HBV-related deaths by year 2030 (see Table A-8). Doubling the current diagnosis rate to 66 percent (HHS 2020

TABLE A-5 Age-Specific Population Level Prevalence Estimate of Chronic Hepatitis B in the United States in 2015

Age Group (years)	HBsAg+	CI (lower bound)	CI (upper bound)
0-19	79,016 (0.10%)	52,597 (0.06%)	141,759 (0.17%)
20-29	160,806 (0.36%)	93,926 (0.21%)	270,006 (0.60%)
30-39	240,381 (0.57%)	161,489 (0.38%)	356,986 (0.85%)
40-49	267,593 (0.65%)	187,482 (0.46%)	387,991 (0.94%)
50-59	244,119 (0.55%)	173,398 (0.39%)	348,416 (0.79%)
60-69	182,157 (0.52%)	116,601 (0.33%)	312,350 (0.89%)
70-79	81,263 (0.41%)	50,177 (0.26%)	127,554 (0.65%)
80+	38,463 (0.32%)	19,492 (0.16%)	73,189 (0.61%)
Total	1,293,798 (0.40%)	855,162 (0.27%)	2,018,251 (0.63%)

NOTE: CHB = chronic hepatitis B; CI = confidence interval; HBeAg = hepatitis B e antigen; HBsAg = hepatitis B surface antigen.

target) without an associated increase in care and treatment would only prevent new cases of hepatocellular carcinoma, cirrhosis, and HBV-related deaths by 2.7, 1.6, and 4.5 percent, respectively, by 2030 (see Table A-9). However, if the HHS 2020 target is accompanied with an increased care and treatment rate of 80 percent, then it would prevent hepatocellular carcinoma, cirrhosis, and HBV-related death by 12, 12.6, and 19 percent, respectively. Compared to the current practice, the hypothetical scenario and WHO 2030 target will prevent new cases of hepatocellular carcinoma, cirrhosis, and HBV-related deaths by 26, 34, and 36 percent and 35, 45, and 50 percent, respectively. And if everyone with chronic HBV is diagnosed, receiving care and treatment (the idealistic scenario), it will prevent 48 and 63 percent of new cases of hepatocellular carcinoma and cirrhosis, respectively, and 70 percent of HBV-related deaths by 2030. In the current practice, the 2015 cohort's lifetime risk for hepatocellular carcinoma, cirrhosis, and HBV-related death risk is 14, 22.5, and 26 percent (see Table A-10), respectively. If diagnosis, care, and treatment rates are increased to 90, 90, and 80 (WHO 2030 target), lifetime risk can drop from 14 to 9 percent for hepatocellular carcinoma, 22.5 to 16 percent for cirrhosis, and 26 to 12 percent for HBV-related death.

The lifetime cost of treatment including drug cost for the current practice is $48,774 and $50,747 with generic and brand entecavir, respectively;

TABLE A-6 Age-Specific Estimates of 1.29 Million Chronic Hepatitis B Cases in the United States by Race/Ethnicity and Nativity in 2015

Age Group	All	White U.S. + Foreign Born	Hispanic U.S. + Foreign Born	Black U.S.	Black Foreign Born	Asian and Pacific Islander U.S.	Asian and Pacific Islander Foreign Born
0-19	79,015	15,595	4,336	2,939	40,670	7,236	8,239
20-59	912,898	109,167	88,805	20,576	123,515	26,327	544,508
≥60	301,880	42,302	23,499	7,973	50,981	6,302	170,823
Total	1,293,793	167,068 (12.9%)	116,640 (9.0%)	31,488 (2.4%)	215,166 (16.6%)	39,865 (3.1%)	723,570 (56.0%)

TABLE A-7 Baseline Population Distribution for the Entry of the Markov Model of Chronic Hepatitis B in the United States

Model Entry Health State	Scenario					
	Current Practice D35/C33/T45	HHS 2020 Target D66/C33/T45	HHS + Improved Rx D66/C80/T80	Hypothetical Scenario D80/C80/T80	WHO 2030 Target D90/C90/T80	Idealistic D100/C100/T100
Inactive (monitor)	8.9%	17.0%	40.7%	49.4%	62.5%	77.2%
Active HBeAg+ treatment	0.2%	0.3%	1.4%	1.6%	2.1%	3.2%
Active HBeAg− treatment	0.9%	1.6%	7.0%	8.5%	10.8%	16.7%
Cirrhosis treatment	0.2%	0.3%	1.3%	1.5%	1.9%	3.0%
Natural history inactive	68.3%	60.2%	36.4%	27.8%	14.7%	0.0%
Natural history active HBeAg+	3.0%	2.9%	1.9%	1.6%	1.1%	0.0%
Natural history active HBeAg−	15.8%	15.0%	9.6%	8.1%	5.9%	0.0%
Natural history cirrhosis	2.8%	2.7%	1.7%	1.4%	1.0%	0.0%

NOTES: D35/C33/T45, 35% diagnosed, 33% in care, 45% in treatment when treatment is appropriate; D66/C33/T45, 66% diagnosed, 33% in care, 45% in treatment when treatment is appropriate; D66/C80/T80, 66% diagnosed, 80% in care, 80% in treatment when treatment is appropriate; D80/C80/T80, 80% diagnosed, 80% in care, 80% in treatment when treatment is appropriate; D90/C90/T80, 90% diagnosed, 90% in care, 80% in treatment when treatment is appropriate; D100/C100/T100, 100% diagnosed, 100% in care, 100% in treatment when treatment is appropriate. HBeAg = hepatitis B e antigen; HHS = Department of Health and Human Services; WHO = World Health Organization.

TABLE A-8 Cumulative Risks of Hepatocellular Carcinoma, Cirrhosis, and HBV-Related Deaths by 2030 in the 2015 Cohort of Chronic HBV-Infected Persons in the United States

	Scenario					
Cumulative Risk	Current Practice D35/C33/T45	HHS 2020 Target D66/C33/T45	HHS + Improved Rx D66/C80/T80	Hypothetical Scenario D80/C80/T80	WHO 2030 Target D90/C90/T80	Idealistic D100/C100/T100
Hepatocellular carcinoma	6.00%	5.84%	5.27%	4.46%	3.91%	3.14%
Cirrhosis	10.31%	10.15%	9.01%	6.84%	5.70%	3.79%
HBV-related death	9.40%	8.98%	7.60%	5.98%	4.66%	2.84%

NOTE: HBV = hepatitis B virus; HHS = Department of Health and Human Services; WHO = World Health Organization.

TABLE A-9 Cumulative Reduction in Hepatocellular Carcinoma, Cirrhosis, and HBV-Related Deaths in the 2015 Cohort of Chronic HBV-Infected Persons with Various Improved Diagnosis, Care, and Treatment Scenarios Compared with the Base Scenario (D35/C33/T45) in 15 Years

	Scenario				
Cumulative Reduction	HHS 2020 Target D66/C33/T45	HHS + Improved Rx D66/C80/T80	Hypothetical Scenario D80/C80/T80	WHO 2030 Target D90/C90/T80	Idealistic D100/C100/T100
Hepatocellular carcinoma cases	2.66%	12.16%	25.66%	34.83%	47.66%
Cirrhosis cases	1.55%	12.60%	33.65%	44.71%	63.23%
HBV-related death	4.46%	19.14%	36.38%	50.42%	69.78%

NOTE: HBV = hepatitis B virus; HHS = Department of Health and Human Services; WHO = World Health Organization.

TABLE A-10 Lifetime Risks of Hepatocellular Carcinoma, Cirrhosis, and HBV-Related Deaths and Discounted Costs, QALYs, and ICERs of Each Target Scenario

Lifetime	Scenario					
	Current Practice D35/C33/T45	HHS 2020 Target D66/C33/T45	HHS + Improved Rx D66/C80/T80	Hypothetical Scenario D80/C80/T80	WHO 2030 Target D90/C90/T80	Idealistic D100/C100/T100
Hepatocellular carcinoma risk	14.03%	13.74%	12.59%	10.65%	9.05%	7.26%
Cirrhosis risk	22.45%	22.35%	21.24%	17.31%	15.68%	13.22%
HBV-related death	25.85%	24.96%	21.69%	16.81%	12.31%	7.32%
QALYs						
Total cohort	17.97	18.09	18.49	18.98	19.45	20.01
Active CHB subgroup	15.53	15.82	17.05	17.61	18.28	19.91
Cirrhosis subgroup	7.42	7.92	11.15	12.62	14.55	18.66
Costs for total cohort ETV (generic)	$48,774	$52,426	$64,233	$66,699	$87,612	$102,723
Costs for total cohort ETV	$50,747	$58,870	$85,854	$94,929	$139,765	$174,382
Costs for total cohort TDF	$49,668	$55,274	$73,789	$79,176	$110,662	$134,394
ICER for total cohort (compared to current practice) ETV (generic)	—	$30,433	$29,729	$17,748	$26,242	$26,446
ICER for total cohort (compared to current practice) ETV	—	$67,692	$67,513	$43,745	$60,147	$60,605
ICER for total cohort (compared to current practice) TDF	—	$46,717	$46,387	$29,216	$41,212	$41,532

NOTE: CHB = chronic hepatitis B; ETV = entecavir; HBV = hepatitis B virus; HHS = Department of Health and Human Services; ICER = incremental cost-effectiveness ratio; QALY = quality-adjusted life year; TDF = tenofovir; WHO = World Health Organization.

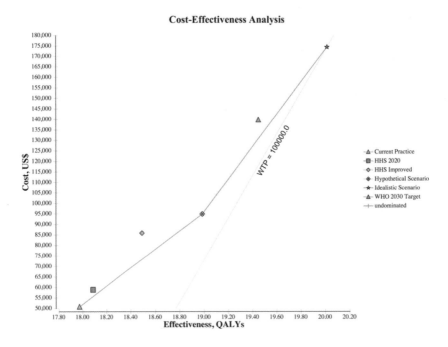

FIGURE A-2 Incremental costs and QALYs for each scenario.

NOTES: The graph plots the incremental discounted life-time costs (y-axis) and the incremental discounted QALYs (x-axis) for each scenario. The solid line represents the cost-effectiveness frontier, those strategies that are potentially cost-effective, and the dotted line represents the WTP, which is a $100,000/QALY. HHS = Department of Health and Human Services; QALY = quality-adjusted life year; WHO = World Health Organization; WTP = willingness to pay.

and $49,668 with tenofovir, and results in 17.97 discounted QALYs per patient (see Table A-10). The hypothetical scenario and WHO 2030 target cost $66,699 to $94,929 and $87,612 to $139,765, respectively. Increasing the cascade of diagnosis, care, and treatment is cost-effective across all the scenarios examined. The ICER for the hypothetical, WHO 2030, and idealistic scenario are $17,748 to $43,745, $26,242 to $60,147, and $26,446 to $60,605, respectively. Figure A-2 shows the cost-effectiveness frontier for all scenarios, those scenarios that are potentially cost-effective depending on the willing to pay per QALY. The hypothetical scenario was the lowest cost alternative and dominated HHS 2020 target and HHS improved scenarios. The idealistic scenario was the next best option, which

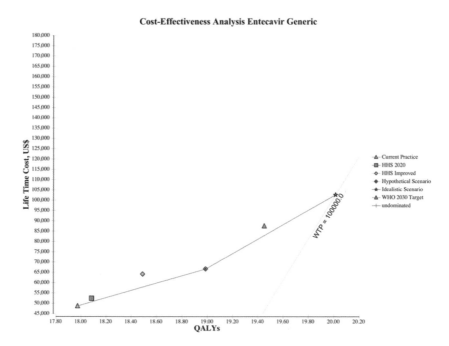

FIGURE A-3 Incremental costs and QALYs for each scenario. Cost-effectiveness frontier with entecavir (generic).
NOTES: The graph plots the incremental discounted life-time costs (y-axis) and the incremental discounted QALYs (x-axis) for each scenario. The solid line represents the cost-effectiveness frontier, those strategies that are potentially cost-effective, and the dotted line represents the WTP, which is a $100,000/QALY. HHS = Department of Health and Human Services; QALY = quality-adjusted life year; WHO = World Health Organization; WTP = willingness to pay.

adds 1.05 QALYs over the hypothetical scenario and 2.04 QALYs over the current practice at a cost of $26,446 for entecavir generic (see Figure A-3), $60,605 for entecavir brand (see Figure A-4), and $41,532 for tenofovir (see Figure A-5) per QALY.

SENSITIVITY ANALYSIS

We performed one-way sensitivity analysis over estimated data ranges for all variables. Monte Carlo probabilistic analysis recalculates expected values in the Markov model numerous times and is used to understand the uncertainties on the model results. The results were sensitive to several

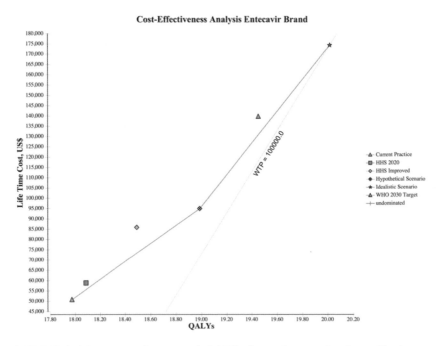

FIGURE A-4 Incremental costs and QALYs for each scenario. Cost-effectiveness frontier with entecavir.

NOTES: The graph plots the incremental discounted life-time costs (y-axis) and the incremental discounted QALYs (x-axis) for each scenario. The solid line represents the cost-effectiveness frontier, those strategies that are potentially cost-effective, and the dotted line represents the WTP, which is a $100,000/QALY. HHS = Department of Health and Human Services; QALY = quality-adjusted life year; WHO = World Health Organization; WTP = willingness to pay.

variables, including the utility of CHB, cirrhosis, and seroclearance (loss of HBsAg), and the probability of transitioning from inactive CHB to hepatocellular carcinoma, from seroclearance to hepatocellular carcinoma, from inactive to active CHB, from inactive CHB to seroclearance, from active hepatitis to hepatocellular carcinoma, and from hepatocellular carcinoma to HBV-related death (see Figures A-6, A-7, A-8, A-9, A-10, and A-11). Sensitivity analysis of the health outcome and lifetime costs, QALYs and ICERs associated with the various increased diagnosis, care, and treatment scenarios is shown in Table A-11 and Table A-12. The sensitivity analysis showed the risk of the 2015 cohort for HBV-related death by 2030 can be

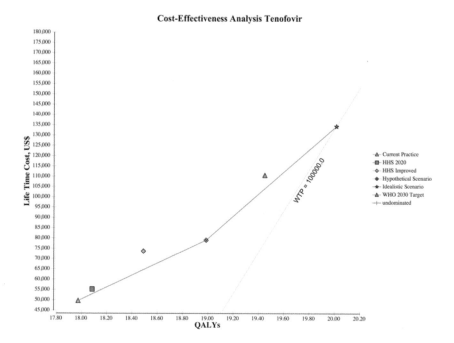

Cost-Effectiveness Analysis Tenofovir

FIGURE A-5 Incremental costs and QALYs for each scenario. Cost-effectiveness frontier with tenofovir.
NOTES: The graph plots the incremental discounted life-time costs (y-axis) and the incremental discounted QALYs (x-axis) for each scenario. The solid line represents the cost-effectiveness frontier, those strategies that are potentially cost-effective, and the dotted line represents the WTP, which is a $100,000/QALY. HHS = Department of Health and Human Services; QALY = quality-adjusted life year; WHO = World Health Organization; WTP = willingness to pay.

as low as 2.7 percent or as high as 10.6 percent with the WHO 2030 target compared with 4.9 to 17.6 percent with current practice. At a willingness to pay threshold of $50,000 per QALY, the hypothetical scenario D80/C80/T80 was optimal (cost-effective) 65 percent of the time while the idealistic scenario was optimal 30 percent of the time. At a willingness to pay threshold of $100,000 per QALY, the idealistic scenario was optimal 100 percent of the time (see Figure A-12). If the idealistic scenario was to be left out of the competing scenarios, the WHO 2030 target is the most optimal scenario at a willingness to pay threshold of $100,000.

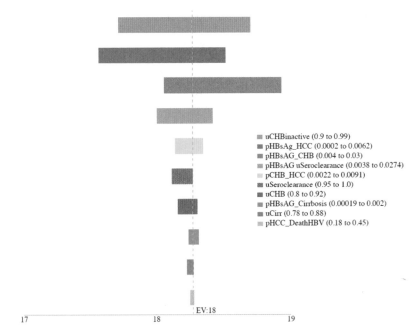

FIGURE A-6 Tornado analysis for net benefits.

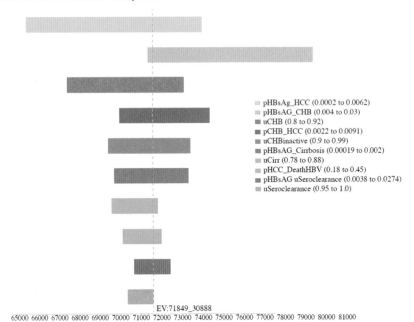

FIGURE A-7 Tornado analysis (ICER) current practice versus HHS 2020 target.

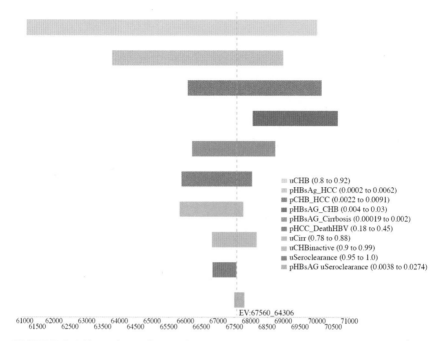

FIGURE A-8 Tornado analysis (ICER) current practice versus HHS improved.

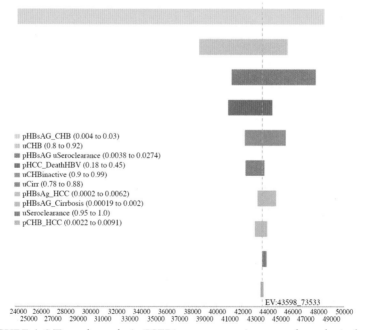

FIGURE A-9 Tornado analysis (ICER) current practice versus hypothetical scenario.

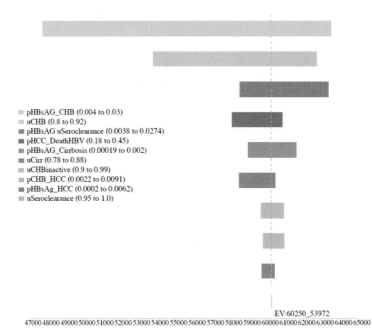

FIGURE A-10 Tornado analysis (ICER) current practice versus WHO 2030 target.

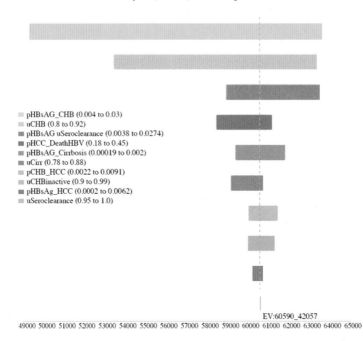

FIGURE A-11 Tornado analysis (ICER) current practice versus idealistic scenario.

TABLE A-11 Sensitivity Analysis of the Best and Worst Case in Cumulative Risks for Hepatocellular Carcinoma, Cirrhosis, and HBV-Related Deaths by 2030 in the 2015 Cohort

Cumulative Risk	Scenario					
	Current Practice D35/C33/T45	HHS 2020 Target D66/C33/T45	HHS + Improved Rx D66/C80/T80	Hypothetical Scenario D80/C80/T80	WHO 2030 Target D90/C90/T80	Idealistic D100/C100/T100
Hepatocellular carcinoma	3.78%-12.63%	3.67%-12.40%	3.40%-11.45%	3.03%-10.49%	2.72%-9.52%	2.33%-8.33%
Cirrhosis	4.30%-14.52%	4.23%-14.24%	4.17%-12.47%	2.96%-9.55%	2.75%-7.68%	2.24%-4.76%
HBV-related death	4.91%-17.61%	4.67%-17.02%	4.03%-14.92%	3.30%-12.70%	2.69%-10.61%	1.85%-8.28%

NOTE: HBV = hepatitis B virus; HHS = Department of Health and Human Services; WHO = World Health Organization.

TABLE A-12 Sensitivity Analysis of the Best and Worst Case in Lifetime Discounted Costs, QALYs, and ICERs of Each Target Scenario

Lifetime	Scenario					
	Current Practice D35/C33/T45	HHS 2020 Target D66/C33/T45	HHS + Improved Rx D66/C80/T80	Hypothetical Scenario D80/C80/T80	WHO 2030 Target D90/C90/T80	Idealistic D100/C100/T100
QALYs	14.98-19.87	15.15-19.93	15.77-20.12	16.50-20.34	17.29-20.52	18.08-20.77
Costs for total cohort ($4,740-19,752 annual)	$16,425-114,197	$18,470-123,465	$25,743-152,993	$24,782-172,822	$35,193-228,392	$43,500-266,642
ICER for total cohort (compared to current practice)	—	$34,083-54,518	$37,272-49,109	$17,781-38,569	$28,874-49,435	$30,083-49,176

NOTE: HHS = Department of Health and Human Services; ICER = incremental cost effectiveness ratio; QALY = quality-adjusted life year; WHO = World Health Organization.

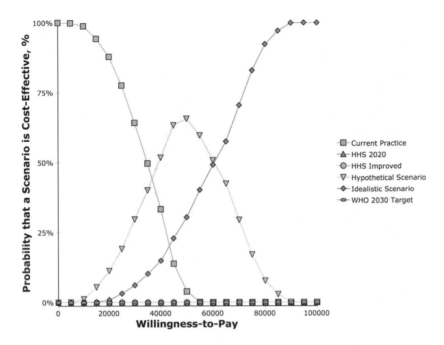

FIGURE A-12 Results of probabilistic sensitivity analysis: cost-effectiveness acceptability curves.
NOTE: HHS = Department of Health and Human Services; WHO = World Health Organization.

DISCUSSION

This is the first study undertaken to model the population health impact and cost-effectiveness of increasing CHB diagnosis, care, and treatment in the United States. The study found implementing programs that would substantially increase rates of CHB diagnosis, care, and viral suppressive therapy with the potent and low-resistance medications can prevent 19 to 70 percent of the HBV-related deaths in 15 years depending on the rates achieved.

In the HHS national action plan for the prevention, care, and treatment of viral hepatitis, among the four overarching goals is to double the number who are aware of their CHB infection to 66 percent by 2020 (HHS, 2015). This study found that merely doubling the number of people diagnosed with CHB to 66 percent would only result in a 4 percent drop in HBV-related death in 15 years if there was no associated increase in care and treatment rates. Increasing care and treatment combined with increased rates of diagnosis could result in a reduction in new cases of hepatocellular carcinoma by 12 to 48 percent, cirrhosis by 13 to 63 percent, and HBV-related death by 19 to 70 percent in 15 years. The WHO target of 90 percent diagnosis and 80 percent treatment would prevent 50 percent of the HBV-related liver deaths. If we can reach an idealistic scenario where almost everyone is diagnosed, cared for and treated if indicated, and adherent to monitoring and treatment, the mortality rate can decrease by 70 percent in 15 years. These estimates would come close to the WHO 2030 target to reduce CHB-related mortality by 65 percent (WHO, 2016).

Increasing the cascade of CHB diagnosis, care, and treatment would also provide high value for money and is cost-effective in all the scenarios examined with an ICER of $17,748 to $30,433 for generic entecavir, $43,745 to $67,692 for brand entecavir, and $29,216 to $46,717 for tenofovir. Increasing the diagnosis and treatment rates to 90 and 80 percent, respectively (WHO 2030 targets), would be cost-effective with an estimated ICER ranging from $26,242 to $60,605, depending on the antiviral drug used. For patients with cirrhosis, great health gain of 7.13 healthy life years can be gained by increasing diagnosis, care, and treatment rates to the WHO 2030 targets compared with current practice. Such an increase in healthy life years is comparable to HIV antiretroviral treatment versus no treatment with a health gain of 8.5 years (Walensky et al., 2013).

This study had several limitations. The model did not include additional program costs (e.g., outreach, campaigns, and awareness programs) for the different scenarios if care, treatment, and adherence to monitoring and treatment were to be increased. In the cost-effectiveness calculations, only medical management (diagnosis, monitoring, managing the disease) and treatment costs were included. Consequently, future research could look into various elements of which type of programs could be implemented locally and nationally and calculate their costs. The model also assumes all the patients who are eligible for treatment received recommended first line suppressive therapy that are highly effective and have very low rates of drug resistance. The broad ranges for some variables in the model come from published cohort studies. These ranges were used for the sensitivity analysis, and, as a result, some ranges in the best and worst case scenarios are broad as well.

According to the National Cancer Institute, liver cancer screening in high-risk patients does not result in reduction in mortality although screening with twice a year ultrasound for early detection of hepatocellular carcinoma is recommended by AASLD for HBsAg+ persons who are at increased risk. The model did not calculate the potential survival benefit of liver cancer screening among CHB patients that received care and the potential survival benefit of antiviral therapy in hepatocellular carcinoma patients.

The estimated prevalence of CHB in 2015 in this study is 1.29 million and ranged from 855,000 to 2.01 million, which is similar to the CDC estimates of 850,000 to 2.2 million. Mitchell et al. estimated 95 percent of new cases of CHB in the United States are imported with an annual increase of 53,800 cases between 2004 and 2008 from immigration (Mitchell et al., 2011). In this study, an estimated 72.5 percent living in the United States in 2015 are foreign born black and Asian and Pacific Islander (see Table A-6). Based on U.S. Census projected migration of blacks and Asian and Pacific Islanders in the next 15 years, the number of new cases of CHB is estimated to increase by 23,370 per year to approximately the 1.64 million by 2030. These estimates did not include migration from the Middle East or Eastern Europe.

The proportion of the 2015 CHB cohort who are HBeAg+, HBeAg+ with active hepatitis, HBeAg– with active hepatitis, and CHB with normal ALT was estimated based on a U.S. multicenter cohort study in adults, but there was no information on cirrhosis (Ghany et al., 2015). Our study has a limitation that we had to estimate the proportion with cirrhosis from two other cohort studies (Iloeje et al., 2006; Kim et al., 2014). By applying the same chronic active hepatitis and cirrhosis estimates in adults to the age group 0 to 19 years, the numbers in the 2015 cohort that would require treatment may be overestimated. However, given that this age group only represents 6.1 percent of the 2015 cohort, the effect would be small.

Recent findings in a United States CHB cohort study (Spradling et al., 2016) found CHB patients were insufficiently monitored for disease status and, among those with cirrhosis, for hepatocellular carcinoma and viremia. In order to convince their patients of the long-term risks of CHB, providers need to be first convinced and educated themselves so that they can manage and increase their patients' adherence to monitoring and treatment. Nationwide programs need to be implemented to increase the rates of diagnosis, care, and treatment for CHB infection in order to eliminate CHB as a public health problem in the United States.

Funding source: This study was commissioned by the National Academies of Sciences, Engineering, and Medicine.

REFERENCES

Arends, P., M. J. Sonneveld, R. Zoutendijk, I. Carey, A. Brown, M. Fasano, D. Mutimer, K. Deterding, J. G. Reijnders, Y. Oo, J. Petersen, F. van Bommel, R. J. de Knegt, T. Santantonio, T. Berg, T. M. Welzel, H. Wedemeyer, M. Buti, P. Pradat, F. Zoulim, B. Hansen, H. L. Janssen, and Virgil Surveillance Study Group. 2015. Entecavir treatment does not eliminate the risk of hepatocellular carcinoma in chronic hepatitis B: Limited role for risk scores in caucasians. *Gut* 64(8):1289-1295.

Arias, E. 2015. United States life tables, 2011. *National Vital Statistics Reports* 64(11). http://www.cdc.gov/nchs/data/nvsr/nvsr64/nvsr64_11.pdf (accessed July 2016).

Bureau of Labor Statistics. n.d. *CPI inflation calculator.* http://www.bls.gov/data/inflation_calculator.htm (accessed July, 2016).

Campsen, J., M. Zimmerman, J. Trotter, J. Hong, C. Freise, R. Brown, A. Cameron, M. Ghobrial, I. Kam, R. Busuttil, S. Saab, C. Holt, J. Emond, J. Stiles, T. Lukose, M. Chang, and G. Klintmalm. 2013. Liver transplantation for hepatitis B liver disease and concomitant hepatocellular carcinoma in the United States with hepatitis B immunoglobulin and nucleoside/nucleotide analogues. *Liver Transplantation* 19(9):1020-1029.

CDC (Centers for Disease Control and Prevention). 2015. *Hepatitis B FAQs for health professionals.* http://www.cdc.gov/hepatitis/hbv/hbvfaq.html#overview (accessed July 2016).

Census Bureau. n.d. *United States Census Bureau.* http://www.census.gov (accessed July 2016).

Chen, Y. C., C. M. Chu, and Y. F. Liaw. 2010. Age-specific prognosis following spontaneous hepatitis B e antigen seroconversion in chronic hepatitis B. *Hepatology* 51(2):435-444.

Chotiyaputta, W., C. Peterson, F. A. Ditah, D. Goodwin, and A. S. Lok. 2011. Persistence and adherence to nucleos(t)ide analogue treatment for chronic hepatitis B. *Journal of Hepatology* 54(1):12-18.

Chu, C. M., and Y. F. Liaw. 2007. HBsAg seroclearance in asymptomatic carriers of high endemic areas: Appreciably high rates during a long-term follow-up. *Hepatology* 45(5): 1187-1192.

Chu, C. M., and Y. F. Liaw. 2009. Incidence and risk factors of progression to cirrhosis in inactive carriers of hepatitis B virus. *American Journal of Gastroenterology* 104(7): 1693-1699.

CMS (Centers for Medicare & Medicaid Services). n.d. *Decision memo for screening for hepatitis B virus (HBV) infection (CAG-00447N).* https://www.cms.gov/medicare-coverage-database/details/nca-decision-memo.aspx?NCAId=283 (accessed February 21, 2017).

Din, E. S., A. Wasley, L. Jacques-Carroll, B. Sirotkin, and S. Wang. 2011. Estimating the number of births to hepatitis B virus-infected women in 22 states, 2006. *Pediatric Infectious Disease Journal* 30(7):575-579.

Fattovich, G., F. Bortolotti, and F. Donato. 2008. Natural history of chronic hepatitis B: Special emphasis on disease progression and prognostic factors. *Journal of Hepatology* 48(2):335-352.

Ghany, M. G., R. Perrillo, R. Li, S. H. Belle, H. L. Janssen, N. A. Terrault, M. C. Shuhart, D. T. Lau, W. R. Kim, M. W. Fried, R. K. Sterling, A. M. Di Bisceglie, S. H. Han, L. M. Ganova-Raeva, K. M. Chang, A. S. Lok, and Hepatitis B Research Network. 2015. Characteristics of adults in the hepatitis B research network in North America reflect their country of origin and hepatitis B virus genotype. *Clinical Gastroenterology and Hepatology* 13(1):183-192.

Heathcote, E. J., P. Marcellin, M. Buti, E. Gane, R. A. De Man, Z. Krastev, G. Germanidis, S. S. Lee, R. Flisiak, K. Kaita, M. Manns, I. Kotzev, K. Tchernev, P. Buggisch, F. Weilert, O. O. Kurdas, M. L. Shiffman, H. Trinh, S. Gurel, A. Snow-Lampart, K. Borroto-Esoda, E. Mondou, J. Anderson, J. Sorbel, and F. Rousseau. 2011. Three-year efficacy and safety of tenofovir disoproxil fumarate treatment for chronic hepatitis B. *Gastroenterology* 140(1):132-143.

HHS (Department of Health and Human Services). 2015. *Action plan for the prevention, care, and treatment of viral hepatitis: 2014-2016.* HHS, Office of the Assistant Secretary for Health, Office of HIV/AIDS and Infectious Disease Policy. https://www.aids.gov/pdf/viral-hepatitis-action-plan.pdf (accessed October 26, 2016).

HRSA (Health Resources and Services Administration). n.d. *Organ Procurement and Transplantation Network.* https://optn.transplant.hrsa.gov/data/view-data-reports/build-advanced (accessed July 2016).

Hu, D. J., J. Xing, R. A. Tohme, Y. Liao, H. Pollack, J. W. Ward, and S. D. Holmberg. 2013. Hepatitis B testing and access to care among racial and ethnic minorities in selected communities across the United States, 2009-2010. *Hepatology* 58(3):856-862.

Hutton, D. W., D. Tan, S. K. So, and M. L. Brandeau. 2007. Cost-effectiveness of screening and vaccinating Asian and Pacific Islander adults for hepatitis B. *Annals of Internal Medicine* 147(7):460-469.

Hyun, C. S., S. Kim, S. Y. Kang, S. Jung, and S. Lee. 2016. Chronic hepatitis B in Korean Americans: Decreased prevalence and poor linkage to care. *BMC Infectious Diseases* 16(1):415.

Iloeje, U. H., H. I. Yang, J. Su, C. L. Jen, S. L. You, and C. J. Chen. 2006. Predicting cirrhosis risk based on the level of circulating hepatitis B viral load. *Gastroenterology* 130(3):678-686.

Juday, T., H. Tang, M. Harris, A. Z. Powers, E. Kim, and G. J. Hanna. 2011. Adherence to chronic hepatitis B treatment guideline recommendations for laboratory monitoring of patients who are not receiving antiviral treatment. *Journal of General Internal Medicine* 26(3):239-244.

Jung, M., M. H. Kuniholm, G. Y. Ho, S. Cotler, H. D. Strickler, B. Thyagarajan, M. Youngblood, R. C. Kaplan, and J. Del Amo. 2016. The distribution of hepatitis B virus exposure and infection in a population-based sample of U.S. Hispanic adults. *Hepatology* 63(2):445-452.

Kanwal, F., M. Farid, P. Martin, G. Chen, I. M. Gralnek, G. S. Dulai, and B. M. Spiegel. 2006. Treatment alternatives for hepatitis B cirrhosis: A cost-effectiveness analysis. *American Journal of Gastroenterology* 101(9):2076-2089.

Kim, L. H., V. G. Nguyen, H. N. Trinh, J. Li, J. Q. Zhang, and M. H. Nguyen. 2014. Low treatment rates in patients meeting guideline criteria in diverse practice settings. *Digestive Diseases and Sciences* 59(9):2091-2099.

Kowdley, K. V., C. C. Wang, S. Welch, H. Roberts, and C. L. Brosgart. 2012. Prevalence of chronic hepatitis B among foreign-born persons living in the United States by country of origin. *Hepatology* 56(2):422-433.

Lin, S. Y., E. T. Chang, and S. K. So. 2007. Why we should routinely screen Asian American adults for hepatitis B: A cross-sectional study of Asians in California. *Hepatology* 46(4):1034-1040.

Lin, X., N. J. Robinson, M. Thursz, D. M. Rosenberg, A. Weild, J. M. Pimenta, and A. J. Hall. 2005. Chronic hepatitis B virus infection in the Asia-Pacific region and Africa: Review of disease progression. *Journal of Gastroenterology and Hepatology* 20(6):833-843.

Liu, S., L. E. Cipriano, M. Holodniy, D. K. Owens, and J. D. Goldhaber-Fiebert. 2012. New protease inhibitors for the treatment of chronic hepatitis C: A cost-effectiveness analysis. *Annals of Internal Medicine* 156(4):279-290.

Lok, A. S., B. J. McMahon, R. S. Brown, Jr., J. B. Wong, A. T. Ahmed, W. Farah, J. Almasri, F. Alahdab, K. Benkhadra, M. A. Mouchli, S. Singh, E. A. Mohamed, A. M. Abu Dabrh, L. J. Prokop, Z. Wang, M. H. Murad, and K. Mohammed. 2016. Antiviral therapy for chronic hepatitis B viral infection in adults: A systematic review and meta-analysis. *Hepatology* 63(1):284-306.

Marcellin, P., E. Gane, M. Buti, N. Afdhal, W. Sievert, I. M. Jacobson, M. K. Washington, G. Germanidis, J. F. Flaherty, R. Aguilar Schall, J. D. Bornstein, K. M. Kitrinos, G. M. Subramanian, J. G. McHutchison, and E. J. Heathcote. 2013. Regression of cirrhosis during treatment with tenofovir disoproxil fumarate for chronic hepatitis B: A 5-year open-label follow-up study. *Lancet* 381(9865):468-475.

Mitchell, T., G. L. Armstrong, D. J. Hu, A. Wasley, and J. A. Painter. 2011. The increasing burden of imported chronic hepatitis B—United States, 1974-2008. *PLoS One* 6(12):e27717.

NASEM (National Academies of Sciences, Engineering, and Medicine). 2016. *Eliminating the public health problem of hepatitis B and C in the United States: Phase one report.* Washington, DC: The National Academies Press.

Papatheodoridis, G. V., H. L. Chan, B. E. Hansen, H. L. Janssen, and P. Lampertico. 2015. Risk of hepatocellular carcinoma in chronic hepatitis B: Assessment and modification with current antiviral therapy. *Journal of Hepatology* 62(4):956-967.

Raffetti, E., G. Fattovich, and F. Donato. 2016. Incidence of hepatocellular carcinoma in untreated subjects with chronic hepatitis B: A systematic review and meta-analysis. *Liver International* 36(9):1239-1251.

Roberts, H., D. Kruszon-Moran, K. N. Ly, E. Hughes, K. Iqbal, R. B. Jiles, and S. D. Holmberg. 2016. Prevalence of chronic hepatitis B virus (HBV) infection in U.S. households: National Health and Nutrition Examination Survey (NHANES), 1988-2012. *Hepatology* 63(2):388-397.

Shuler, C. M., A. E. Fiore, R. Neeman, B. P. Bell, W. Kuhnert, S. Watkins, K. Kilgour, and K. E. Arnold. 2009. Reduction in hepatitis B virus seroprevalence among U.S.-born children of foreign-born Asian parents—Benefit of universal infant hepatitis B vaccination. *Vaccine* 27(43):5942-5947.

Spradling, P. R., J. Xing, L. B. Rupp, A. C. Moorman, S. C. Gordon, E. T. Teshale, M. Lu, J. A. Boscarino, C. M. Trinacty, M. A. Schmidt, and S. D. Holmberg. 2016. Infrequent clinical assessment of chronic hepatitis B patients in United States general healthcare settings. *Clinical Infectious Diseases* 63(9):1205-1208.

Stanaway, J. D., A. D. Flaxman, M. Naghavi, C. Fitzmaurice, T. Vos, I. Abubakar, L. J. Abu-Raddad, R. Assadi, N. Bhala, B. Cowie, M. H. Forouzanfour, J. Groeger, K. Mohd Hanafiah, K. H. Jacobsen, S. L. James, J. MacLachlan, R. Malekzadeh, N. K. Martin, A. A. Mokdad, A. H. Mokdad, C. J. Murray, D. Plass, S. Rana, D. B. Rein, J. H. Richardus, J. Sanabria, M. Saylan, S. Shahraz, S. So, V. V. Vlassov, E. Weiderpass, S. T. Wiersma, M. Younis, C. Yu, M. El Sayed Zaki, and G. S. Cooke. 2016. The global burden of viral hepatitis from 1990 to 2013: Findings from the Global Burden of Disease Study 2013. *The Lancet* 388(10049):1081-1088.

Tanaka, J., T. Koyama, M. Mizui, S. Uchida, K. Katayama, J. Matsuo, T. Akita, A. Nakashima, Y. Miyakawa, and H. Yoshizawa. 2011. Total numbers of undiagnosed carriers of hepatitis C and B viruses in Japan estimated by age- and area-specific prevalence on the national scale. *Intervirology* 54(4):185-195.

Tenney, D. J., R. E. Rose, C. J. Baldick, K. A. Pokornowski, B. J. Eggers, J. Fang, M. J. Wichroski, D. Xu, J. Yang, R. B. Wilber, and R. J. Colonno. 2009. Long-term monitoring shows hepatitis B virus resistance to entecavir in nucleoside-naive patients is rare through 5 years of therapy. *Hepatology* 49(5):1503-1514.

Terrault, N. A., N. H. Bzowej, K. M. Chang, J. P. Hwang, M. M. Jonas, and M. H. Murad. 2016. AASLD guidelines for treatment of chronic hepatitis B. *Hepatology* 63(1):261-283.

Thiele, M., L. L. Gluud, A. D. Fialla, E. K. Dahl, and A. Krag. 2014. Large variations in risk of hepatocellular carcinoma and mortality in treatment naive hepatitis B patients: Systematic review with meta-analyses. *PLoS One* 9(9):e107177.

Toy, M., J. A. Salomon, H. Jiang, H. Gui, H. Wang, J. Wang, J. H. Richardus, and Q. Xie. 2014. Population health impact and cost-effectiveness of monitoring inactive chronic hepatitis B and treating eligible patients in Shanghai, China. *Hepatology* 60(1):46-55.

Truven Health Analytics. 2016. *Red Book.* http://micromedex.com/products/product-suites/clinical-knowledge/redbook (accessed July 2016).

Ugwu, C., P. Varkey, S. Bagniewski, and T. Lesnick. 2008. Sero-epidemiology of hepatitis B among new refugees to Minnesota. *Journal of Immigrant and Minority Health* 10(5):469-474.

USPSTF (U.S. Preventive Services Task Force). 2016. *USPSTF A and B recommendations.* http://www.uspreventiveservicestaskforce.org (accessed January 9, 2017).

Walensky, R. P., P. E. Sax, Y. M. Nakamura, M. C. Weinstein, P. P. Pei, K. A. Freedberg, A. D. Paltiel, and B. R. Schackman. 2013. Economic savings versus health losses: The cost-effectiveness of generic antiretroviral therapy in the United States. *Annals of Internal Medicine* 158(2):84-92.

WHO (World Health Organization). 2016. *Global health sector strategy on viral hepatitis, 2016-2021: Towards ending viral hepatitis.* Geneva, Switzerland: WHO. http://apps.who.int/iris/bitstream/10665/246177/1/WHO-HIV-2016.06-eng.pdf (accessed July 19, 2016).

Wong, G. L., H. L. Chan, C. W. Mak, S. K. Lee, Z. M. Ip, A. T. Lam, H. W. Iu, J. M. Leung, J. W. Lai, A. O. Lo, H. Y. Chan, and V. W. Wong. 2013. Entecavir treatment reduces hepatic events and deaths in chronic hepatitis B patients with liver cirrhosis. *Hepatology* 58(5):1537-1547.

Woo, G., G. Tomlinson, C. Yim, L. Lilly, G. Therapondos, D. K. Wong, W. J. Ungar, T. R. Einarson, M. Sherman, J. E. Heathcote, and M. Krahn. 2012. Health state utilities and quality of life in patients with hepatitis B. *Canadian Journal of Gastroenterology and Hepatology* 26(7):445-451.

Appendix B

Modeling the Elimination of Hepatitis C in the United States

Homie Razavi
Center for Disease Analysis

Chronic hepatitis C virus infection (HCV) is a leading cause of cirrhosis, hepatocellular carcinoma (HCC) and liver transplantation in the United States (NIDDK, 2016; HRSA, 2016; Yang et al., 2012). The advent of direct-acting antiviral (DAA) therapies in recent years means that HCV can be treated with sustained viral response (SVR) rates in excess of 90 percent, and treatment regimens continue to become more efficacious and easier to tolerate for patients (Martinello and Dore, 2016). Achieving SVR has positive health, quality of life, and economic implications for cured patients (Smith-Palmer et al., 2015). This analysis considers the impact of treatment uptake on disease burden at the national level under four different scenarios. Understanding future disease burden and potential strategies to mitigate burden is critical for the elimination of HCV in the United States (NASEM, 2016).

METHODS

Model

The HCV disease progression model has been described in detail previously (Blach et al., 2016; Razavi et al., 2014). The model was designed using Microsoft Excel® (Microsoft Corp., Redmond, Washington) to track the viremic HCV infected population by disease stage through 2030. The model estimated the annual number of incident HCV infections, after accounting for spontaneous cure (Seeff, 2002). Fibrosis progression of all cases was followed over time through 2030. The number of cases at any stage of liver disease was calculated and tracked by age and gender. The population was aged in 1 year age cohorts through age 84 and cases aged ≥85 years were tracked as a single cohort. The population in each age group, except for the ≥85 year cohort, was moved to the next age each year to simulate aging. Background population data for the United States were obtained from the United Nations' population database by age, gender, and one year age cohort (United Nations, 2015).

Disease progression was estimated through fibrosis and liver disease stages with annual adjustment for background mortality (United Nations, 2015). Cases by disease stage were calculated by multiplying the progression rate and the total cases at previous stages of the disease in the previous year. Background mortality was adjusted to account for increased mortality among the portion of the viremic population who are people who inject drugs (PWID) and people with a history of blood transfusion. Based on U.S. data showing that 0.3 percent of individuals aged ≥13 years were active PWID and that 43.126 percent were anti-HCV positive (Lansky et al., 2014), it was estimated that there are 251,900 viremic active PWID, assuming a 75 percent viremia rate (Edlin et al., 2015; Seeff, 2002). A standardized mortality ratio (SMR) of 10.0 was estimated (Bjornaas et al., 2008; Engstrom et al., 1991; Frischer et al., 1997; Hickman et al., 2003; Oppenheimer et al., 1994; Perucci et al., 1991) and applied to background mortality rates for the 7.3 percent of viremic cases who are active PWID aged 15-44 years. In addition, an estimated 6.5 percent of the infected population reported a history of transfusion (Daniels et al., 2009); an SMR of 1.5 (Kamper-Jørgensen et al., 2008) was applied to background mortality rates for these cases.

HCV Prevalence

Based on data from the 2003-2010 National Health and Nutrition Examination Survey (NHANES), there were an estimated 3.6 million individuals positive for HCV antibody and approximately 75 percent (Edlin et al., 2015; Seeff, 2002) were HCV RNA-positive (viremic), equivalent to 2.7 million chronically infected individuals (Denniston et al., 2014). NHANES potentially undersamples several groups with elevated risk for HCV infection, including incarcerated people, homeless people, hospitalized patients, nursing home residents, active-duty military, and Native Americans living on reservations. Analyses that accounted for these high-risk groups, in addition to data from NHANES, resulted in updated prevalence estimates of 4.6 million individuals who are HCV antibody positive and 3.5 million individuals who are HCV-RNA positive (Edlin et al., 2015). The HCV model tracked only viremic individuals, and assumed a prevalent popula-

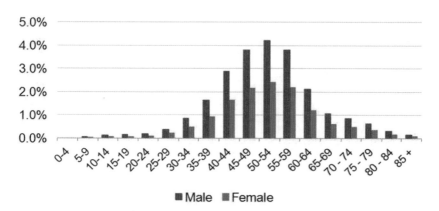

FIGURE B-1 Model input: hepatitis C virus prevalence rates by age and gender, United States, 2010.

tion of 3.5 million viremic cases in 2010, at the end of the NHANES data period analysis.

The distribution of cases by age and gender was based on data reported from NHANES (2003-2010) by age and gender, where the proportion of viremic cases among males (63.6 percent) exceeded that of females (36.4 percent) by a factor of 1.75 (Denniston et al., 2014). The reported distribution of viremic cases by age group was extrapolated to the national level with the assumption of decreasing prevalence among persons aged <20 years not represented in NHANES (see Figure B-1). The age of prevalent cases was further validated by estimating the projected proportion of cases by birth cohort in 2010 and comparing that to published estimates, demonstrating that approximately three-quarters of infected persons in the United States were born during 1945-1965 (Smith et al., 2012). The genotype distribution of the prevalent population in the United States was based upon NHANES laboratory data files (CDC, 2015). Genotype data from survey cycles during 2003-2014 were summed and the distribution was input as 57.0 percent (G1a), 22.1 percent (G1b), 0.5 percent (G1 other), 10.9 percent (G2), 8.1 percent (G3), 0.8 percent (G4) and 0.5 percent (G6). Prevalent cases were described by subpopulation; reported proportions of cases captured by NHANES, and underrepresented groups were extrapolated to model outputs in 2015 (Edlin et al., 2015). Similarly, reported proportions of infected persons by insurance coverage category were applied to prevalent cases in 2015 (Fitch et al., 2013).

HCV Incidence

Total HCV cases in a given year were assumed to be the sum of existing and new HCV cases after adjustment for mortality and spontaneous cure. The number of new infections was back-calculated using a two-step process that first calculated the annual number of new infections, followed by the age and gender distribution of these cases. The annual number of new cases was calibrated to the estimated prevalence of HCV in 2010 (Edlin et al., 2015). Annual relative incidence values were used to describe changes in the annual number of new HCV infections, and were based upon published estimates that were available from 1982 to 2014 (CDC, 2016). Based on the number of reported acute infections with an underascertainment multiplier, the Centers for Disease Control and Prevention (CDC) estimated that 180,000 new infections occurred in 1982 increasing to a peak of 291,000 new infections in 1989. In 2014, there were an estimated 30,500 (24,200-104,200) new HCV infections (CDC, 2016). Excel® Solver was used to determine a constant that, when multiplied by the relative incidence, resulted in the sum of all new cases since 1950 achieving the target model prevalence of HCV in 2010, after adjustment for mortality.

Diagnosed/Treated

The number of diagnosed cases was calculated in the model in order to better understand potential constraints on treatment uptake. Analyses of NHANES data have demonstrated that 51 percent of infected cases were already aware of their infection (Denniston et al., 2014; Volk et al., 2009). However, this may be an underestimate due to the underrepresentation of high risk groups in NHANES (Edlin et al., 2015). For modeling purposes, it was assumed that 45 percent of the viremic population was previously diagnosed in 2010, equivalent to 1,575,000 diagnosed viremic cases. In addition, it was assumed that 110,000 new cases would be diagnosed annually based on reported acute cases in sentinel centers (Klevens et al., 2009), along with an underascertainment multiplier adjusting for undercounting based on the proportions of infected persons developing symptoms and seeking care, as well as the proportion of those diagnosed who were reported to surveillance systems (Klevens et al., 2014).

The annual number of treated patients was based on sales unit data reported for pegylated interferon during 2004-2012. During this time period, annual treated ranged from 124,800 cases (2005) to 59,000 cases (2012). In later years, expert feedback and published estimates were used to estimate total treated patients. Assumptions for treatment efficacy varied by scenario, as described below.

The total number of annual liver transplants by diagnostic category was available from the Organ Procurement and Transplantation Network for the years 1988 to 2015. All transplants in five diagnostic categories (acute hepatic necrosis [AHN] with HCV, AHN with hepatitis B virus [HBV] and HCV, alcoholic cirrhosis with HCV, cirrhosis with HBV and HCV, and cirrhosis with HCV) were assumed to be HCV-related, and 23.6 percent to 41.6 percent (Yang et al., 2012) of transplants in two additional categories (HCC, HCC and cirrhosis) were assumed to be HCV-related. These were summed to estimate total HCV-related transplants in a given year. In 2015, there were 7,127 liver transplants performed in the United States (HRSA, 2016) and 2010 (28 percent) were attributed to HCV.

Sensitivity Analysis

For key model inputs, low and high ranges were entered based on published ranges and expert input (see Table B-1). Model generated uncertainty intervals (UIs) were calculated using high/low Beta-PERT distributions around inputs and conducting Monte Carlo analysis using Oracle Crystal Ball® (Oracle Corp., Redwood City, California). Uncertainty around total viremic cases and liver deaths during 2015-2030 under the 2015 Base scenario were calculated. In addition, leading drivers of uncertainty for viremic prevalence, incident decompensated cirrhosis, incident HCC and HCV-related mortality in 2030 were identified.

Model Validation

To validate model outputs, the annual number of incident HCC cases attributable to chronic HCV infection was considered. Total annual incident cases of liver and intrahepatic bile duct cancer are reported by the Surveillance, Epidemiology, and End Results Program (SEER) (SEER Program, 2015). Based on an analysis of SEER data collected during 2000-2010, it was assumed that 72 percent of liver and intrahepatic duct cancers would be classified as HCC (Altekruse et al., 2014). Analysis of incident HCC cases in Olmsted County, Minnesota, reported HCC attributable to HCV alone and to HCV and alcohol in combination (Yang et al., 2012), during 1991-2000 and 2001-2008. For the purposes of validating the model, it was assumed that 100 percent of HCC cases attributed to HCV alone, and 80 percent of cases attributed to HCV and alcohol, would be HCV-related. It was calculated that 23.6 percent of incident HCC cases would be attributed to HCV during 1991-2000, increasing to 41.6 percent of incident HCC during 2001-2008. It was estimated that there were 1869 incident HCV-related HCC cases at the national level in 1991, increasing to 7,582 cases by 2008. These data were plotted and compared to model estimated HCC incident cases during 1991-2008 (see Figure B-2). The annual number of

TABLE B-1 Sensitivity Analysis Inputs, United States, 2015 Base Scenario

Category	Low	High	Source
Annual new infections (2017-2030)	2,760	217,000	Expert input, Massachusetts Department of Public Health, 2016; Onofrey et al., 2015
Viremic cases (2010)	2,500,000	4,700,000	Edlin et al., 2015
Annual treated (2017-2030)	65,000	260,000	Drug unit sales, expert input
Mild to moderate fibrosis – Transition probability multiplier	0.59	1.53	Harris et al., 2014
Mod to cirrhosis – Transition probability multiplier	0.57	1.9	Harris et al., 2014
Transfusion SMR	1.3	17.6	Kamper-Jørgensen et al., 2008
Injection Drug Use SMR	9.5	29.9	Bjornaas et al., 2008; Engstrom et al., 1991; Frischer et al., 1997; Hickman et al., 2003; Oppenheimer et al., 1994; Perucci et al., 1991
Cirrhosis to HCC – Transition probability multiplier	0.74	1.32	Harris et al., 2014
Cirrhosis to decompensated cirrhosis – Transition probability multiplier	0.70	1.36	Harris et al., 2014
HCC to liver death (year 1) – Transition probability	58.9%	74.2%	Bernfort et al., 2006; Ries et al., 2007
HCC to liver death (subsequent years) – Transition probability	13.5%	19.5%	Ries et al., 2007
Decompensated cirrhosis to liver death – Transition probability multiplier	0.80	1.20	Harris et al., 2014
Annual diagnosed (2017-2030)	27,500	110,000	Klevens et al., 2014; Klevens et al., 2009

NOTE: HCC = hepatocellular carcinoma; SMR = standardized mortality ratio.

liver-related deaths was calculated in the model and compared to national estimates for the number of HCV-related deaths based on death certificates during 2010-2014 (CDC, 2016) (see Figure B-2).

Scenarios

Four scenarios were developed to estimate the disease burden associated with varying levels of treatment efficacy, treatment and screening levels, and new infections. Changes occurred over time waves and were based on estimates reported in the literature and national reports, as well as expert input (see Table B-2).

2013 Base

The 2013 Base scenario was based on data from historical treatment regimens of pegylated interferon and ribavirin. This scenario was considered in order to show the impact of recent increases in treatment with more efficacious regimens. Under this scenario, it was assumed that 60 percent of diagnosed patients would be medically eligible for treatment (see Table B-2). Treated patients experienced SVR rates of 55 percent (G1), 70 percent (G2/G3), 48 percent (G4) and 55 percent (other and mixed genotypes). The annual number of treated patients was held constant at 32,000, and annual diagnosed patients gradually declined from 110,000 cases during 2013-2015 to 55,000 cases during 2025-2030. The number of new infections was held relatively constant at approximately 30,000 new infections annually.

2015 Base

The 2015 Base scenario was based upon the latest treatment data, and reflects the recent uptake of DAA regimens. In 2015, it was estimated that the treated population increased to 260,000 treated cases (see Figure B-3). It was assumed that annual treatment would gradually decline by 50 percent to 130,000 annual treated cases by 2020. The efficacy of treatment was assumed to increase from 55 percent (2013) to 95 percent (2017), and treatment eligibility also reached 95 percent. Treatment eligibility was restricted to people with moderate fibrosis (≥F2) beginning in 2014 as new regimens were introduced. It was assumed that individuals aged 15-64 years were eligible for treatment until 2020, when treatment was expanded to individuals aged 15-74 years (see Table B-2). Assumptions for annual diagnosed cases and new infections were identical to the 2013 Base scenario.

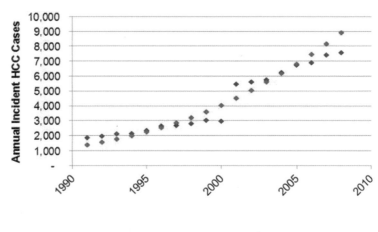

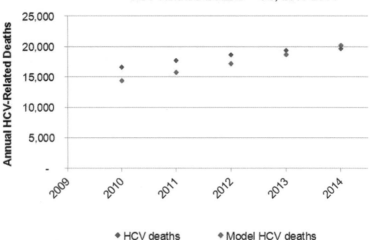

FIGURE B-2 Model validation: HCV-related HCC incidence, United States, 1991-2008, and HCV-related deaths, United States, 2010-2014.
NOTE: HCC = hepatocellular carcinoma; HCV = hepatitis C virus.
SOURCES: Altekruse et al., 2014; CDC, 2016; SEER Program, 2015; Yang et al., 2012.

Aggressive ≥F0

The Aggressive ≥F0 scenario was based on a continuation of the high levels of treatment observed in 2015 continuing into the future. This scenario applied the same assumptions as the 2015 Base scenario for treatment efficacy and eligibility, but assumed that treatment continued at a high level (260,000 annually treated) through 2030. In addition, the number diagnosed was calculated so that 80 percent of all prevalent cases would be diagnosed by 2030 (see Figure B-4). To achieve this, annual diagnosed decreased from 110,000 annually to 71,700 annually by 2025. Under this scenario, new infections were assumed to decline sharply as a result of dramatically increased treatment and reduced transmission. A reduction from 30,000 new infections to 2,700 new infections annually by 2025 was modeled. In order to assess the impact of treating less advanced cases, treatment was expanded to ≥F1 cases in 2015 and ≥F0 cases in 2017.

Aggressive ≥F2

The Aggressive ≥F2 scenario applied the same assumptions as the Aggressive ≥F0 scenario, but assumed that treatment was limited to ≥F2 patients for the entirety of the time period. As cases with no/minimal fibrosis were not treated in this scenario, it was assumed that HCV transmission would not decline substantially and annual new cases remained constant at approximately 30,000 cases. Applying an 80 percent limit on total diagnosed in 2030, the number of newly diagnosed was estimated to decline to 83,700 cases by 2025. Annual treated was held constant at 260,000, but fibrosis restrictions resulted in the model running out of diagnosed eligible patients to treat beginning in 2026. By 2030, there were an estimated 118,600 treated patients due to depletion of the eligible pool of potential patients.

RESULTS

Scenarios

For each scenario, annual estimates for prevalence and incidence (total and by disease stage) were plotted through 2030. The relative increase or decrease in cases by 2030 was compared to the caseload in 2015. Outputs from the 2015 Base scenario were compared against results from the other scenarios. Finally, the cumulative number of incident decompensated cirrhosis, incident HCC, and liver-related deaths during 2015-2030 were calculated and compared against values for the 2015 Base scenario to estimate percentage reductions in disease burden as compared to the current

TABLE B-2 Scenario Assumptions, United States, 2013-2030

Scenario	Assumption	Wave 1	Wave 2	Wave 3	Wave 4	Wave 5
Base 2013	Years	2013-2015	2016-2017	2018-2019	2020-2024	2025-2030
	Annual Treated	32,000	32,000	32,000	32,000	32,000
	Annual Newly Diagnosed	110,000	110,000	77,780	55,000	55,000
	Fibrosis Stage	≥F0	≥F0	≥F0	≥F0	≥F0
	Annual New Infections	29,690	30,270	30,100	29,980	29,800
	Treated Age	15-64	15-64	15-64	15-64	15-64
	SVR	58%	58%	58%	58%	58%
Base 2015	Years	2013-2014	2015-2016	2017-2019	2020-2024	2025-2030
	Annual Treated	32,000	260,000	183,800	130,000	130,000
	Annual Newly Diagnosed	110,000	110,000	77,780	55,000	55,000
	Fibrosis Stage	≥F0	≥F2	≥F2	≥F2	≥F2
	Annual New Infections	29,690	30,340	30,160	29,980	29,830
	Treated Age	15-64	15-64	15-74	15-74	15-74
	SVR	58%	90%	95%	95%	95%

Aggressive ≥F0	Years	2013-2014	2015-2016	2017-2019	2020-2024	2025-2030
	Annual Treated	32,000	260,000	260,000	260,000	260,000
	Annual Newly Diagnosed	110,000	110,000	110,000	88,790	71,660
	Fibrosis Stage	≥F0	≥F1	≥F0	≥F0	≥F0
	Annual New Infections	29,690	30,340	22,620	11,150	2,730
	Treated Age	15-64	15-64	15-74	15-74	15-74
	SVR	58%	90%	95%	95%	95%
Aggressive ≥F2	Years	2013-2014	2015-2016	2017-2019	2020-2024	2025-2030
	Annual Treated	32,000	260,000	260,000	260,000	260,000
	Annual Newly Diagnosed	110,000	110,000	110,000	95,940	83,670
	Fibrosis Stage	≥F0	≥F2	≥F2	≥F2	≥F2
	Annual New Infections	29,690	30,330	30,150	29,960	29,800
	Treated Age	15-64	15-64	15-74	15-74	15-74
	SVR	58%	90%	95%	95%	95%

NOTE: SVR = sustained virologic response.

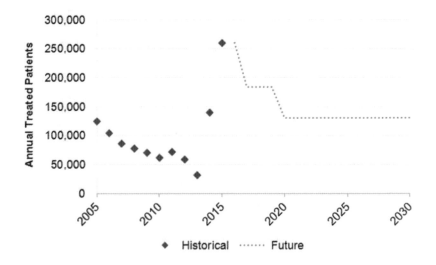

FIGURE B-3 Annual treated patients, 2015 Base scenario, 2005-2030.

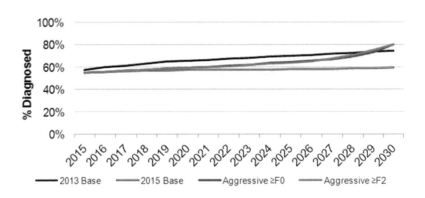

FIGURE B-4 Proportion of viremic cases diagnosed by scenario, United States, 2015-2030.

treatment paradigm. The results for the 2013 Base scenario were included only for illustration purposes as this scenario was not considered a likely future option (treatment with the older therapies).

2015 Base

There were an estimated 3,117,000 viremic cases in 2015, declining over 10 percent from 3,500,000 cases in 2010. Viremic cases decreased from 3,117,000 (UI: 2,290,000-3,892,000) in 2015 to 1,495,000 (762,000-2,116,000) in 2030, a decrease of 50 percent (see Figures B-5 and B-6). Under this scenario, prevalent compensated and decompensated cirrhotic cases declined 35 percent during 2015-2030, to 302,800 and 28,900 cases, respectively. Prevalent HCC decreased 40 percent between 2015 and 2030 to 13,600 cases in 2030. Cumulative incident decompensated cirrhosis and HCC were estimated at 188,000 and 188,800 cases, respectively. An-

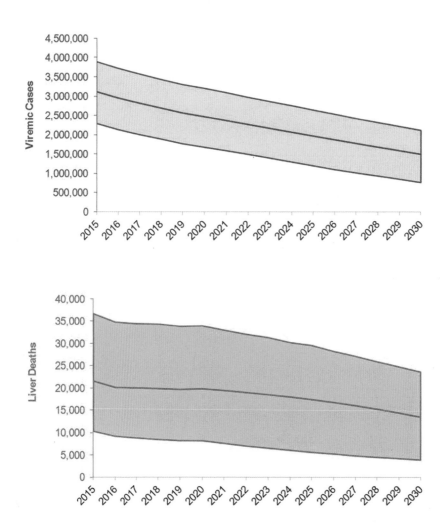

FIGURE B-5 Viremic cases and liver deaths with uncertainty intervals, 2015 Base scenario, 2015-2030.

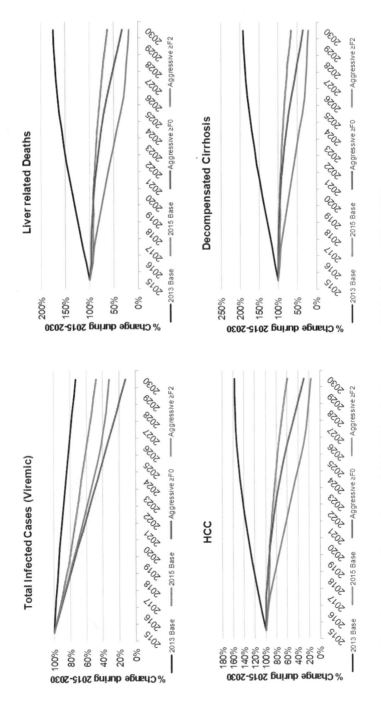

FIGURE B-6 Percentage change during 2015-2030 value by scenario, United States, 2015-2030.

NOTE: HCC = hepatocellular carcinoma.

nual liver deaths were estimated at 13,500 (UI: 3900-23,600) for 2030, a decline of 40 percent from 2015 when there were 21,600 (10,300-36,700) deaths (see Figure B-5), while cumulative deaths over the time period were estimated at 289,200 deaths. The 2015 treatment and diagnosis rate has averted 215,100 deaths relative to the treatment and diagnosis rate in 2013 Base scenario (see Table B-3). This represents a 55 percent decrease as compared to the 2013 Base scenario.

Viremic cases were characterized using model outputs under the 2015 Base Scenario. In 2015, there were an estimated 1,290,000 cases in the 50-59 year old age group, over 40 percent of all cases (see Figure B-7). The burden of advanced fibrosis and cirrhosis was concentrated in older age groups with 85 percent and 95 percent of F3 and F4 (compensated cirrhosis, decompensated cirrhosis, HCC and liver transplant) cases among persons aged ≥50 years, respectively. The prevalent number of F4 cases declined 35 percent during 2015-2030 from 565,700 cases to 356,500 cases, but the proportion of total cases classified as F4 increased from 20 percent to 25 percent (see Figure B-7).

The distribution of viremic cases by subpopulation in 2015 calculated how many cases would be represented by the NHANES sample, and how many additional cases would occur in underrepresented groups. In 2015, subpopulations were estimated at 2,404,800 NHANES (77 percent), 361,000 incarcerated people (12 percent), 158,700 homeless people (5 percent), 88,000 Native Americans living on reservations (2.8 percent), 53,300

TABLE B-3 Key Model Output Summary by Scenario, United States, 2015-2030

Scenario:	Base 2015	Aggressive ≥F0	Aggressive ≥F2
Relative to:	Base 2013	Base 2015	Base 2015
Reduction in viremic infections	910,000	1,105,100	515,500
Liver deaths averted	215,000	28,800	98,500
Total new HCC cases averted (2015-2030)	123,000	19,000	57,700
Total new decompensated cirrhosis cases averted (2015-2030)	124,000	19,000	58,200
Total number of new infections averted (2015-2030)	(200)	279,400	0

NOTE: HCC = hepatocellular carcinoma.

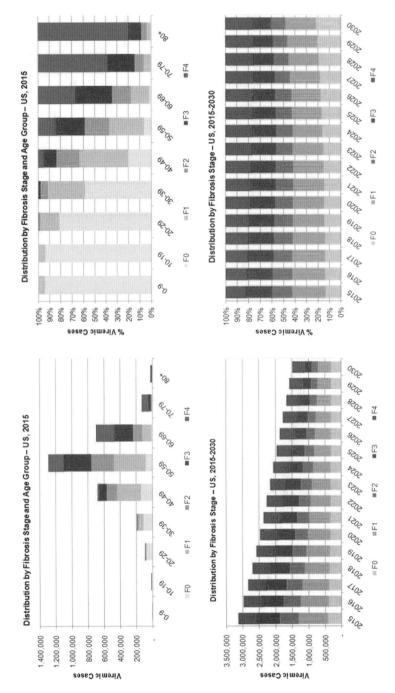

FIGURE B-7 Distribution of viremic HCV cases by fibrosis stage and age group, United States, 2015, and distribution by fibrosis stage, United States, 2015-2030.

hospitalized patients (1.7 percent), 46,500 nursing home residents (1.5 percent) and 5000 active-duty military (0.2 percent) (see Figure B-8). Insurance type in 2015 was extrapolated at 997,900 uninsured (32 percent), 767,400 privately insured (25 percent), 371,400 Medicaid (12 percent), 361,000 incarcerated (12 percent), 307,400 Veterans Affairs or other military (10 percent), 198,000 dual Medicare and Medicaid (6 percent) and 115,300 Medicare (4 percent) (see Figure B-8).

2013 Base

Under the 2013 Base scenario, the number of prevalent cases was projected to decline 25 percent from 3,302,000 cases in 2015 to 2,406,000 cases in 2030, largely due to aging of the population and mortality (see Figure B-9). Prevalent compensated cirrhosis cases were projected to increase 45 percent from 520,900 to 764,900 cases during 2015-2030, while decompensated cirrhosis cases were projected to increase from 45,300 to 86,900 (90 percent increase) as shown in Figure B-9. Prevalent HCC cases increase from 24,300 to 38,000, a 55 percent increase. Cumulative incidence of decompensated cirrhosis and HCC during 2015-2030 was estimated at 311,700 and 312,100 incident cases, respectively. Under this scenario, annual liver-related deaths were projected to increase 75 percent from 21,800 in 2015 to 38,000 in 2030, and cumulative deaths during the time period were estimated at 504,300 deaths.

Aggressive ≥F0

Under the Aggressive ≥F0 scenario, viremic cases decline 85 percent to 390,000 cases by 2030 (see Figure B-9). Prevalent compensated and decompensated cirrhosis decline 70 percent and 65 percent, to 145,000 and 15,200 prevalent cases in 2030, respectively. Prevalent HCC also declines 70 percent to 6,600 cases in 2030, while annual liver deaths decline 65 percent to 7,100 deaths in 2030. As compared to the 2015 Base scenario, there were 75 percent fewer viremic cases in 2030, 50 percent fewer compensated cirrhosis, decompensated cirrhosis and HCC cases (see Figure B-10). Liver-related deaths also declined to 50 percent of level expected in the 2015 Base scenario, and cumulative liver deaths were estimated at 260,400, a 10 percent decrease from the 2015 Base scenario (see Figure B-11). Cumulative incident decompensated cirrhosis and HCC both declined by 10 percent as compared to the 2015 Base scenario with a total of 168,900 and 169,900 cases, respectively. By 2030, this scenario had achieved the greatest reduction in viremic prevalence.

Distribution of Viremic Cases by Subpopulation

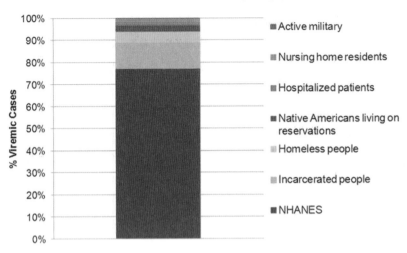

Distribution of Viremic Cases by Insurance Category

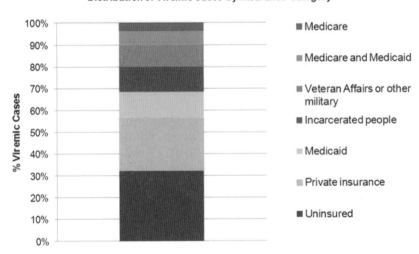

FIGURE B-8 Distribution of viremic cases by subpopulation and insurance category.
NOTE: NHANES = National Health and Nutrition Examination Survey.

253

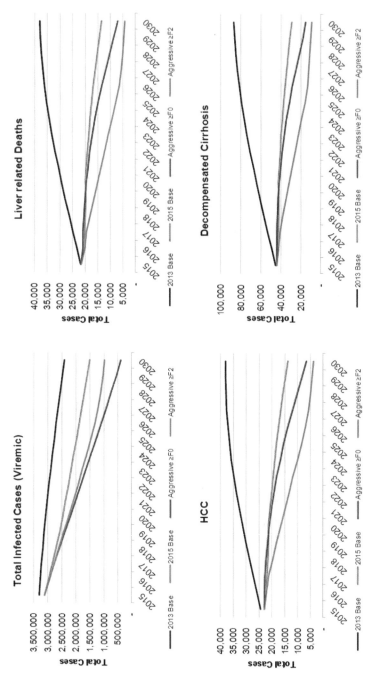

FIGURE B-9 Total cases by scenario, United States, 2015–2030.
NOTE: HCC = hepatocellular carcinoma.

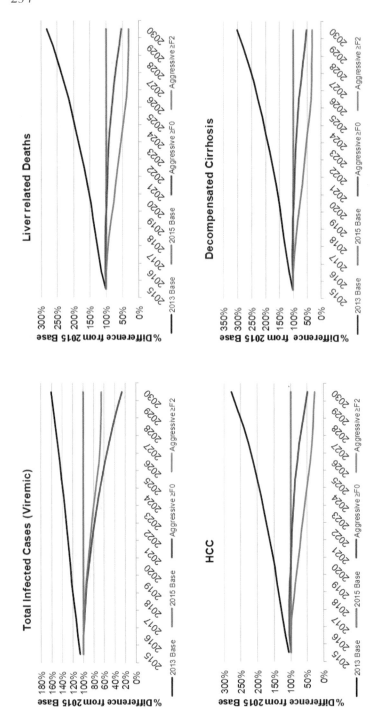

FIGURE B-10 Percentage difference from 2015 Base scenario, United States, 2015-2030.
NOTE: HCC = hepatocellular carcinoma.

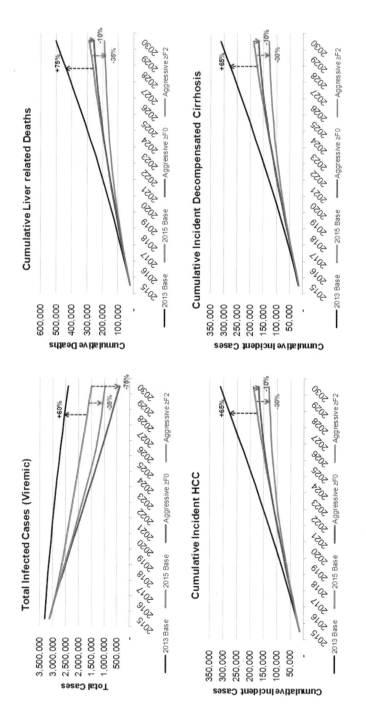

FIGURE B-11 Cumulative disease burden by scenario with percentage reduction from 2015 Base scenario in 2030, United States, 2015-2030.

NOTE: HCC = hepatocellular carcinoma.

256

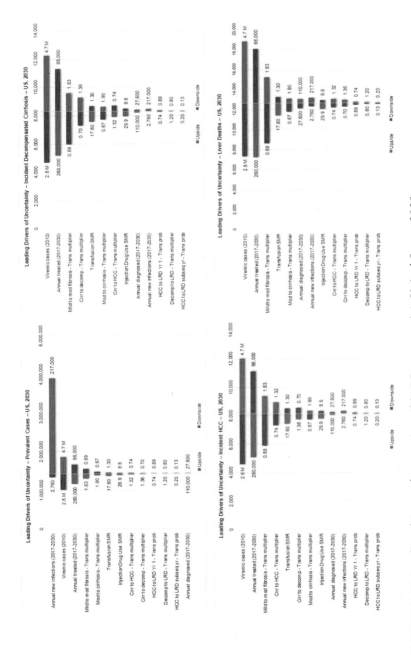

FIGURE B-12 Leading drivers of uncertainty (2015 Base scenario), United States, 2030.
NOTE: HCC = hepatocellular carcinoma; LRD = liver-related death; SMR = standardized mortality ratio.

Aggressive ≥F2

The Aggressive ≥F2 scenario resulted in a 70 percent reduction in cases to 980,000 viremic infections in 2030 (see Figures B-9 and B-6). Prevalent compensated and decompensated cirrhosis cases declined 80 percent over the time period to 87,300 and 9,300 cases in 2030, while HCC cases declined 85 percent to 3,700 cases. Liver-related deaths declined 80 percent to 4,100 deaths in 2030 (see Figure B-9). As compared to the 2015 Base scenario, there were 35 percent fewer viremic cases in 2030, as well as 70 percent fewer compensated cirrhotic, decompensated cirrhotic, and HCC cases (see Figure B-10). Liver deaths in 2030 declined 70 percent as compared to the 2015 Base scenario, and cumulative liver deaths declined by 35 percent (190,700 deaths) (see Figure B-11). Cumulative incident decompensated cirrhosis and HCC during 2015-2030 were estimated at 129,800 and 131,100 cases, respectively, and were 30 percent less than estimates for the 2015 Base scenario. The Aggressive ≥F2 scenario had the largest impact in reducing end stage liver disease and liver-related mortality.

Sensitivity Analysis

For total viremic infections in 2030, inputs for annual new infections, base prevalence and annual treated were the greatest drivers of uncertainty, together accounting for >95 percent of uncertainty (see Figure B-12). For incident decompensated cirrhosis, HCC, and liver deaths in 2030, inputs for base prevalence, annual treated, and the mild to moderate fibrosis transition probability multiplier were found to have the largest impact on uncertainty, with these factors accounting for approximately 95 percent of uncertainty (see Figure B-12).

DISCUSSION

The analysis presented here provides a range of future outcomes under different scenarios, but does not define a specific future scenario. Key insights are derived by comparing scenarios and identifying the factors that are important. Specific measures at different points in time were examined as a function of all uncertainties—viremic infections, liver-related deaths, number of individuals with HCV-related HCC and the number of decompensated cirrhosis cases. Although cirrhotic cases have been used as a measure of disease burden in the past, this disease stage can contain individuals with compensated and decompensated cirrhosis. The latter was selected since it is associated with a high mortality rate and potentially more accurate reporting.

The uncertainties considered as part of this analysis had a different level of impact on the measures we considered. For example, of all the uncertainties considered, incidence had the largest impact on the forecasted total number of viremic HCV cases (prevalent cases) in the United States in 2030 (see Figure B-12). In 2011, the CDC estimated 16,500 (7,200-43,400) new HCV infections. This figure increased to 30,500 (24,200-104,200) new infections per year by 2014 (CDC, 2016). The increase in new HCV infections is explained by the rapid rise of PWID in the United States and this population is not distributed homogeneously across the country (Suryaprasad et al., 2014). When HCV incidence rates in Massachusetts were applied to the United States population, an estimated 217,000 new HCV infections could be occurring in the United States (Massachusetts Department of Public Health, 2016; Onofrey et al., 2015) (see Figure B-12). Thus, the biggest driver of uncertainty in the future prevalence of HCV is the uncertainty in the number of new infections. The number of people diagnosed, treated, or progressing to advanced liver disease had a much smaller impact on total viremic infections in the United States. As a result, this analysis indicated that future HCV infection forecasts in the United States would benefit from important studies to develop more accurate estimates of current and future new infections in the United States and developing strategies to minimize new infections.

As injection drug use is the leading risk factor for new infections (CDC, 2016), it is important to consider requirements to reduce HCV infections among PWID. New PWID tend to be young (ages 15-35) and are infected by sharing needles and injection paraphernalia with those already infected (CDC, 2011). HCV disease progression is a function of age and duration of infection (Poynard et al., 2001), which would mean that the majority of this population has no fibrosis (F0) or early stage fibrosis (F1-F2). Studies have shown that an increase in harm reduction programs (opioid substitution therapy and syringe exchange programs) are effective in reducing the number of new HCV infections (Martin et al., 2013b; Nolan et al., 2014; Tsui et al., 2014; Turner et al., 2011; White et al., 2014). In the absence of vaccines, treatment of this population can also reduce the viral pool of this population resulting in a reduction in total and new infections over time (Martin et al., 2013a). However, current policies in a number of states do not provide access to HCV treatment for PWID and/or those in early stages of fibrosis. A reduction in the number of new HCV infections will require programs to reduce the number of people starting injection drug use, expanding harm reduction programs for those already injecting, and providing HCV treatment to PWID and those in early stages of fibrosis (F0-F2) (Bruggmann and Grebely, 2015).

Reducing incidence of new infections is among the World Health Organization (WHO) targets for eliminating HCV as a public health threat (WHO, 2016) (see Figure B-13). In addition, countries are required to re-

Target areas			Baseline 2015	2020 target	2030 target
Service coverage	Prevention	1 Three-dose hepatitis B vaccine for infants (coverage %)	82%	90%	90%
		2 Prevention of mother-to-child transmission of HBV: hepatitis B birth-dose vaccination or other approaches (coverage %)	38%	50%	90%
		3 Blood and injection safety (coverage %) — Blood safety: donations screened with quality assurance	89%	95%	100%
		3 Blood and injection safety (coverage %) — Injection safety: use of engineered devices	5%	50%	90%
		4 Harm reduction (sterile syringe/needle set distributed per person per year for people who inject drugs [PWID])	20	200	300
	5 Treatment	5a Diagnosis of HBV and HCV (coverage %)	<5%	30%	90%
		5b Treatment of HBV and HCV (coverage %)	<1%	5 million (HBV) 3 million (HCV)	80% eligible treated
Impact leading to elimination		Incidence of chronic HBV and HCV infections	6-10 million	30% reduction	90% reduction
		Mortality of chronic HBV and HCV infections	1.46 million	10% reduction	65% reduction

FIGURE B-13 WHO: Service coverage targets that would eliminate HBV and HCV as public health threats, 2015-2030.
NOTE: HBV = hepatitis B virus; HCV = hepatitis C virus; WHO = World Health Organization.
SOURCE: WHO, 2016.

duce mortality from HCV infections. To meet this requirement, a reduction in advanced liver disease (HCC and decompensated cirrhosis) is needed.

The sensitivity analysis showed that the number of new infections has a very small impact on the forecasted number of liver-related deaths in 2030 (see Figure B-12). Individuals newly infected with HCV will not progress to advanced liver disease for a long period (Pradat et al., 2007), and the impact of new HCV infections on mortality is unseen for several decades. Instead, to meet the reduction in mortality target, we have to manage those already infected with HCV. The key drivers of uncertainty in the number of liver-related deaths in 2030 is the number of individuals already infected with HCV, the number of patients treated per year, and the progression probability from mild to moderate fibrosis (see Figure B-12). The HCV prevalence estimates provided by NHANES (Denniston et al., 2014) may underestimate the total number of infections due to undersampling in some populations (homeless people, incarcerated people, etc.). However, a number of studies have examined these populations and report a higher number of infections (Chak et al., 2011; Edlin et al., 2015). The key driver of uncertainty in our forecast of the number of liver-related deaths in 2030 is the total number of HCV infections; additional studies to narrow this range can improve the quality of our forecast. The next driver of uncertainty is how many people will be treated annually. Achieving SVR is effective in halting or slowing progression to advanced liver disease and it is not surprising that treatment has a substantive impact on liver-related deaths (Simmons et al., 2015).

The last variable that had a large impact on forecasted liver related deaths was the rate of progression from mild to moderate fibrosis. This progression rate is influenced by alcohol consumption and body mass (Hourigan et al., 1999; Poynard et al., 1997). Additional longitudinal studies in the U.S. population are needed to reduce this uncertainty, especially given ongoing high rates of obesity (Ogden et al., 2014) and associated risk of fibrosis development (Poynard et al., 2010).

The above discussion focused on quantifying the main drivers of uncertainties for total infections and liver-related deaths. As part of this analysis, we also examined what is required to achieve WHO targets. Relative to the treatment paradigm represented by the 2013 Base scenario, great advances have already been made. Increased treatment and higher SVR will result in 215,000 averted deaths and 910,000 fewer HCV infections (see Table B-3). Here, we assume the total number of treated patients will decline to 130,000 per year (50 percent of 2015 value) and the number of newly diagnosed will also decline by 50 percent as it will become more difficult to find undiagnosed individuals.

However, maintaining the annual number of treated patients at 260,000 and expansion of screening to diagnose 80 percent of HCV infections by 2030 would have even greater impact in averting liver deaths and reducing total infections. Under this scenario, treatment restrictions will have a large impact on outcomes. With a continued focus on treating ≥F2 patients, 98,500 deaths may be averted by 2030 relative to the 2015 base scenario (see Table B-3). Those with advanced fibrosis are more likely to progress to advanced liver disease, thus concentrating treatment on these individuals will have a large impact on averting HCC and decompensated cirrhosis cases. Yet most new infections are occurring among younger individuals infected by those with no or early stages of fibrosis (F0-F2). Therefore, focusing treatment on ≥F2 will have minimal impact on new infections (see Table B-3). To reduce new infections, treatment has to be expanded to all. Under this scenario (Aggressive ≥F0), we project 28,000 deaths averted and >90 percent reduction in the number of new infections in the United States corresponding to 279,400 total new infections averted (see Table B-3). This scenario will require expansion of HCV screening as well as expansion of harm reduction programs for PWID. Although the number of treated patients in 2015 indicates that the healthcare system in the United States can already treat 260,000 patients per year, expansion of HCV treatment to general practitioners will be required to provide access to patients without access to major treatment centers and specialists.

In conclusion, the only way to achieve WHO targets is to remove treatment restrictions and provide access to all, expand screening to diagnose 80 percent of infected persons by 2030, and continue to treat 260,000 patients per year. This strategy will reduce infections by 90 percent and avert nearly a quarter million deaths in the next 14 years.

REFERENCES

Altekruse, S. F., S. J. Henley, J. E. Cucinelli, and K. A. McGlynn. 2014. Changing hepatocellular carcinoma incidence and liver cancer mortality rates in the United States. *American Journal of Gastroenterology* 109(4):542-553.

Bernfort, L., K. Sennfält, and O. Reichard. 2006. Cost-effectiveness of peginterferon alfa-2b in combination with ribavirin as initial treatment for chronic hepatitis C in Sweden. *Scandinavian Journal of Infectious Diseases* 38(6-7):497-505.

Bjornaas, M. A., A. S. Bekken, A. Ojlert, T. Haldorsen, D. Jacobsen, M. Rostrup, and O. Ekeberg. 2008. A 20-year prospective study of mortality and causes of death among hospitalized opioid addicts in Oslo. *BMC Psychiatry* 8(1).

Blach, S., S. Zeuzem, M. Manns, I. Altraif, A.-S. Duberg, D. H. Muljono, I. Waked, S. M. Alavian, M.-H. Lee, F. Negro, F. Abaalkhail, A. Abdou, M. Abdulla, A. A. Rached, I. Aho, U. Akarca, I. Al Ghazzawi, S. Al Kaabi, F. Al Lawati, K. Al Namaani, Y. Al Serkal, S. A. Al-Busafi, L. Al-Dabal, S. Aleman, A. S. Alghamdi, A. A. Aljumah, H. E. Al-Romaihi, M. I. Andersson, V. Arendt, P. Arkkila, A. M. Assiri, O. Baatarkhuu, A. Bane, Z. Ben-Ari, C. Bergin, F. Bessone, F. Bihl, A. R. Bizri, M. Blachier, A. J. Blasco, C. E. B. Mello, P. Bruggmann, C. R. Brunton, F. Calinas, H. L. Y. Chan, A. Chaudhry, H. Cheinquer, C.-J. Chen, R.-N. Chien, M. S. Choi, P. B. Christensen, W.-L. Chuang, V. Chulanov, L. Cisneros, M. R. Clausen, M. E. Cramp, A. Craxi, E. A. Croes, O. Dalgard, J. R. Daruich, V. de Ledinghen, G. J. Dore, M. H. El-Sayed, G. Ergör, G. Esmat, C. Estes, K. Falconer, E. Farag, M. L. G. Ferraz, P. R. Ferreira, R. Flisiak, S. Frankova, I. Gamkrelidze, E. Gane, J. García-Samaniego, A. G. Khan, I. Gountas, A. Goldis, M. Gottfredsson, J. Grebely, M. Gschwantler, M. G. Pessôa, J. Gunter, B. Hajarizadeh, O. Hajelssedig, S. Hamid, W. Hamoudi, A. Hatzakis, S. M. Himatt, H. Hofer, I. Hrstic, Y.-T. Hui, B. Hunyady, R. Idilman, W. Jafri, R. Jahis, N. Z. Janjua, P. Jarčuška, A. Jeruma, J. G. Jonasson, Y. Kamel, J.-H. Kao, S. Kaymakoglu, D. Kershenobich, J. Khamis, Y. S. Kim, L. Kondili, Z. Koutoubi, M. Krajden, H. Krarup, M.-s. Lai, W. Laleman, W.-c. Lao, D. Lavanchy, P. Lázaro, H. Leleu, O. Lesi, L. A. Lesmana, M. Li, V. Liakina, Y.-S. Lim, B. Luksic, A. Mahomed, M. Maimets, M. Makara, A. O. Malu, R. T. Marinho, P. Marotta, S. Mauss, M. S. Memon, M. C. M. Correa, N. Mendez-Sanchez, S. Merat, A. M. Metwally, R. Mohamed, C. Moreno, F. H. Mourad, B. Müllhaupt, K. Murphy, H. Nde, R. Njouom, D. Nonkovic, S. Norris, S. Obekpa, S. Oguche, S. Olafsson, M. Oltman, O. Omede, C. Omuemu, O. Opare-Sem, A. L. H. Øvrehus, S. Owusu-Ofori, T. S. Oyunsuren, G. Papatheodoridis, K. Pasini, K. M. Peltekian, R. O. Phillips, N. Pimenov, H. Poustchi, H. Prabdial-Sing, H. Qureshi, A. Ramji, D. Razavi-Shearer, K. Razavi-Shearer, B. Redae, H. W. Reesink, E. Ridruejo, S. Robbins, L. R. Roberts, S. K. Roberts, W. M. Rosenberg, F. Roudot-Thoraval, S. D. Ryder, R. Safadi, O. Sagalova, R. Salupere, F. M. Sanai, J. F. S. Avila, V. Saraswat, R. Sarmento-Castro, C. Sarrazin, J. D. Schmelzer, I. Schréter, C. Seguin-Devaux, S. R. Shah, A. I. Sharara, M. Sharma, A. Shevaldin, G. E. Shiha, W. Sievert, M. Sonderup, K. Souliotis, D. Speiciene, J. Sperl, P. Stärkel, R. E. Stauber, C. Stedman, D. Struck, T.-H. Su, V. Sypsa, S.-S. Tan, J. Tanaka, A. J. Thompson, I. Tolmane, K. Tomasiewicz, J. Valantinas, P. Van Damme, A. J. van der

Meer, I. van Thiel, H. Van Vlierberghe, A. Vince, W. Vogel, H. Wedemeyer, N. Weis, V. W. S. Wong, C. Yaghi, A. Yosry, M.-f. Yuen, E. Yunihastuti, A. Yusuf, E. Zuckerman, and H. Razavi. 2016. Global prevalence and genotype distribution of hepatitis C virus infection in 2015: A modelling study. *The Lancet Gastroenterology & Hepatology* 2(3): 161-176.

Bruggmann, P., and J. Grebely. 2015. Prevention, treatment and care of hepatitis C virus infection among people who inject drugs. *International Journal of Drug Policy* 26:S22-S26.

CDC (Centers for Disease Control and Prevention). 2011. Hepatitis C virus infection among adolescents and young adults: Massachusetts, 2002-2009. *Morbidity and Mortality Weekly Report* 60(17):537-541.

CDC. 2015. *National Health and Nutrition Examination Survey data, 2003-2014.* https://www.cdc.gov/nchs/nhanes (accessed January 11, 2017).

CDC. 2016. *Viral hepatitis–Statistics & surveillance.* https://www.cdc.gov/hepatitis/statistics (accessed November 11, 2016).

Chak, E., A. H. Talal, K. E. Sherman, E. R. Schiff, and S. Saab. 2011. Hepatitis C virus infection in USA: An estimate of true prevalence. *Liver International* 31(8):1090-1101.

Daniels, D., S. Grytdal, and A. Wasley. 2009. Surveillance for acute viral hepatitis, United States, 2007. *Morbidity and Mortality Weekly Report* 58(S S03):1-27.

Denniston, M. M., R. B. Jiles, J. Drobeniuc, R. M. Klevens, J. W. Ward, G. M. McQuillan, and S. D. Holmberg. 2014. Chronic hepatitis C virus infection in the United States, National Health and Nutrition Examination Survey, 2003 to 2010. *Annals of Internal Medicine* 160(5):293-300.

Edlin, B. R., B. J. Eckhardt, M. A. Shu, S. D. Holmberg, and T. Swan. 2015. Toward a more accurate estimate of the prevalence of hepatitis C in the United States. *Hepatology* 62(5):1353-1363.

Engstrom, A., C. Adamsson, P. Allebeck, and U. Rydberg. 1991. Mortality in patients with substance abuse: A follow-up in Stockholm County, 1973-1984. *International Journal of the Addictions* 26(1):91-106.

Fitch, K., K. Iwasaki, B. Pyenson, and T. Engel. 2013. *Health care reform and hepatitis C: A convergence of risk and opportunity.* New York: Milliman, Inc.

Frischer, M., D. Goldberg, M. Rahman, and L. Berney. 1997. Mortality and survival among a cohort of drug injectors in Glasgow, 1982–1994. *Addiction* 92(4):419-427.

Harris, R. J., B. Thomas, J. Griffiths, A. Costella, R. Chapman, M. Ramsay, D. De Angelis, and H. E. Harris. 2014. Increased uptake and new therapies are needed to avert rising hepatitis C-related end stage liver disease in England: Modelling the predicted impact of treatment under different scenarios. *Journal of Hepatology* 61(3):530-537.

Hickman, M., Z. Carnwath, P. Madden, M. Farrell, C. Rooney, R. Ashcroft, A. Judd, and G. Stimson. 2003. Drug-related mortality and fatal overdose risk: Pilot cohort study of heroin users recruited from specialist drug treatment sites in London. *Journal of Urban Health* 80(2):274-287.

Hourigan, L. F., G. A. Macdonald, D. Purdie, V. H. Whitehall, C. Shorthouse, A. Clouston, and E. E. Powell. 1999. Fibrosis in chronic hepatitis C correlates significantly with body mass index and steatosis. *Hepatology* 29(4):1215-1219.

HRSA (Health Resources and Services Administration). 2016. *Organ Procurement and Transplantation Network.* https://optn.transplant.hrsa.gov/data (accessed October 28, 2016).

Kamper-Jørgensen, M., M. Ahlgren, K. Rostgaard, M. Melbye, G. Edgren, O. Nyrén, M. Reilly, R. Norda, K. Titlestad, and E. Tynell. 2008. Survival after blood transfusion. *Transfusion* 48(12):2577-2584.

Klevens, R. M., J. Miller, C. Vonderwahl, S. Speers, K. Alelis, K. Sweet, E. Rocchio, T. Poissant, T. M. Vogt, and K. Gallagher. 2009. Population-based surveillance for hepatitis C virus, United States, 2006–2007. *Emerging Infectious Diseases* 15(9):1499-1502.

Klevens, R. M., S. Liu, H. Roberts, R. B. Jiles, and S. D. Holmberg. 2014. Estimating acute viral hepatitis infections from nationally reported cases. *American Journal of Public Health* 104(3):482-487.

Lansky, A., T. Finlayson, C. Johnson, D. Holtzman, C. Wejnert, A. Mitsch, D. Gust, R. Chen, Y. Mizuno, and N. Crepaz. 2014. Estimating the number of persons who inject drugs in the United States by meta-analysis to calculate national rates of HIV and hepatitis C virus infections. *PLoS One* 9(5):e97596.

Martin, N., P. Vickerman, A. Clements, M. Cramp, D. De Angeles, J. Dillon, S. Fahey, G. Foster, D. Goldberg, and F. Gordon. 2013a. Are current treatment rates sufficient to reduce HCV prevalence among people who inject drugs? Model projections in seven UK settings. *Journal of Hepatology* 58(Suppl 1):S356.

Martin, N. K., M. Hickman, S. J. Hutchinson, D. J. Goldberg, and P. Vickerman. 2013b. Combination interventions to prevent HCV transmission among people who inject drugs: Modeling the impact of antiviral treatment, needle and syringe programs, and opiate substitution therapy. *Clinical Infectious Diseases* 57(Suppl 2):S39-S45.

Martinello, M., and G. J. Dore. 2016. Editorial commentary: Interferon-free hepatitis C treatment efficacy from clinical trials will translate to "real world" outcomes. *Clinical Infectious Diseases* 62(7):927-928.

Massachusetts Department of Public Health. 2016. *Bureau of Infectious Disease*. http://www.mass.gov/eohhs/gov/departments/dph/programs/id (accessed November 1, 2016).

NASEM (National Academies of Sciences, Engineering, and Medicine). 2016. *Eliminating the public health problem of hepatitis B and C in the United States: Phase one report*. Washington, DC: The National Academies Press.

NIDDK (National Institute of Diabetes and Digestive and Kidney Diseases). 2016. *Cirrhosis*. https://www.niddk.nih.gov/health-information/liver-disease/cirrhosis (accessed November 15, 2016).

Nolan, S., V. Dias Lima, N. Fairbairn, T. Kerr, J. Montaner, J. Grebely, and E. Wood. 2014. The impact of methadone maintenance therapy on hepatitis C incidence among illicit drug users. *Addiction* 109(12):2053-2059.

Ogden, C. L., M. D. Carroll, B. K. Kit, and K. M. Flegal. 2014. Prevalence of childhood and adult obesity in the United States, 2011-2012. *JAMA* 311(8):806-814.

Onofrey, S., J. Aneja, G. A. Haney, E. H. Nagami, A. DeMaria, G. M. Lauer, K. Hills-Evans, K. Barton, S. Kulaga, and M. J. Bowen. 2015. Underascertainment of acute hepatitis C virus infections in the U.S. surveillance system: A case series and chart review. *Annals of Internal Medicine* 163(4):254-261.

Oppenheimer, E., C. Tobutt, C. Taylor, and T. Andrew. 1994. Death and survival in a cohort of heroin addicts from London clinics: A 22-year follow-up study. *Addiction* 89(10):1299-1308.

Perucci, C. A., M. Davoli, E. Rapiti, D. D. Abeni, and F. Forastiere. 1991. Mortality of intravenous drug users in Rome: A cohort study. *American Journal of Public Health* 81(10):1307-1310.

Poynard, T., P. Bedossa, and P. Opolon. 1997. Natural history of liver fibrosis progression in patients with chronic hepatitis C. *The Lancet* 349(9055):825-832.

Poynard, T., V. Ratziu, F. Charlotte, Z. Goodman, J. McHutchison, and J. Albrecht. 2001. Rates and risk factors of liver fibrosis progression in patients with chronic hepatitis C. *Journal of Hepatology* 34(5):730-739.

Poynard, T., P. Lebray, P. Ingiliz, A. Varaut, B. Varsat, Y. Ngo, P. Norha, M. Munteanu, F. Drane, and D. Messous. 2010. Prevalence of liver fibrosis and risk factors in a general population using non-invasive biomarkers (FibroTest). *BMC Gastroenterology* 10(40).

Pradat, P., N. Voirin, H. L. Tillmann, M. Chevallier, and C. Trépo. 2007. Progression to cirrhosis in hepatitis C patients: An age-dependent process. *Liver International* 27(3):335-339.

Razavi, H., I. Waked, C. Sarrazin, R. Myers, R. Idilman, F. Calinas, W. Vogel, M. Correa, C. Hézode, P. Lázaro, U. Akarca, S. Aleman, I. Balık, T. Berg, F. Bihl, M. Bilodeau, A. Blasco, C. Brandão Mello, P. Bruggmann, M. Buti, J. Calleja, H. Cheinquer, P. Christensen, M. Clausen, H. Coelho, M. Cramp, G. Dore, W. Doss, A. Duberg, M. El-Sayed, G. Ergör, G. Esmat, K. Falconer, J. Félix, M. L. G. Ferraz, P. Ferreira, S. Frankova, J. García-Samaniego, J. Gerstoft, J. Giria, F. J. Gonçales, E. Gower, M. Gschwantler, M. Guimarães Pessôa, S. J. Hindman, H. Hofer, P. Husa, M. Kåberg, K. Kaita, A. Kautz, S. Kaymakoglu, M. Krajden, H. Krarup, W. Laleman, D. Lavanchy, R. Marinho, P. Marotta, S. Mauss, C. Moreno, K. Murphy, F. Negro, V. Nemecek, N. Örmeci, A. Øvrehus, J. Parkes, K. Pasini, K. Peltekian, A. Ramji, N. Reis, S. Roberts, W. Rosenberg, F. Roudot-Thoraval, S. Ryder, R. Sarmento-Castro, D. Semela, M. Sherman, G. Shiha, W. Sievert, J. Sperl, P. Stärkel, R. Stauber, A. Thompson, P. Urbanek, P. Van Damme, I. van Thiel, H. Van Vlierberghe, D. Vandijck, H. Wedemeyer, N. Weis, J. Wiegand, A. Yosry, A. Zekry, M. Cornberg, B. Müllhaupt, and C. Estes. 2014. The present and future disease burden of hepatitis C virus (HCV) infection with today's treatment paradigm. *Journal of Viral Hepatitis* 21(Suppl 1):34-59.

Ries, L. A. G., J. L. Young, Jr., G. E. Keel, M. P. Eisner, Y. D. Lin, and M.-J. D. Horner. 2007. *SEER Survival Monograph: Cancer survival among adults: U.S. SEER Program, 1988-2001, patient and tumor characteristics. NIH pub. no. 07-6215.* Bethesda, MD: National Cancer Institute, SEER Program.

Seeff, L. B. 2002. Natural history of chronic hepatitis C. *Hepatology* 36(5 Suppl 1):S35-S46.

SEER (Surveillance, Epidemiology, and End Results) Program. 2015. *SEER*Stat Database: Incidence - SEER 9 Regs Research Data, Nov 2015 Sub (1973-2013).*

Simmons, B., J. Saleem, K. Heath, G. S. Cooke, and A. Hill. 2015. Long-term treatment outcomes of patients infected with hepatitis C virus: A systematic review and meta-analysis of the survival benefit of achieving a sustained virological response. *Clinical Infectious Diseases* 61(5):730-740.

Smith, B. D., R. L. Morgan, G. A. Beckett, Y. Falck-Ytter, D. Holtzman, and J. W. Ward. 2012. Hepatitis C virus testing of persons born during 1945–1965: Recommendations from the Centers for Disease Control and Prevention. *Annals of Internal Medicine* 157(11):817-822.

Smith-Palmer, J., K. Cerri, and W. Valentine. 2015. Achieving sustained virologic response in hepatitis C: A systematic review of the clinical, economic and quality of life benefits. *BMC Infectious Diseases* 15(19).

Suryaprasad, A. G., J. Z. White, F. Xu, B.-A. Eichler, J. Hamilton, A. Patel, S. B. Hamdounia, D. R. Church, K. Barton, C. Fisher, K. Macomber, M. Stanley, S. Guilfoyle, K. Sweet, S. Liu, K. Iqbal, R. Tohme, U. Sharapov, B. Kupronis, J. Ward, and S. Holmberg. 2014. Emerging epidemic of hepatitis C virus infections among young non-urban persons who inject drugs in the United States, 2006–2012. *Clinical Infectious Diseases* 59(10):1411-1419.

Tsui, J. I., J. L. Evans, P. J. Lum, J. A. Hahn, and K. Page. 2014. Association of opioid agonist therapy with lower incidence of hepatitis C virus infection in young adult injection drug users. *JAMA Internal Medicine* 174(12):1974-1981.

Turner, K. M. E., S. Hutchinson, P. Vickerman, V. Hope, N. Craine, N. Palmateer, M. May, A. Taylor, D. De Angelis, and S. Cameron. 2011. The impact of needle and syringe provision and opiate substitution therapy on the incidence of hepatitis C virus in injecting drug users: Pooling of U.K. evidence. *Addiction* 106(11):1978-1988.

United Nations. 2015. *World population prospects: The 2015 revision, key findings and advance tables. Working paper no. ESA/P/WP.241.* New York: United Nations, Department of Economic and Social Affairs, Population Division.

Volk, M. L., R. Tocco, S. Saini, and A. S. Lok. 2009. Public health impact of antiviral therapy for hepatitis C in the United States. *Hepatology* 50(6):1750-1755.

White, B., G. J. Dore, A. R. Lloyd, W. D. Rawlinson, and L. Maher. 2014. Opioid substitution therapy protects against hepatitis C virus acquisition in people who inject drugs: The HITS-c study. *Medical Journal of Australia* 201(6):326-329.

WHO (World Health Organization). 2016. *Combating hepatitis B and C to reach elimination by 2030.* Geneva, Switzerland: WHO.

Yang, J. D., B. Kim, S. O. Sanderson, J. L. S. Sauver, B. P. Yawn, R. A. Pedersen, J. J. Larson, T. M. Therneau, L. R. Roberts, and W. R. Kim. 2012. Hepatocellular carcinoma in Olmsted County, Minnesota, 1976-2008. *Mayo Clinic Proceedings* 87(1):9-16.

Appendix C

Public Meeting Agenda

COMMITTEE ON A NATIONAL STRATEGY FOR
THE ELIMINATION OF HEPATITIS B AND C

National Academy of Sciences Building, 2100 Constitution Avenue NW
Washington, DC 20001

June 8, 2016
Room 120

PHASE TWO ORIENTATION

9:00-9:15   Welcome and Introductions
                Brian Strom, *Committee Chair*

9:15-10:15   Sponsor Orientation to Phase Two
                John Ward, *Director, Division of Viral Hepatitis,* Centers
                for Disease Control and Prevention (CDC)
                Nadine Gracia, *Deputy Assistant Secretary for Minority
                Health,* Office of Minority Health, Department of Health
                and Human Services (HHS)
                Michael Fried, *Board Member,* American Association for
                the Study of Liver Diseases
                Ryan Clary, *Executive Director,* National Viral Hepatitis
                Roundtable

10:15-10:30   Break

SCREENING AND REFERRALS TO CARE

10:30-12:00   Panel Discussion on Novel Strategies for Testing and
Follow-Up
Kathleen Maurer, *Moderator*
- **Sabrina Assoumou,** *Assistant Professor of Medicine,*
Boston University
- **Alicia Ifkovic-Mau,** *Correctional Counselor
Supervisor, Department of Corrections,* State of
Connecticut
- **William Stauffer,** *Professor of Medicine and
Pediatrics, Division of Infectious Diseases and
International Medicine,* University of Minnesota
- **David Thomas,** *Director, Division of Infectious
Diseases,* Johns Hopkins School of Medicine

12:00-1:00   Lunch

INNOVATIVE FINANCING FOR HEPATITIS C TREATMENTS

1:00-2:30   Panel Discussion on Paying for Cures
Neeraj Sood, *Moderator*
- **Tim Gronniger,** *Deputy Chief of Staff,* Centers for
Medicare & Medicaid Services
- **Steve Miller,** *Chief Medical Officer,* Express Scripts
- **Coy Stout,** *Vice President, Managed Markets,* Gilead

2:30-2:45   Break

2:45-4:15   Panel Discussion on Hepatitis C Treatment in
Government Programs
Brian Strom, *Moderator*
- **John Coster,** *Director, Division of Pharmacy,* Center
for Medicaid and Children's Health Insurance
Program (CHIP) Services, Centers for Medicare &
Medicaid Services
- **Kimberley Lenz,** *Clinical Pharmacy Manager,*
MassHealth
- **Robert Zavoski,** *Medical Director,* Connecticut
Department of Social Services

4:15-4:45   Public Health and Drug Pricing: Policy Solutions for
Population Coverage
Joshua Sharfstein, *Professor of the Practice,* Johns
Hopkins Bloomberg School of Public Health

5:00   Adjourn

6:30   Working dinner for committee and staff at Circle Bistro

June 9, 2016
Members' Room

INTERNATIONAL PROGRAMS ON VIRAL HEPATITIS

9:00-9:05   Welcome
Brian Strom, *Committee Chair*

9:05-9:35   Global Momentum for Viral Hepatitis Elimination
Stefan Wiktor, *Team Lead, Global Hepatitis Program,*
World Health Organization (WHO)

9:40-10:10   An Australian Perspective on Hepatitis Elimination
Ben Cowie, *Director, WHO Collaborating Centre for
Viral Hepatitis,* The Doherty Institute, University of
Melbourne

10:10-10:30   Break

HARM REDUCTION AND NEEDLE EXCHANGE

10:30-12:00   Panel Discussion on Harm Reduction in Rural Areas and
Small Towns
Shruti Mehta, *Moderator*
- **Jerome Adams,** *Health Commissioner,* Indiana State
Department of Health
- **Jennifer Havens,** *Associate Professor,* Center for Drug
and Alcohol Research, University of Kentucky College
of Medicine
- **Robin Pollini,** *Senior Research Scientist,* Pacific
Institute for Research and Evaluation

12:00-1:00   Lunch

INTEGRATING CLINICAL AND PUBLIC HEALTH DATA

1:00-2:30   Panel Discussion on Using Electronic Records for
                 Clinical Medicine and Public Health
                 Grace Wang, *Moderator*
                 • **Jeff Duchin,** *Professor in Medicine, Division of*
                   Allergy and Infectious Diseases, University of
                   Washington
                 • **Michael Klompas,** *Associate Professor and Infectious*
                   Diseases Specialist, Harvard Medical School and
                   Harvard Pilgrim Health Care Institute
                 • **Chia Wang,** *Infectious Diseases Specialist and Clinical*
                   Associate Professor of Medicine, Virginia Mason
                   Medical Center, International Community Health
                   Services and University of Washington

Appendix D

Committee Biographies

Brian L. Strom, M.D., M.P.H., is the inaugural chancellor of Rutgers Biomedical and Health Sciences (RBHS) and the executive vice president for health affairs at Rutgers University. RBHS is composed of eight schools and five centers/institutes, and includes academic, patient care, and research facilities. Dr. Strom was formerly the executive vice dean of institutional affairs, founding chair of the Department of Biostatistics and Epidemiology, founding director of the Center for Clinical Epidemiology and Biostatistics, and founding director of the Graduate Program in Epidemiology and Biostatistics, all at the Perelman School of Medicine of the University of Pennsylvania (Penn).

Dr. Strom earned a B.S. in Molecular Biophysics and Biochemistry from Yale University, and an M.D. from the Johns Hopkins University School of Medicine. He was an intern and resident in Internal Medicine, then a National Institutes of Health (NIH) Fellow in Clinical Pharmacology at the University of California, San Francisco. He simultaneously earned an M.P.H. in Epidemiology at the University of California, Berkeley. He has been on the faculty of the University of Pennsylvania School of Medicine since 1980. The Center for Clinical Epidemiology and Biostatistics (CCEB) that he created at Penn includes more than 550 faculty, research and support staff, and trainees. At the time Dr. Strom stepped down, CCEB research received nearly $49 million/year in extramural support.

Although Dr. Strom's interests span many areas of clinical epidemiology, his major research interest is in the field of pharmacoepidemiology, that is, the application of epidemiologic methods to the study of drug use and effects. He is recognized as a founder of this field and for his pioneer work in using large automated databases for research. He is editor of the field's major text (now in its fifth edition) and editor in chief for *Pharmacoepidemiology and Drug Safety*, the official journal of the International Society for Pharmacoepidemiology. As one of many specific contributions, his research was pivotal in prompting the American Heart Association and American Dental Association to reverse 50 years of guidelines, and recommend against use of antibiotics to prevent infective endocarditis, instead of recommending for this widespread practice. In addition to writing more than 600 papers and 12 books, he has been principal investigator (PI) for more than 275 grants, including more than $115 million in direct costs alone.

Dr. Strom is also a nationally recognized leader in clinical research training. At the Perelman School of Medicine, he developed graduate training programs in epidemiology and biostatistics. More than 625 clinicians have been trained or are in training through the largest of these training programs, which leads to a Master of Science in Clinical Epidemiology degree. Dr. Strom was PI or Co-PI of 11 NIH-funded training grants (T32, D43, K12, and K30), each of which supported clinical epidemiology trainees in different specialties and subspecialties. He has been the primary mentor for more than 65 former and current clinical research trainees and numerous junior faculty members. Internationally, Dr. Strom was a key contributor to the conceptualization and planning that led to the development of the International Clinical Epidemiology Network (INCLEN), created in 1979 with support provided by the Rockefeller Foundation to provide clinical research training to clinicians from selected developing country sites.

Dr. Strom was a member of the Board of Regents of the American College of Physicians, the Board of Directors of the American Society for Clinical Pharmacology and Therapeutics, and the Board of Directors for the American College of Epidemiology. He is currently a member of the Board of Directors for the Association for Patient-Oriented Research. He was previously president of the International Society for Pharmacoepidemiology and the Association for Clinical Research Training. Dr. Strom was on the Drug Utilization Review Committee and the Gerontology Committee of the U.S. Pharmacopoeia; served on the Drug Safety and Risk Management Advisory Committee for the Food and Drug Administration; chaired the Institute of Medicine (IOM) Committee to Assess the Safety and Efficacy of the Anthrax Vaccine; chaired the IOM Committee on Smallpox Vaccine Program Implementation, the IOM Committee to Review the National Institute for Occupational Safety and Health's Traumatic Injury Program, and the IOM Committee on the Consequences of Reducing Sodium in the Population; and was a member of the IOM Committee to Review the Centers for Disease Control and Prevention Anthrax Vaccine Safety and Efficacy

Research Program, and the IOM Committee on Standards for Developing Trustworthy Clinical Practice Guidelines.

Dr. Strom is also a member of the American Epidemiology Society, and is one of a handful of clinical epidemiologists ever elected to The American Society for Clinical Investigation and American Association of Physicians. He is an elected member of the National Academy of Medicine and National Academy of Science. Dr. Strom received the 2003 Rawls-Palmer Progress in Medicine Award from the American Society for Clinical Pharmacology & Therapeutics, the Naomi M. Kanof Clinical Investigator Award of the Society for Investigative Dermatology, the George S. Pepper Professorship of Public Health and Preventive Medicine, and the Sustained Scientific Excellence Award from the International Society for Pharmaco-epidemiology. In addition, Dr. Strom was the 2008 recipient of the John Phillips Memorial Award for Outstanding Work in Clinical Medicine. This award is from the American College of Physicians and is considered to be one of the highest awards in Internal Medicine. Dr. Strom also received the 2013 Association for Clinical and Translational Science/American Federation for Medical Research National Award for Career Achievement and Contribution to Clinical and Translational Science for translation from clinical use into public benefit and policy. Penn awards that Dr. Strom received include the Class of 1992 Class Teaching Award and the Samuel Martin Health Evaluation Sciences Research Award. Dr. Strom received the 2004 Christian R. and Mary F. Lindback Award, the University's most prestigious teaching award, in recognition of the contribution he has made in his career to clinical research teaching. The 2016 Oscar B. Hunter Career Award in Therapeutics was awarded to Dr. Strom for his outstanding contributions to clinical pharmacology and therapeutics.

Jon Kim Andrus, M.D., joined the faculty at the University of Colorado's Division of Vaccines and Immunization of the Center for Global Health as Adjoint Professor and Senior Investigator in February 2017. Based in Washington, D.C., Jon leads the University of Colorado's efforts to advocate for the evidence-based use of life-saving vaccines in the world's poorest communities. Dr. Andrus has more than 30 years of experience working in global health at all levels of the health system.

Prior to coming to the University of Colorado, Dr. Andrus was Executive Vice President of the Sabin Vaccine Institute. He also served as Deputy Director at the Pan American Health Organization (PAHO). At PAHO, among several duties, he oversaw departments of Emergency Preparedness and Disaster Relief; and Knowledge Management and Communication. Prior to that, he was the lead technical advisor for PAHO's immunization program, providing oversight and guidance for PAHO's technical cooperation to member countries. He also served as polio focal point for polio eradication in Southeast Asia and regional advisor for immunization during the 1990s.

Dr. Andrus also holds faculty appointments at the University of California, San Francisco, and the Johns Hopkins Bloomberg School of Public Health. He began his global health career as a Peace Corps volunteer, serving as a district medical officer in Malawi and has since held positions in the Centers for Disease Control and Prevention's (CDC's) Global Immunization Division, as head of the Vaccinology and Immunization Program at the Institute for Global Health at the Universities of California at San Francisco and Berkeley, and as director and professor of the Global Health M.P.H. Program at George Washington University.

Currently Dr. Andrus is the co-chair of the Global Polio Partners Group and a member of the International Monitoring Board for the Polio Transition. Dr. Andrus serves on numerous World Health Organization advisory committees, including PAHO's Technical Advisory Group for Vaccine Preventable Diseases, and SEARO's Verification Commission for Measles and Rubella Elimination. He also has been an active member of the ROTA Council.

Dr. Andrus has published more than 100 scientific peer-reviewed papers on topics covering disease eradication, the introduction of new vaccines and primary care. He has received numerous awards, including the 2013 Transformational Leadership Award of the University of California, the 2011 Global Leadership Award of the Pneumococcal Awareness Council of Experts, and the 2000 Distinguished Service Medal—the highest award of the United States Public Health Service—for his leadership in working to eradicate polio in Southeast Asia. He has received awards for his leadership in the eradication of measles, rubella and congenital rubella syndrome, as well as the introduction of new vaccines in developing countries.

Dr. Andrus holds a B.S. from Stanford University, obtained an M.D. from the University of California, Davis, and completed his residencies in family medicine at the University of California, San Francisco School of Medicine and preventive medicine at the CDC.

Andrew Aronsohn, M.D., is a specialist in the diagnosis and treatment of liver disease, including medical management of liver transplantation. He is an associate professor at the University of Chicago Center for Liver Diseases, and a faculty member at the MacLean Center for Clinical Medical Ethics. Dr. Aronsohn's research interests involve investigation of ethical issues surrounding hepatitis C therapy which include fair distribution of resources and linkage to care. He is currently leading the HCV curriculum of ECHO Chicago, which aims to educate and empower primary care providers to effectively manage hepatitis C in a local primary care setting.

Dr. Aronsohn also serves as a co-lead in the AASLD/IDSA guidance for hepatitis C treatment.

Daniel R. Church, M.P.H., is a senior epidemiologist in the Bureau of Infectious Disease and Laboratory Sciences at the Massachusetts Department of Health. He has helped to develop and implement the statewide viral hepatitis program, including disease surveillance; medical management services; counseling and testing programs; adult vaccination programs; educational campaigns for providers, patients, and communities; and project evaluation. He was a member of the Institute of Medicine committee that authored the report *Hepatitis and Liver Cancer: A National Strategy for Prevention and Control of Hepatitis B and C.* Mr. Church received his M.P.H. in Epidemiology and Biostatistics from the Boston University School of Public Health.

Seymour S. Cohen, Ph.D., has worked on bacterial viruses since 1945, offering the first systematic exploration of the biochemistry of virus-infected cells and of how viruses multiply. His subsequent research included delineating the phenomenon of thymineless death, developing derivatives of ara-A compound, working on RNA synthesis, studying the effects of polyamines on metabolic systems, and studying plant viruses (including viral cations). Much of his research has contributed to the chemical treatment of cancer and viral infections.

Alison A. Evans, Sc.D., is an associate professor in the Department of Epidemiology and Biostatistics at Drexel University Dornsife School of Public Health. She is also on the adjunct research faculty in the public health program of the Hepatitis B Foundation, Doylestown, Pennsylvania. Prior to joining Drexel, she was an associate member at the Fox Chase Cancer Center. Her research interests include the epidemiology and natural history of the hepatitis B virus (HBV) and other chronic viral infections, the association of chronic viral infections with cancer, and public health interventions to decrease the global burden of HBV infection. She received her Sc.D. in Epidemiology from the Harvard School of Public Health.

Paul Kuehnert, D.N.P., R.N., is a nurse and public health expert who currently oversees Robert Wood Johnson Foundation's work in building bridges among the health care system, public health, and other community services and agencies to improve overall population health. As a former county health officer in Illinois and former deputy state health officer in Maine, he brings extensive public health experience to the group. He has an acute awareness of the strengths of local and state public health agencies in combating conditions such as hepatitis B and C as well as the challenges they face. He is very familiar with the topics of surveillance, implementation of disease control programs, screening, epidemiology, and community-based program implementation, including in the area of HIV/AIDS.

Vincent Lo Re, M.D., M.S.C.E., is an assistant professor of medicine (infectious diseases) and epidemiology at the University of Pennsylvania, senior scholar in the Penn Center for Clinical Epidemiology and Biostatistics, and co-director of the Penn Center for AIDS Research HIV/Viral Hepatitis Scientific Working Group. Dr. Lo Re leads a nationally recognized research program that examines the epidemiology of acute and chronic liver diseases in HIV-infected patients. He has conducted population-based and mechanistic studies that have helped to move the field of chronic viral hepatitis and HIV/viral hepatitis coinfection forward in a unique way. Recent research has evaluated end-stage liver disease and liver cancer events among HIV/hepatitis C–coinfected patients; examined how chronic viral hepatitis and HIV/viral hepatitis coinfection influence extra-hepatic outcomes, particularly metabolic bone disease; determined the impact that medications have on acute liver injury and progression of chronic viral hepatitis; and evaluated adherence and adverse effects of antiviral therapies of chronic hepatitis B and C. He has particular expertise in evaluating liver-related and other health outcomes among viral hepatitis-infected patients within large electronic data sources, such as the Veterans Health Administration, Kaiser Permanente Northern California, Medicaid, Medicare, and Sentinel. His research has been funded by the National Institute of Allergy and Infectious Diseases, National Institute of Diabetes and Digestive and Kidney Diseases, National Cancer Institute, Agency for Healthcare Research and Quality, Department of Veterans Affairs, and the Food and Drug Administration (FDA). Additionally, Dr. Lo Re has been a standing member of FDA's Antiviral Drug (now Anti-Infective) Advisory Committee since 2014 and co-chair of the Liver Core of the Veterans Aging Cohort Study since 2009. He maintains an active clinical practice devoted to the care of patients with chronic viral hepatitis, particularly those coinfected with HIV.

Kathleen Maurer, M.D., M.P.H., M.B.A., is the Connecticut Department of Correction's (DOC's) director of health and addiction services and medical director. Before assuming her current post in 2011, she was assistant medical director at Correctional Managed Health Care, a division of the University of Connecticut Health Center, which contracts with DOC for offender medical care. Dr. Maurer has provided hands-on clinical care and medical program management in the private sector. In correctional care, she is particularly interested in the quality of patient care, in the role of correctional health care in the broader scope of public health such as in the treatment of hepatitis C virus in offender-patients, and in facilitating reentry programs through integration of community and correctional health care. Her initiatives have included working to expand Medicaid access to halfway house residents and to integrate Medicaid usage management with the correctional system. She is also developing a systemwide medication-assisted therapy program for the Connecticut DOC. Dr. Maurer is the primary author of the monograph entitled *Hepatitis C in Correctional Settings: Challenges and Opportunities*, published by the American Correctional Association. Dr. Maurer earned her M.D. from Yale University School of Medicine. She also earned an M.P.H. from Yale. She holds an M.B.A. from the University of Connecticut and is Board certified in Internal Medicine, Occupational and Environmental Medicine, and Addiction Medicine.

Randall R. Mayer, M.S., M.P.H., serves as chief of the Bureau of HIV, STD, and Hepatitis at the Iowa Department of Public Health. In this capacity, he oversees prevention, care, and public health surveillance programs. He currently serves on the Infectious Disease Policy Committee of the Association of State and Territorial Health Officials. In 2010, he served as a panel member on the Institute of Medicine's Committee on Viral Hepatitis, which produced the report entitled, *Hepatitis and Liver Cancer: A National Strategy for Prevention and Control of Hepatitis B and C*. From 2012 to 2013, Mr. Mayer served as Chair of the National Alliance of State and Territorial AIDS Directors (NASTAD). In 2013, Mr. Mayer received NASTAD's Nicholas A. Rango Leadership award, and in 2014, he received a NASTAD Program Excellence Award for his work in addressing HIV criminalization and stigma. Earlier positions in the Department included HIV Surveillance Coordinator and Interim Director for the Division of Behavioral Health. He received his M.P.H. in Epidemiology from the University of Minnesota and his M.S. in Plant Cell Physiology from Purdue University.

Shruti Mehta, Ph.D., M.P.H., is a professor in the Johns Hopkins University Bloomberg School of Public Health. Her primary research interests include helping hard-to-reach populations to understand the epidemiology and natural and treated history of HIV, hepatitis C virus (HCV), and HIV/HCV coinfection. Populations of interest include injection drug users and men who have sex with men as well as their sexual partners in both Baltimore and international settings, particularly India. Dr. Mehta has a special interest in identifying and overcoming barriers to care and treatment of HIV and HCV among such populations.

Stuart C. Ray, M.D., serves as vice chair of medicine for data integrity and analytics and associate fellowship program director and professor in the Division of Infectious Diseases within the Department of Medicine, with secondary appointments in Viral Oncology and Health Sciences Informatics at the Johns Hopkins University School of Medicine. He directs the virology laboratory and is a Clinical Investigator in the Center for Viral Hepatitis Research in the Division of Infectious Diseases. He is a faculty member of the graduate Immunology program, the graduate Pharmacology program, and the Janeway Firm of the Osler Medical Service. Dr. Ray received his M.D. from Vanderbilt University School of Medicine. After an internship and residency at Johns Hopkins Hospital, he continued as an assistant chief of service and Fellow in Infectious Diseases. During his Fellowship, he studied the immunology and sequence variation of HIV in the laboratory of Dr. Robert Bollinger. During that time, he developed an interest in HIV sequence variation during antiretroviral therapy in a productive collaboration with Dr. Robert Siliciano that continues to the present.

In 1997, Dr. Ray joined the Johns Hopkins faculty, and under the mentorship of Dr. David Thomas, shifted his primary research focus to hepatitis C virus (HCV). His laboratory work has focused on the sequence variation of HCV during acute and chronic infection, and developing and applying computational and molecular biology tools to underlying mechanisms, including stochastic variation, immune selection, and viral fitness. He continues to care for inpatients and outpatients with HIV, HCV, and other infectious diseases.

Arthur L. Reingold, M.D., is the Edward Penhoet Distinguished Professor of Global Health and Infectious Diseases at the School of Public Health, University of California, Berkeley (UCB). He is also professor of epidemiology and biostatistics and clinical professor of medicine at the University of California, San Francisco (UCSF). His research interests include emerging and reemerging infections and vaccine-preventable diseases in the United States and developing countries. Dr. Reingold serves on the World Health Organization's Strategic Advisory Group of Experts on vaccines and vaccine policy as vice chair. He is also director of the California Emerging Infections Program, and of the National Institutes of Health's Fogarty AIDS International Training and Research Program at UCB/UCSF. His recent publications include articles on the impact of the introduction of pneumococcal conjugate vaccine in the United States and related topics. Before joining the UCB faculty, Dr. Reingold worked for 8 years at the Centers for Disease Control and Prevention. He is a member of the National Academy of Medicine.

Samuel So, M.D., is a professor of surgery and the Lui Hac Minh Professor at Stanford University. He is also the director of the Asian Liver Center and director of the Multidisciplinary Liver Cancer Program at the same institution. He has published numerous studies on solid organ transplantation and gastric and liver cancers. Dr. So is well known for his work on hepatitis B and liver cancer education and prevention programs. Through his research, Dr. So has identified the need for a public health approach to liver cancer prevention among recent Asian immigrants and first and second generation Asians living in the United States. These populations have not been the typical focus of U.S. screening and prevention programs. Dr. So is listed among the *Best Doctors in America* published by Woodward/White Inc. For his work in education and prevention, he received the 2005 National Leadership Award from the New York University Center for the Study of Asian American Health and the 2008 American Liver Foundation Salute to Excellence Award. He is a member of the National Academies of Sciences, Engineering, and Medicine Board on Population Health and Public Health Practice. Dr. So received his M.B.B.S. in Medicine and Surgery from the University of Hong Kong, and did postdoctoral and Clinical Fellowships at the University of Minnesota.

Neeraj Sood, Ph.D., is the vice dean for research at the University of Southern California (USC) Price School of Public Policy. In addition, he is director of research at the Leonard D. Schaeffer Center for Health Policy and Economics and an associate professor at the Price School and the School of Pharmacy's Department of Pharmaceutical and Health Economics. His prior work focused on the economics of innovation, HIV/AIDS, health care financing, and global health.

His research has been published in several peer-reviewed journals and books, including leading journals in economics, medicine, and health policy. He has testified frequently on health policy issues before state legislators. His work also has been featured in media outlets such as *The New York Times*, *Washington Post*, *U.S. News & World Report*, and *Scientific American*. Dr. Sood was the finalist for the 16th and 21st Annual National Institute for Health Care Management Health Care Research Award, recognizing outstanding research in health policy. He was also the 2009 recipient of the Eugene Garfield Economic Impact Prize, recognizing outstanding research demonstrating how medical research impacts the economy.

Dr. Sood is on the editorial boards of Health Services Research and Forum for Health Economics and Policy and is a research associate at the National Bureau of Economic Research. Prior to joining USC, Dr. Sood was a senior economist at RAND and professor at the Pardee RAND Graduate School.

Grace Wang, M.D., M.P.H., is a board-certified family physician for International Community Health Services in Seattle. Dr. Wang graduated from the University of Michigan with a degree in Early Childhood Education. She received her medical training at Cornell University Medical College in New York City and has an M.P.H., also from the University of Michigan.

Dr. Wang has worked in primary care and public health in New York City and Seattle. She is a member of the Executive Committee for the National Association of Community Health Centers Board of Directors and serves on the boards for Project Access Northwest and Kin On.

Lucy E. Wilson, M.D., Sc.M., is a medical epidemiologist and infectious disease physician at the Maryland Department of Health and Mental Hygiene, where she serves as chief of the Center for Surveillance, Infection Prevention, and Outbreak Response. Dr. Wilson implements surveillance and prevention of reportable infectious diseases (including hepatitis B and C infections), consults on infection control issues across the health care continuum and in the general community, and oversees Maryland's outbreak responses, including food-related outbreaks, novel influenza pandemic response, and Ebola virus disease response. Dr. Wilson is the Principal Investigator of the Healthcare Associated Infections (HAI) branch of the Centers for Disease Control and Prevention (CDC)/Maryland Emerging Infections Program, conducting HAI surveillance and prevention research. She is also the medical advisor for the CDC grant "Community-based Programs to Test and Cure Hepatitis C" in Maryland. Dr. Wilson is an adjunct assistant professor at the Johns Hopkins University School of Medicine. Previously, she was on the Johns Hopkins School of Medicine Division of Infectious Diseases faculty as medical director of the Johns Hopkins HIV County Program. Her research focused on the natural history of hepatitis C in injection drug users and HIV clinical outcomes.